Adult Malnutrition

Malnutrition is a global health problem and results in significant clinical and financial consequences for people, communities, and healthcare institutions. Causes of malnutrition are often complex and multifactorial, and can include acute illness or injury, chronic disease, and a variety of socioeconomic factors.

While many professional articles have been published on malnutrition, there is no single source of information that encompasses all aspects of the condition. *Adult Malnutrition: Diagnosis and Treatment* reviews the risk factors and etiologies of malnutrition, as well as screening, assessment, diagnosis, and treatment to aid healthcare professionals in the identification and successful care of individuals with this condition in a variety of settings.

FEATURES

- Discusses how to identify malnutrition risks through the use of validated nutrition screening tools in diverse settings
- Provides detailed instructions on conducting a nutrition-focused physical exam, including illustrations depicting differing degrees of muscle wasting and fat loss
- Presents information on risk factors, diagnosis, and treatment of vitamin and mineral deficiencies, including photos illustrating signs of deficiency to aid in diagnosis
- Details treatments for malnutrition related to acute illness/injury, chronic illness, social/environmental circumstances, or starvation
- Reviews challenges and potential solutions to malnutrition identification and treatment in healthcare institutions

Edited by Jennifer Doley, MBA, RDN, CNSC, FAND, and Mary J. Marian, DCN, RDN, CSO, FAND, FASPEN, this book serves as a key text for registered dietitian nutritionists, health practitioners, and clinicians.

Adult Malnutrition
Diagnosis and Treatment

Edited by
Jennifer Doley, MBA, RDN, CNSC, FAND
Mary J. Marian, DCN, RDN, CSO, FAND, FASPEN

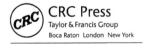

CRC Press
Taylor & Francis Group
Boca Raton London New York

CRC Press is an imprint of the
Taylor & Francis Group, an **informa** business

First edition published 2023
by CRC Press
6000 Broken Sound Parkway NW, Suite 300, Boca Raton, FL 33487-2742

and by CRC Press
4 Park Square, Milton Park, Abingdon, Oxon, OX14 4RN

CRC Press is an imprint of Taylor & Francis Group, LLC

© 2023 Taylor & Francis Group, LLC

Library of Congress Cataloging-in-Publication Data
Names: Doley, Jennifer, editor. | Marian, Mary J., editor.
Title: Adult malnutrition : diagnosis and treatment / edited by Jennifer Doley, MBA, RDN, CNSC, FAND, and Mary J. Marian, DCN, RDN, CSO, FAND, FASPEN.
Description: First edition. | Boca Raton : CRC Press, 2023. |
Includes bibliographical references and index. |
Summary: "This is the first book to offer a comprehensive overview of adult malnutrition in one volume. Written by the top malnutrition experts in the field, this is an invaluable resource for registered dietitian nutritionists, nurses and other healthcare professionals involved in identifying and treating malnutrition. This timely volume covers malnutrition's definition, identification, diagnosis, treatment and clinical and financial implications. Numerous photographs assist in the identification of malnutrition. This resource addresses both inpatient hospital and community care settings"– Provided by publisher.
Identifiers: LCCN 2022016691 (print) | LCCN 2022016692 (ebook) |
ISBN 9781032011868 (hardback) | ISBN 9781032000954 (paperback) |
ISBN 9781003177586 (ebook)
Subjects: LCSH: Malnutrition–Diagnosis. | Malnutrition–Treatment. | Nutrition disorders.
Classification: LCC RC623 .A38 2023 (print) | LCC RC623 (ebook) |
DDC 362.1963/9–dc23/eng/20220601
LC record available at https://lccn.loc.gov/2022016691
LC ebook record available at https://lccn.loc.gov/2022016692

ISBN: 9781032011868 (hbk)
ISBN: 9781032000954 (pbk)
ISBN: 9781003177586 (ebk)

DOI: 10.1201/9781003177586

Typeset in Times
by Newgen Publishing UK

Contents

Contributors

Michelle Bratton, RDN, CSO
University of Arizona Cancer Center
Tucson, AZ

Christan Bury, MS, RD, LD, CNSC
Cleveland Clinic
Cleveland, OH

Jennifer Doley, MBA, RDN, CNSC, FAND
Carondelet St. Mary's Hospital
Tucson, AZ

Laura D. Howenstine, MS, RD, LDN, NWCC
Duke University Hospital
Durham, NC

Maureen Janowski, RDN, LDN, CSG, FAND
Morrison Healthcare
Chicago, IL

Kavitha Krishnan, MS, RD, LD, CNSC
Cleveland Clinic
Cleveland, OH

Mary Kronik, RDN, LD, CNSC
Cleveland Clinic
Cleveland, OH

Gisele Leger, MS, RDN, LDN, CNSC, FAND
Morrison Healthcare
Boston, MA

Ainsley Malone, MS, RDN, LD, CNSC, FAND, FASPEN
Mt. Carmel East Hospital
Columbus, OH

Diane Nowak, RD, LD, CNSC
Cleveland Clinic
Cleveland, OH

Wendy Phillips, MS, RD, CLE, NWCC, FAND
Morrison Healthcare
Cleveland, OH

Angela Prinzo, MS, RD, LD
Cleveland Clinic
Cleveland, OH

Mary Krystofiak Russell, MS, RDN, LDN, FAND, FASPEN
Rosalind Franklin University of Medicine and Science
Chicago, IL

Terese Scollard, MBA, RDN, LD, FAND
MySurgeryPlate LLC
Beaverton, OR

Julianne Werner, MS, RD, LD, CNSC
Cleveland Clinic
Cleveland, OH

Sunitha Zechariah, PHD, RDN, LD, CNSC, FAND
Morrison Healthcare
Atlanta, GA

1 History and Consequences

Mary Krystofiak Russell

CONTENTS

I INTRODUCTION

Although malnutrition has been recognized for centuries as a condition that impedes recovery from, or in some cases causes, disease or illness, the widespread recognition of its myriad effects on not only the immune system and quality of life but also on clinical outcomes (such as cost of care, length of stay, infection, and mortality) has come only in the last half-century. This chapter will describe selected historical milestones in the identification and understanding of clinical malnutrition and highlight selected data published since ~2000 that define the significant outcome consequences associated with it. The intent of this chapter is to provide an introduction and background to the topic and set the stage for the detailed information in subsequent chapters.

II HISTORY

Interest in the value of food and nutrition and, by extension, malnutrition dates to the 5th century BCE, in which Hippocrates stated, "The patient ought likewise to be consider'd, whether he is able to hold out with the prescribed diet, even in the height of disease; for if the diet is not sufficient, the patient will grow too faint, and be overcome by the disease".[1,2] Sprengel and others for decades attributed the maxim "let food be thy medicine and medicine be thy food" to Hippocrates. Subsequent research by Cardenas and others notes that in spite of its ubiquity as a citation, this quote cannot be found in any of the writings of Hippocrates; the attribution began in the mid-1920s and peaked in the 1970s.[3] Hippocrates was likely one of the first people on record to note a connection between food and nutrition and health and disease. However, he suggested that although food may be closely linked to health and disease, the concept of food was not to be confused with that of medication.[4]

DOI: 10.1201/9781003177586-1

Malnutrition in individuals who are ill, and especially those who require hospitalization, has been extensively documented and established as a significant concern for over 150 years. Florence Nightingale noted "Every careful observer of the sick will agree in this that thousands of patients are annually starved in the midst of plenty, from want of attention to the ways alone which make it possible for them to take food".[5]

In 1887, the American Medical Association (AMA) appointed a Committee on Dietetics and noted "We should give the physician as much knowledge about the preparation of food for the sick as the trained nurse. Which American college will be the first to have a Professor of Gastronomy, or if preferred, of Dietetics?"[6] The American Dietetic Association, now the Academy of Nutrition and Dietetics (Academy), officially launched in 1917 with appropriate feeding of war victims and hospitalized patients a major priority.

A   EARLY IDENTIFICATION, SIGNIFICANCE, AND PREVALENCE

A call to action about the serious effect of malnutrition on the care and progress of hospitalized patients came in 1974, with Butterworth's seminal piece "The Skeleton in the Hospital Closet".[7] In his article, Dr. Butterworth referred to "physician-induced malnutrition" as being "one of the most serious nutritional problems of our time" and noted that that "one of the largest pockets of unrecognized malnutrition in America exists … in the private rooms and wards of big city hospitals".[7] This call to action was the first time in the current era that physicians and other care providers were alerted to the fact that malnutrition contributed to morbidity, mortality and longer length of stay (LOS), or in other words, nutritional status had an effect on clinical outcomes.[8]

In the same year, 1974, Bistrian and Blackburn[9] alerted the medical community to the fact that over 50% of the patients on a major hospital's general surgical ward had moderate to severe protein calorie malnutrition, assessed by common techniques used at the time: triceps skinfold and arm muscle circumference measurements. The authors commented that their observation suggested that "nutritional support of hospitalized patients has been neglected".[9] Other observations they reference used serum albumin (a very frequently used measure at the time) rather than skinfold and arm muscle circumference as a malnutrition indicator.[10,11]

In 1976, Bistrian and Blackburn[12] turned their attention to general medical patients and noted that at least 44% of the patients studied showed signs of protein calorie malnutrition (based on weight/height, triceps skinfold measurements, arm muscle circumference, serum albumin, and hematocrit). Compared with the surgical patients they studied earlier, the medical patients were noted to be more calorically depleted but with better protein status; however, they noted that all of these patients exhibited concerning degrees of malnutrition. Harking back to the AMA comment in 1887, they noted the lack of nutrition education in medical schools and issued a call to correct that deficiency.[12]

In the first issue of the *Journal of Parenteral and Enteral Nutrition*, published in 1977, Bistrian and Blackburn[13] laid out a comprehensive plan for the nutritional and metabolic assessment of the hospitalized patient. This paper noted that malnutrition treatment required regular monitoring to confirm the effects of such treatment. They also noted that a nutrition assessment must be effective in naming those characteristics that establish the presence of malnutrition, particularly malnutrition that would influence clinical outcomes.[13]

Awareness of the prevalence and consequences of compromised nutritional status (malnutrition) in hospitalized patients clearly took off in the mid-70s and has continued. A glance at the reference list following any article on malnutrition reveals a remarkably large number of publications, often authored by physicians in the later 1970s and 1980s (sometimes with registered dietitian nutritionists (RDNs) or registered nurses as collaborators) and later published with RDNs as primary authors.

B DIAGNOSIS

The use of serum albumin as an indicator of nutritional status was first described by Blackburn and colleagues in 1977.[14] Those investigators also discussed the use of serum transferrin and total iron-binding capacity as nutrition assessment tools. In 1996, Mears[15] reported that serum prealbumin was a more sensitive indicator of nutrition status than serum albumin. At about the same time, Charney[16] noted that the synthesis and degradation of hepatic proteins were significantly altered during critical illness, and that those factors made the use of these proteins as nutrition assessment indicators challenging at best. In 2004, Fuhrman et al.[15] reported that hepatic proteins were correlated with severity of illness, morbidity and mortality, and were useful as prognostic indicators for the development of malnutrition, but not indicators of malnutrition per se or of the success of nutritional repletion.

Recently, the American Society of Parenteral and Enteral Nutrition (ASPEN) published a position paper noting that albumin and prealbumin are inflammatory markers associated with nutrition risk and not helpful monitoring parameters for nutrition therapy.[14] Because of the work of Charney, Fuhrman, Mueller and many others, clinicians realized that identification of malnutrition required an entirely new perspective.

A crucial step in the identification and standardization of undernutrition was initiated by Detsky and colleagues in the late 1980s and early 1990s, with the development and dissemination of the Subjective Global Assessment (SGA) tool.[18–21] Also in the late 1980s, Dempsey, Mullen and Buzby asserted that many clinicians understood that there was a connection between malnutrition in surgical patients and poor outcomes.[22] They published a review of studies that related increased surgical morbidity to poor nutritional status. The article discussed options for proactive identification of surgical patients with relevant nutrition and concluded that there were data to support the potential role for preoperative nutrition support of some malnourished patients. They also called for a large clinical trial to test this hypothesis.[20] Over the next decades, many studies in hospitalized patients correlated malnutrition identified by the SGA with increased mortality, and the SGA was used as a comparator for nutrition screening tools.[21,23,24]

The contemporary work in defining and assessing consequences of malnutrition took a new turn with the publication of a proposal for the etiology-based diagnosis of malnutrition.[25] Chapter 2 will review the iterations of this etiology-based process, including the Academy/ASPEN clinical characteristics[25] and the Global Leadership on Malnutrition (GLIM) criteria recommended for the identification of adult malnutrition,[26] malnutrition diagnosis and prevalence, and the evolution of the rise of clinical malnutrition to a globally focused issue of concern.

III CONSEQUENCES

That malnutrition is associated with both metabolic and clinical consequences is indisputable, as the work of the early researchers and clinicians clearly demonstrates. Many investigators have published clinical studies and review articles that highlight the consequences of malnutrition, and suggestions for managing it; these reviews reference many valuable studies, which cannot be fully described here. New publications about the incidence, treatment and consequences of malnutrition are published weekly; readers should prioritize staying up to date on the literature. This section will limit its primary scope to selected studies published since 2000.

Interesting to those who may think that the concept of health economic outcomes as connected to nutritional status is a relatively contemporary issue, consider the work of Tucker and Miguel, published in 1996, which examined the topic of cost containment through nutrition intervention.[27] Their detailed review referenced many studies carried out in the 1980s through early 1990s that documented a relationship between risk of malnutrition and outcomes such as LOS and cost of care.[27] The authors noted that many of the studies mentioned in their review determine malnutrition status based on medical and diet history, anthropometric variables such as height/weight and/or weight loss, and laboratory values such as serum albumin and total lymphocyte count – reflecting the clinical focus and "wisdom" at the time.

Note that it was over *25 years ago* when the Tucker and Miguel's[27] work described the "predictable penalties of hospital malnutrition" in detail: impaired immune and inflammatory responses, inability to fight infections, negative effects of vitamin and mineral deficiencies on wound healing and pressure injury development and longer hospital stays. They called these the "cost penalties for malnutrition" which they contend are often "hidden" from accounting systems. They advocated for, among other things, robust nutrition screening programs and much more widespread awareness of the risks posed by altered nutritional status.[27] Their closing words could have been written today and are a clarion call, encouraging action by all those seeking to reduce the negative consequences and outcomes of inpatient malnutrition. They called for improvement in nutrition services, monitoring of its effects, and careful documentation of the subsequent cost savings.[27]

In 2000, Allison cited this work, noting that patients with a high nutrition risk score had a LOS five to six days longer than those at low risk, and that 80% of that difference was related to disease severity rather than malnutrition itself. He noted that Tucker's work showed that for every two days of early nutrition intervention, LOS was reduced by one day.[28]

Kubrack and Jensen's[29] detailed narrative review of the issues associated with malnutrition in acute care patients offers a thorough description of consequences, as reported by dozens of researchers. This review is another excellent source of references spanning over 20 years. Consequences of malnutrition that are mentioned include loss of lean body mass, reduced respiratory, renal and cardiac function, reduced intestinal absorption of a variety of nutrients, reduced psychological responses leading to fatigue and apathy, altered immunity leading to delayed wound healing and increased risk of infection, increased use of hospital resources, longer LOS and more frequent readmissions.[29]

A few years later, Barker, Gout and Crowe[30] published a very detailed review of the adverse outcomes of malnutrition, for both the patient and the healthcare system. Although their work specifically referenced consequences for patients in Australia, the issues highlighted, and references cited, make this publication crucial for anyone seeking a comprehensive overview of the consequences of malnutrition. The authors cite 15 studies that note various negative outcomes of malnutrition, including higher infection and complication rates, muscle loss, slow wound healing, longer LOS, and higher rates of morbidity and mortality.[30]

A detailed study published in 2018 by the Agency for Healthcare Research and Quality (AHRQ) noted that data on adult inpatient stays for those diagnosed with malnutrition (vs. data on other inpatient stays) reflected a longer LOS, higher costs, increased comorbidities, and a five-fold increase in likelihood of death.[31] This study includes detailed information on patient characteristics, outcomes, and most common principal diagnoses. Malnutrition is identified using a broad set of diagnostic codes that includes the following six categories.[31] (Note that these categories do not align directly with the Consensus Statement of the Academy/ASPEN characteristics[25] recommended for the identification and documentation of adult malnutrition.)

- Post-surgical non-absorption
- Nutritional neglect
- Cachexia
- Protein-calorie malnutrition
- Weight loss or failure to thrive
- Underweight

Regarding consequences of malnutrition, the report noted that costs of non-maternal, non-neonatal inpatient stays related to six types of malnutrition except underweight ranged from twice as much for protein-calorie malnutrition to 17 times as much for weight loss or failure to thrive diagnoses when compared to stays that did not involve malnutrition. Further, the report commented the malnutrition-related stays for all six types (except postsurgical non-absorption) in 2016 had a higher proportion of in-hospital deaths, ranging from 3.6% for an underweight diagnosis to 11.2% for cachexia. Regarding LOS, malnutrition-related inpatient stays were longer than the average 5-day LOS for all inpatients, ranging from 6.2 days for an underweight diagnosis to 11.2 days for a diagnosis of protein-calorie malnutrition. Regarding average cost of both "index stays" and readmission, cost for both was highest among stays involving protein-calorie malnutrition and postsurgical non-absorption, compared with other types of malnutrition.[31]

TABLE 1.1

Malnutrition Consequences: Effects on Wound Healing

Source	Patient population	Sample size	Malnutrition definition	Results
Harris[32] 2004	Review	—	—	Loss of 10% of lean body mass leads to impaired immunity, but the body prioritizes the need for protein for healing. Healing of existing wounds decreases by 20%, and new wounds develop from loss of collagen, decreased zinc absorption, edema, weakness, and infection
Campos[33] 2008	Review	—	—	Malnutrition prolongs inflammatory phase, decreasing fibroblast proliferation and collagen synthesis; increases infection risk by decreasing T-cell function, phagocytic activity, and antibody levels. Some studies show immunonutrition beneficial for wound healing
Fry[34] 2010	Surgical	887,189 cases from 1368 hospitals	Coded as a secondary diagnosis	Malnutrition / weight loss associated with 4× increased likelihood of PI development
Stechmiller[35] 2010	Review	—	—	Weight loss, low BMI, reduced dietary protein intake, and eating difficulties associated with PI development or impaired healing

Abbreviations: PI = pressure injury; BMI = body mass index.

Tables 1.1 to 1.6 highlight data from selected studies on adults that report negative consequences of malnutrition on specific, relevant outcomes. As mentioned earlier, the number of studies in the literature is significant, and many earlier efforts used serum albumin or other less accurate determinants of malnutrition. These tables are meant to give the reader an idea of the breadth and extent of literature on the topic and to invite further review and analysis.

TABLE 1.2

Malnutrition Consequences: Effects on Infection

Source	Patient population	Sample size	Malnutrition definition	Results
Correia[36] 2003	Inpatient	709	SGA	Moderately and severely malnourished infection rate 19.4% vs. 10.1% in well nourished
Schneider[37] 2004	Inpatient	1637	NRI (weight, albumin)	Nosocomial infection prevalence 8.8% overall: 4.4% in non-malnourished, 7.6% in moderately malnourished, 14.6% in severely malnourished. Malnutrition is an independent risk factor for nosocomial infections
Fry[34] 2010	Surgical	887,189 Cases from 1368 hospitals	Coded as a secondary diagnosis	Malnutrition / weight loss associated with 3× increased incidence in of mediastinitis after CABG 2× surgical site infection, 4× catheter associated urinary tract infection, 16× intravascular device infection, 3× postoperative pneumonia
Shpata[38] 2014	Surgical	694	NRS-2002	Malnutrition independent risk factor for total complications and infectious complications

Abbreviations: SGA = Subjective Global Assessment; NRI = Nutritional Risk Index; CABG = coronary artery bypass graft; NRS-2002 = Nutritional Risk Screening 2002.

TABLE 1.3

Malnutrition Consequences: Effects on Mortality

Source	Patient population	Sample size	Malnutrition definition	Results
Correia[36] 2003	Inpatient	709	SGA	Mortality rate 12.4% for moderately and severely malnourished vs. 4.7% for well-nourished
Ben-Ishay[39] 2011	General surgery patients	96	MUST	Mortality in the high-risk group was higher overall, in hospital, and after six months and one year of follow-up
Agarwal[40] 2013	Inpatients in 56 hospitals	3122	SGA	The odds of 90-day in-hospital mortality were twice greater for malnourished patients and those consuming ≤ 25% of offered food

(Continued)

TABLE 1.3 (Continued)
Malnutrition Consequences: Effects on Mortality

Source	Patient population	Sample size	Malnutrition definition	Results
Shpata[38] 2014	Surgical	694	NRS-2002	Malnutrition independent risk factor for mortality
Felder[41] 2015	Medical	887	NRS-2002	Strong association of higher NRS-2002 score with mortality
Mosquera[42] 2016	Inpatients with major abdominal surgery	490	Academy/ASPEN criteria	Malnourished mortality 7.5% vs. well-nourished 2.3%
Ceniccola[43] 2018	ICU	375	NRS-2002 and Academy/ASPEN criteria	Mortality risk 2.5 × higher in moderate and severe malnutrition
Hudson[44] 2018	Inpatients referred for nutrition assessment	3907	Academy/ASPEN criteria	Malnourished mortality 8% vs. non-malnourished 5%
Mogensen[45] 2018	ICU patients with SIRS or sepsis	85	Inadequate intake, muscle wasting, weight loss, edema, underweight	38% malnourished at ICU admission. Malnourished 3× odds of 28-day mortality vs. those not malnourished
Mogensen[45] 2018	ICU	23,575	RDN clinical judgment based on inadequate energy and/or protein intake, muscle and/or subcutaneous fat wasting and unintentional weight loss	Odds of 90-day post-discharge mortality in patients at risk for malnutrition, non-specific malnutrition, or any protein-energy malnutrition were 1.4, 2.4, and 5-fold higher, respectively vs. patients without malnutrition. Malnutrition associated with increased post-discharge mortality, hospital readmission and discharge to a care facility
Ceniccola[46] 2020	Trauma patients in ICU	4114	Academy/ASPEN criteria	Malnourished mortality risk 1.96 times higher than non-malnourished
Hiura[47] 2020	Inpatients with an ICU stay	5606	Academy/ASPEN criteria	Severely malnourished had significantly higher mortality rates than those without severe malnutrition

Abbreviations: SGA = Subjective Global Assessment; MUST = Malnutrition Universal Screening Tool; NRS-2002 = Nutritional Risk Screening 2002; Academy/ASPEN = Academy of Nutrition and Dietetics/American Society of Parenteral and Enteral Nutrition; ICU = intensive care unit; SIRS = systemic inflammatory response syndrome; RDN = Registered Dietitian Nutritionist.

TABLE 1.4

Malnutrition Consequences: Effects on Length of Stay, Acute Care

Source	Patient population	Sample size	Malnutrition definition	Results
Correia[36] 2003	Inpatient	709	SGA	Malnourished longer LOS (16.7 ± 24.5 days) vs. well-nourished (10.1 ± 11.7 days)
Gout[48] 2009	Inpatient	275	SGA	Malnourished longer LOS (13.3 days) vs. well-nourished (8.8 days)
Ben-Ishay[39] 2011	General surgery patients	96	MUST	At nutrition risk longer LOS (18.8 ± 11.5 days) vs. not at risk (7 ± 5.3 days)
Lim[49] 2012	Inpatient	818	SGA	Malnourished longer LOS (6.9 ± 7.3 days) vs. well nourished (4.6 ± 5.6 days). Malnourished more likely to be readmitted within 15 days
Agarwal[40] 2013	Inpatient	3122	SGA	Malnourished longer LOS and readmission rates (15 days and 36%) vs. well-nourished (10 days and 30%)
Shpata[38] 2014	Surgical	694	NRS-2002	Malnutrition independent risk factor for longer ICU LOS and longer time on mechanical ventilation
Jeejeebhoy[50] 2015	Medical and surgical	1022	SGA, NRS-2002, weight, mid-arm and calf circumference, serum albumin, HGS, patient self-assessment of food intake	HGS and reduced food intake during 1st week of hospitalization were independent predictors of LOS in severely malnourished
Allard[51] 2016	Inpatient	1015	SGA	Malnutrition at admission was independently associated with prolonged LOS.
Curtis[52] 2017	Medical and surgical	958	SGA	Average LOS 3.2 days longer for moderately malnourished and 3.3 days longer for severely malnourished. Moderate malnutrition associated with 27% increase LOS and severe malnutrition 44% increase. Medical patients: 40% increase LOS for moderate malnutrition and 50% for severe malnutrition. Surgical patients: 28% increase LOS for moderate malnutrition and 27% for severe malnutrition

(Continued)

TABLE 1.4 (Continued)
Malnutrition Consequences: Effects on Length of Stay, Acute Stay

Source	Patient population	Sample size	Malnutrition definition	Results
Mosquera[42] 2016	Inpatients with major abdominal surgery	490	Academy/ASPEN criteria	Malnourished postoperative LOS 13.3 days vs. not malnourished 7.4 days
Hiller[53] 2017	Inpatient	404	Academy/ASPEN criteria	Malnourished LOS 9.8 days vs. not malnourished 4.38 days Malnourished 4.3 times more likely to have a LOS > 7 days vs. not malnourished
Hudson[44] 2018	Inpatients referred for nutrition assessment	3907	Academy/ASPEN criteria	Malnourished patients longer LOS (14.99 ± 17.82 days) vs. not malnourished (11.85 ± 11.13 days)
Hiura[47] 2020	Inpatients with an ICU stay	5606	Academy/ASPEN criteria	Severely malnourished LOS 18 days vs. without severe malnutrition 8 days

Abbreviations: SGA = Subjective Global Assessment; LOS = length of stay; MUST = Malnutrition Universal Screening Tool; NRS-2002 = Nutritional Risk Screening 2002; ICU = intensive care unit; HGS = hand grip strength; Academy/ASPEN = Academy of Nutrition and Dietetics/American Society of Parenteral and Enteral Nutrition.

TABLE 1.5
Malnutrition Consequences: Effects on Cost of Care

Source	Patient population	Sample size	Malnutrition definition	Results
Braunschweig[54] 2000	Inpatients LOS > 7 d	404	SGA at admission and discharge	Patients who declined nutritionally had higher hospital charges ($45,762 ± $4021) vs. those who did not decline ($28,631 ± $1835); odds of complications significantly higher
Correia[36] 2003	Inpatient	709	SGA	Mean daily expense per patient for malnourished $228 vs. well-nourished $138
Lim[49] 2012	Inpatient	818	SGA	The average cost of hospitalization 24% higher for malnourished

TABLE 1.5 (Continued)
Malnutrition Consequences: Effects on Cost of Care

Source	Patient population	Sample size	Malnutrition definition	Results
Guerra[55] 2016	Medical and surgical	637	MUST, NRS-2002, Academy/ ASPEN criteria, PG-SGA	NRS-2002: Malnutrition risk increased average costs by €452 MUST: High malnutrition risk increased costs by €617 Academy/ASPEN and PG-SGA: Severe malnutrition increased costs by €416 and €589, respectively Overall, malnutrition increased costs 19–29%
Curtis[52] 2017	Medical and surgical	958	SGA	Moderate and severe malnutrition associated with 45% and 54% increase in total costs, 55% and 68% increase in medical costs, and 52% and 51% increase in surgical costs, respectively. Total cost (Canadian $) for surgical patients increased by $2857 for moderately malnourished and $2915 for severely malnourished. Total cost for medical patients was increased by $2986 for moderately malnourished and $2984 for severely malnourished
Mosquera[42] 2016	Inpatients undergoing major abdominal surgery	490	Academy/ ASPEN criteria	Moderate/severe malnutrition associated with $20,000 higher cost per patient

Abbreviations: LOS = length of stay; SGA = Subjective Global Assessment; MUST = Malnutrition Universal Screening Tool; NRS-2002 = Nutritional Risk Screening 2002; PG-SGA = Patient Generated Subjective Global Assessment; Academy/ASPEN = Academy of Nutrition and Dietetics/American Society of Parenteral and Enteral Nutrition.

TABLE 1.6

Malnutrition Consequences: Effects on 30-Day Readmission to Hospital

Source	Patient population	Sample size	Malnutrition definition	Results
Jeejeebhoy[50] 2015	Medical and surgical	733	SGA, NRS-2002, weight, mid-arm and calf circumference, serum albumin, HGS, patient self-assessment of food intake	Severe malnutrition per SGA and HGS independent predictors of 30-day readmission
Mosquera[42] 2016	Inpatients with major abdominal surgery	490	Academy/ASPEN criteria	Malnourished patients, compared to well nourished, had higher rate of readmission (22.6% vs. 16.1%) and mortality (7.5% vs. 2.3%)
Hiller[53] 2017	Inpatient	404	Academy/ASPEN criteria	108 malnourished patients (53%) readmitted within 30 days or died within 90 days of discharge vs. 36 normally well patients (18%)
Hudson[44] 2018	Inpatients referred for nutrition assessment	3907	Academy/ASPEN criteria	Malnourished likelihood of readmission 40% vs. well nourished 23%

Abbreviations: SGA = Subjective Global Assessment; NRS-2002 = Nutritional Risk Screening 2002; HGS = hand grip strength; Academy/ASPEN = Academy of Nutrition and Dietetics/American Society of Parenteral and Enteral Nutrition.

IV   CONCLUSION

Malnutrition in individuals who are ill has been recognized for over 2500 years. For at least 150 of those years, experts have exhorted the medical community to identify and treat this condition, with less than satisfactory results. The call to action for all healthcare professionals is clear – we must make this issue a priority.

The consequences of untreated malnutrition are serious: Longer LOS, increased infections, higher mortality, and more frequent readmissions within 30 days of discharge.[40] This text will inform readers about all things malnutrition: the diagnosis, prevalence, etiology, screening process, assessment techniques, treatment and monitoring, reimbursement, next steps including enhancements to regulatory and documentation processes, and measuring success.

The perfect outcome: Realizing the vision of the pioneers who called on clinicians to identify malnutrition early, and treat it effectively, to maximize the health outcomes of all individuals in their care.

REFERENCES

1. Sprengell C. *Hippocrates: The Aphorisms of Hippocrates, and the Sentence of Celsus: with Explanations and References to the Most Considerable Writers.* 2nd ed. Gale Ecco; 2010.
2. Reber E, Gomes F, Bally L, Scheutz P, Stanga Z. Nutritional management of medical inpatients. *J Clin Med.* 2019; 8(8):1130–1140.
3. Dr. Goodfood. Published July 18, 2018. Accessed January 24, 2021. www.drgoodfood.org/en/news/let-food-be-thy-medicine-hippocrates.
4. Cardenas D. Let not thy food be confused with thy medicine: The Hippocratic misquotation. *ESPEN Journal.* 2013; 8(6):E260–E262.
5. Nightingale F. *Notes on Nursing: What It Is and What It Is Not.* Appleton and Company; 1860.
6. Barber M. *History of the American Dietetic Association 1917–1959.* JB Lippincott and Company; 1959.
7. Butterworth C. The skeleton in the hospital closet. *Nutrition Today.* 1974;9:4–8.
8. Taylor B, Rice T. Must our malnourished patients eat right or die? *Crit Care Med.* 2015;43(12):2689–2690.
9. Bistrian B, Blackburn G, Hallowell E, Heddell R. Protein status of general surgical patients. *JAMA.* 1974;230(6):858–860.
10. Bollet AJ, Owns SO. Evaluation of nutritional status of selected hospitalized patients. *Am J Clin Nutr.* 1973;26(9):931–938.
11. Prevost EA, Butterworth CE. Nutrition care of hospitalized patients (abstract). *Am J Clin Nutr.* 1974;27:432.
12. Bistrian B, Blackburn G, Vitale J, Cochran D, Naylor J. Prevalence of malnutrition in general medical patients. *JAMA.* 1976;235(15):1567–1570.
13. Bistrian B, Blackburn G, Maini B, Schlamm H, Smith M. Nutritional and metabolic assessment of the hospitalized patient. *JPEN J Parenter Enteral Nutr.* 1977;1(1):11–22.
14. Evans D, Corkins M, Malone A, et al. The use of visceral proteins as nutrition markers: an ASPEN position paper. *Nutr Clin Pract.* 2021;36(1):22–28.
15. Mears E. Outcomes of continuous process improvement of a nutritional care program incorporating serum prealbumin measurements. *Nutrition.* 1996;12(7–8):479–484.
16. Charney P. Nutrition assessment in the 1990s: Where are we now? *Nutr Clin Pract.* 1995;10(4):131–139.
17. Furhman MP, Charney P, Mueller C. Hepatic proteins and nutrition assessment. *J Am Diet Assoc.* 2004;104(8):1258–1264.
18. Detsky AS, McLaughlin JR, Baker JP, et al. What is subjective global assessment of nutritional status? *JPEN J Parenter Enteral Nutr.* 1987;11(1):8–13.
19. Detsky AS, Smalley PS, Chang J. The rational clinical examination: is this patient malnourished? *JAMA.* 1994;271(1):54–58.
20. Detsky AS, McLaughlin JR, Baker JP, et al. What is subjective global assessment of nutritional status? 1987. Classical article. *Nutr Hosp.* 2008;23(4):400–407.
21. Compher C, Mehta N. Diagnosing malnutrition: where are we and where do we need to go? *J Acad Nutr Diet.* 2016;116(5):779–784.
22. Dempsey GT, Mullen JL, Buzby GP. The link between nutritional status and clinical outcome: can nutritional intervention modify it? *Am J Clin Nutr.* 1988;47(2 Suppl):352–356.
23. Skipper A, Ferguson M, Thompson K, Castellanos VH, Porcari J. Nutrition screening tools: an analysis of the evidence. *JPEN J Parenter Enteral Nutr.* 2012;36(3):292–298.

24. Skipper A, Coltman A, Tomesko J, et al. Position of the Academy of Nutrition and Dietetics: malnutrition (undernutrition) screening tools for all adults. *J Acad Nutr Diet.* 2020;120(4):709–713.

25. Jensen GL, Mirtallo J, Compher C, et al. Adult starvation and disease-related malnutrition: A proposal for an etiology-based diagnosis in the clinical practice setting from the International Consensus Guideline Committee. *Clin Nutr.* 2010;29(2):151–153.

26. De van der Schueren MAE, Keller H, GLIM Consortium. Global Leadership Initiative on Malnutrition (GLIM): guidance on validation of the operational criteria for the diagnosis of protein-energy malnutrition in adults. *Clin Nutr.* 2020;39(9):2872–2880.

27. Tucker H, Miguel SG. Cost containment through nutrition intervention. *Nutr Rev.* 1996;54(4 Pt 1):111–121.

28. Allison SP. Malnutrition, disease and outcome. *Nutrition.* 2000;16(7–8):590–593.

29. Kubrak C, Jensen L. Malnutrition in acute care patients. A narrative review. *Int J Nurs Stud.* 2007;44(6):1036–1054.

30. Barker L, Gout B, Crowe T. Hospital malnutrition: prevalence, identification and impact on patients and the healthcare system. *Int J Environ Res Public Health.* 2011;8(2):514–527.

31. Fingar KR, Weiss AJ, Barrett ML, et al. All-cause readmissions following hospital stays for patients with malnutrition, 2013. *Agency for Healthcare Research and Quality, Statistical Brief.* #218, December 2016. Accessed February 23, 2021. https://hcup-us.ahrq.gov/reports/statbriefs/sb218-Malnutrition-Readmissions-2013.jsp.

32. Harris CL, Fraser C. Malnutrition in the institutionalized elderly: the effect on wound healing. *Ostomy Wound Manage.* 2004;50(10):54–63.

33. Campos ACL, Groth AK, Branco AB. Assessment and nutritional aspects of wound healing. *Curr Opin Clin Nutr Metab Care.* 2008;11(3):281–288.

34. Fry D, Pine M Jones B, Meimban R. Patient characteristics and occurrence of never events. *Acrh Surg.* 2010;145(2):148–151.

35. Stechmiller J. Understanding the role of nutrition and wound healing. *Nutr Clin Pract.* 2010;25(1):61–68.

36. Correia MI, Waitzberg DL. The impact of malnutrition on morbidity, mortality, length of hospital stay, and costs evaluated through a multivariate model analysis. *Clin Nutr.* 2003;22(3):235–239.

37. Schneider S, Veyres P, Pivot X, et al. Malnutrition is an independent factor associated with nosocomial infections. *Br J Nutr.* 2004;92(1):105–111.

38. Shpata V, Prendushi X, Kreka M, Kla I, Kurti F, Ohn I. Malnutrition at the time of surgery affects negatively the clinical outcome of critically ill patients with gastrointestinal cancer. *Med Arch.* 2014;68(4):263–267.

39. Ben-Ishay O, Mashiach T, Kluger Y, Chermish Y. Malnutrition in surgical wards: a plea for concern. *Gastroenterol Res Pract.* 2011;2011:840512.

40. Agarwal E, Ferguson M, Banks M, et al. Malnutrition and poor food intake are associated with prolonged hospital stay, frequent readmissions, and greater in-hospital mortality: results from the Nutrition Care Day Survey 2010. *Clin Nutr.* 2013;32(5):737–745.

41. Felder S, Lechtenboehmer C, Bally M, et al. Association of nutritional risk and adverse medical outcomes across different medical inpatient populations. *Nutrition.* 2015;31(11–12):1385–1393.

42. Mosquera C, Koutlas NJ, Edwards KC, et al. Impact of malnutrition on gastrointestinal surgery patients. *J Surg Res.* 2016;205(1):95–101.

43. Ceniccola GD, Holanda TP, Pequeno RDF, et al. Relevance of AND-ASPEN criteria of malnutrition to predict hospital mortality in critically ill patients: A prospective study. *J Crit Care.* 2018;44:398–403.

44. Hudson L, Chittams J, Griffith C, Compher C. Malnutrition identified by Academy of Nutrition and Dietetics/American Society for Parenteral and Enteral Nutrition is associated with more 30-day readmission, greater hospitality mortality, and longer hospital stays: a retrospective analysis of nutrition assessment data in a major medical center. *JPEN J Parenter Enteral Nutr.* 2018;42(5):892–897.

45. Mogensen KM, Horkan CM, Purtle SW, et al. Malnutrition, critical illness survivors and post-discharge outcomes: a cohort study. *JPEN J Parenter Enteral Nutr.* 2018;42(3):557–565.

46. Ceniccola GD, Okamura AB, Neta JDS, et al. Association between AND-ASPEN malnutrition criteria and hospital mortality in critically ill trauma patients: a prospective cohort study. *JPEN J Parenter Enteral Nutr.* 2020;44(7):1347–1354.

47. Hiura G, Lebwohl B, Seres D. Malnutrition diagnosis in critically ill patients using 2012 Academy of Nutrition and Dietetics/American Society for Parenteral and Enteral Nutrition standardized diagnostic characteristics is associated with longer hospital and intensive care unit length of stay and increased in-hospital mortality. *JPEN J Parenter Enteral Nutr.* 2020;44(2):256–264.

48. Gout BS, Barker LA, Crowe TC. Malnutrition identification, diagnosis, and dietetic referrals: are we doing a good enough job? *Nutr Diet.* 2009;66(4):206–211.

49. Lim SL, Ong KCB, Chan YH, Loke WC, Ferguson M, Daniels L. Malnutrition and its impact on cost of hospitalization, length of stay, readmissions and 3-year mortality. *Clin Nutr.* 2012;31(3):345–350.

50. Jeejeebhoy KN, Keller H, Gramlich L, et al. Nutritional assessment: comparison of clinical assessment and objective variables for the prediction of length of hospital stay and readmission. *Am J Clin Nutr.* 2015;101(5):956–965.

51. Allard JP, Keller H, Jeejeebhoy K, et al. Malnutrition at hospital admission-contributors and effect on length of stay: a prospective cohort study from the Canadian Malnutrition Task Force. *JPEN J Parenter Enteral Nutr.* 2016;40(4):487–497.

52. Curtis L, Bernier P, Jeejeebhoy K, et al. Costs of hospital malnutrition. *Clin Nutr.* 2017;36(5):1391–1396.

53. Hiller LD, Shaw RF, Fabri PJ. Difference in composite end point of readmission and death between malnourished and nonmalnourished veterans assessed using Academy of Nutrition and Dietetics/American Society for Parenteral and Enteral Nutrition clinical characteristics. *JPEN J Parenter Enteral Nutr.* 2017;41(8):1316–1324.

54. Braunschweig C, Gomez S, Sheean P. Impact of declines in nutritional status on outcomes in adult patients hospitalized more than 7 days. *J Am Diet Assoc.* 2000;100(1):1316–1322.

55. Guerra RS, Sousa AS, Fonseca I, Pichel F, et al. Comparative analysis of undernutrition screening and diagnostic tools as predictors of hospitalisation costs. *J Human Nutr Diet.* 2016;29(2):165–173.

2 Diagnosis

Gisele Leger

CONTENTS

I INTRODUCTION

Although malnutrition is a global problem, there is lack of consensus on how it should be defined.[1–3] The word malnutrition means "bad" nutrition, which can refer to both undernutrition and overnutrition. Dozens of definitions for malnutrition have been published by medical dictionaries, as well as expert committees representing national and international organizations. Some definitions solely focus on the imbalance of nutrients that are consumed in the diet. Other definitions are more complex and address the physiological influences that increase demand or decrease utilization of nutrients, or the clinical consequences that follow malnutrition.[4]

When defining malnutrition there are several factors that should be considered. Any nutrient may be deficient, not just energy and protein, and can contribute to malnutrition. Additionally, clinicians must understand that the consumption of nutrients does not only imply intake via the oral route, but also nutrition provided by enteral and parenteral means. Clinicians must recognize the role of malabsorption, excessive losses, inflammatory status and increased metabolic demands in creating the nutrition deficit. Clinical outcomes of malnutrition must also be recognized. Finally, clinicians must appreciate that the need for nutrients can greatly vary for individuals throughout their lifespan based on various physiological and environmental circumstances.[4] Considering this complexity, it is not surprising that there is considerable lack of consensus and misunderstanding of malnutrition.[2,4]

Unlike the difficulties in defining malnutrition, diagnosis of many medical diseases is more straightforward. A clinician evaluating a patient for diabetes can

DOI: 10.1201/9781003177586-2

follow an established criterion for diagnosis such as the presence of fasting plasma glucose ≥ 126 mg/dL.[5] Hypertension stage 2 is diagnosed when a person's systolic blood pressure is ≥ 140 mmHg and/or their diastolic blood pressure is ≥ 90 mmHg.[6] Unfortunately, the diagnosis of malnutrition is not so simple. Despite the existence of many validated nutrition screening tools to identify patients at risk of malnutrition, in many cases this is where the diagnostic process ends. This chapter will review some historical publications that have led efforts toward defining malnutrition, as well as more recently published malnutrition criteria in the adult population.

A WORLD HEALTH ORGANIZATION (WHO)

The World Health Organization is a specialized agency of the United Nations responsible for global public health. As described in its constitution, ratified in 1948, the objective of the WHO "shall be the attainment by all peoples of the highest possible level of health".[7] To achieve this objective, one of the many functions of the WHO is to promote improvement of peoples' nutrition status worldwide.[7]

1 Severe Protein-Energy Malnutrition

The WHO recognizes severe protein-energy malnutrition as a major contributing factor to infant mortality in some countries. They urge that clinically identifiable syndromes such as kwashiorkor, nutritional marasmus, pellagra, and keratomalacia be reported.[8]

In 1981, medical experts from across the world contributed to the creation of a WHO publication titled "The Treatment and Management of Severe Protein-Energy Malnutrition".[9] Its purpose was to provide guidelines for the treatment of severe protein-energy malnutrition in children. In this document, protein-energy malnutrition was classified as marasmus, kwashiorkor, or a mixed form, marasmic kwashiorkor.[9] The leading diagnostic signs for marasmus were described as those of starvation: an "old man's face", an emaciated body that is "only skin and bones", accompanied by "irritability and fretfulness".[9] Kwashiorkor was described as edema and apathy, often accompanied by discoloration of the hair and, especially if the edema is severe, by "flaky paint" dermatosis.[9] The WHO publication also classified protein-energy malnutrition in children by the presence of edema and the degree of underweight as defined by the National Center for Health Statistics (NCHS) classification "weight for length" reference values.[9] This definition became the basis for the diagnosis of malnutrition in children and is listed in the International Classification of Diseases (ICD), also published by the WHO.

2 Body Mass Index (BMI)

An article from the WHO in 1995 stated that BMI in adults (weight in kg/(height in m)^2) is indicated as a measure of adult nutritional status.[10] BMI values <16, 17 and 18.5 (severe, moderate, and mild) were described as a measure of thinness or underweight.[10] The authors cite a modest chance that a low BMI could be related to constitutional thinness; however, they evaluate this at less than 5%.[10] See Table 2.1.[11]

TABLE 2.1
Classification of Malnutrition in Adults by Body Mass Index

Body mass index	Nutritional status
≥18.5	Normal
17.0–18.49	Mild malnutrition
16.0–16.99	Moderate malnutrition
<16.0	Severe malnutrition

Source: Reprinted with permission from World Health Organization, *Management of Severe Malnutrition: A Manual for Physicians and Other Senior Health Workers* (Geneva, 1999).[11]

B   SUBJECTIVE GLOBAL ASSESSMENT (SGA)

The SGA, first developed by Baker et al.[14] in 1982, has long been recognized as the gold standard in diagnosing malnutrition.[12–14] Researchers assessed the nutritional status of 59 hospitalized surgical patients based on history and physical examination.[14] Factors included an evaluation of weight history, changes in oral intake, gastrointestinal symptoms, functional capacity, muscle and fat wasting, edema, ascites, and chronic illness. Trained examiners developed a tool to classify patients as mildly malnourished, severely malnourished, or well nourished. The interobserver reproducibility, or the level of agreement between examiners, was considered substantial. The tool correlated well with objective evaluations which included laboratory and anthropometric measures. Severity of malnutrition also correlated with an increase in the incidence of infection, use of antibiotics, and hospital length of stay, which were chosen as markers of clinical morbidity. A later publication of these data provided more information on the accuracy of the SGA and indicated a sensitivity of 82% and specificity of 72%.[15]

In 1987, the group published subsequent research which provided more details regarding the history and physical examination indicators included in the SGA (see Table 2.2).[16] They further explored the validity for 202 surgical patients with similar results. In this cohort, it was found that the percentage of measured weight loss was an important predictor of the severity of malnutrition. The study investigators stated that the variable "disease and its relation to nutritional requirements" was difficult to define for most clinicians (Table 2.2). Clinicians struggled to classify the metabolic stress of the patient's condition as either low, moderate, high, or no stress. They also found that the clinicians were not influenced by this variable when deciding on the SGA rating of well nourished, moderately or severely malnourished. Although it was speculated that it may be dropped from the SGA, the evaluation of metabolic requirements remains part of the tool.[16]

Since the original publication, the SGA has been used and validated in multiple patient populations, such as oncology, acute and chronic kidney disease, HIV, pancreatitis, transplant and pediatrics.[17–21] More recently, the Canadian Malnutrition Task Force has adopted the SGA as their tool for the bedside malnutrition diagnosis of hospitalized patients.[22]

TABLE 2.2
1987 Subjective Global Assessment Tool[16]

A. History
  1. Weight change
        Overall loss in past 6 months: amount = #_____ kg; % loss = #_____
        Change in past 2 weeks: _____ increase,
                            _____ no change,
                            _____ decrease.
  2. Dietary intake change (relative to normal)
      _____ No change,
      _____ Change _____duration = #_____ weeks.
              _____ type: _____suboptimal solid diet, _____full liquid diet
                          _____ hypocaloric liquids, _____ starvation.
  3. Gastrointestinal symptoms (that persisted for >2 weeks)
      _____ none, _____ nausea, _____ vomiting, _____ diarrhea, _____ anorexia.
  4. Functional capacity
      _____ No dysfunction (e.g., full capacity),
      _____ dysfunction _____ duration = #_____ weeks.
                  _____ type: _____ working suboptimally,
                          _____ ambulatory,
                          _____ bedridden.
  5. Disease and its relation to nutritional requirements
      Primary diagnosis (specify)_____
      Metabolic demand (stress): _____ no stress,   _____ low stress,
                        _____ moderate stress, _____ high stress.
B. Physical (for each trait specify: 0 = normal, 1+ = mild, 2+ = moderate, 3+ = severe).
  #_____ loss of subcutaneous fat (triceps, chest)
  #_____ muscle wasting (quadriceps, deltoids)
  #_____ ankle edema
  #_____ sacral edema
  #_____ ascites
C. SGA rating (select one)
      _____ A = Well nourished
      _____ B = Moderately (or suspected of being) malnourished
      _____ C = Severely malnourished

Source: Reprinted with permission from World Health Organization, *Management of Severe Malnutrition: A Manual for Physicians and Other Senior Health Workers*

Note: Users would select the appropriate category with a checkmark, or enter numerical value where indicated by "#". (Geneva, 1999).

TABLE 2.3
Etiology-Based Terminology for Nutrition Diagnosis in Clinical Practice[23]

Terminology	Description	Examples
Starvation-related malnutrition	Chronic starvation without inflammation	Anorexia nervosa
Chronic illness-related malnutrition	Inflammation is chronic and of mild to moderate degree	Organ failure, pancreatic cancer, rheumatoid arthritis or sarcopenic obesity
Acute illness- or injury-related malnutrition	Inflammation is acute and of severe degree	Major infection, burns, trauma or closed head injury

C INTERNATIONAL CONSENSUS GUIDELINE COMMITTEE

In 2010, a group of international clinical nutrition experts proposed an etiology-based approach to diagnosing adult malnutrition in the clinical setting where the committee recognized the important role of inflammation in disease-related malnutrition (see Table 2.3).[23] Inflammation elevates resting energy expenditure and nitrogen excretion, which affects energy and protein requirements.[23] Acute inflammation that results from critical illness or injury has a severe catabolic influence on lean mass. In chronic illness, the inflammatory process is influenced by the progression and severity of illness. When severity of illness/persistence of inflammation results in a decrease in lean mass that causes functional impairment, malnutrition is considered disease-related.[23]

The consensus guideline committee state that patients may be diagnosed with more than one etiology of malnutrition, and may also change from one etiology to another.[23] Of particular risk is the patient with starvation or chronic disease state-related malnutrition, as their nutritional status can rapidly deteriorate further during an acute disease or injury-related event. The committee acknowledged that the application of this diagnostic approach in clinical practice would require validation and that criteria to support these diagnoses would need further development.[23]

D ACADEMY OF NUTRITION AND DIETETICS AND THE AMERICAN SOCIETY FOR PARENTERAL AND ENTERAL NUTRITION CONSENSUS STATEMENT

In 2009, the Academy of Nutrition and Dietetics (Academy) and the American Society of Parenteral and Enteral Nutrition (ASPEN) created a work group to identify and standardize markers of nutritional status versus the inflammatory response associated with diseases and/or conditions. The work group determined that these markers should have the following attributes: be few in number, support a nutrition diagnosis, characterize severity of malnutrition, change as nutritional status changes, be evidence-based when possible or consensus-derived when insufficient evidence exists, and be able to change over time as evidence of validity accrues.[24]

TABLE 2.4
Academy/ASPEN Clinical Characteristics Supporting a Diagnosis of Malnutrition[24]

Clinical characteristic	Malnutrition in the context of acute illness or injury		Malnutrition in the context of chronic illness		Malnutrition in the context of social or environmental circumstances	
	Non-severe (moderate) malnutrition	Severe malnutrition	Non-severe (moderate) malnutrition	Severe malnutrition	Non-severe (moderate) malnutrition	Severe malnutrition
Energy intake	<75% of estimated energy requirement for >7 days	≤50% of estimated energy requirement for ≥5 days	<75% of estimated energy requirement for ≥1 month	<75% of estimated energy requirement for ≥1 month	<75% of estimated energy requirement for ≥3 months	≤50% of estimated energy requirement for ≥1 month
Interpretation of weight loss	1–2% in 1 wk; 5% in 1 mo; 7.5% in 3 mos	>2% in 1 wk; >5% in 1 mo; >7.5% in 3 mos	5% in 1 mo; 7.5% in 3 mos; 10% in 6 mos; 20% in 1 yr	>5% in 1 mo; >7.5% in 3 mos; >10% in 6 mos; >20% in 1 yr	5% in 1 mo; 7.5% in 3 mos; 10% in 6 mos; 20% in 1 yr	>5% in 1 mo; >7.5% in 3 mos; >10% in 6 mos; >20% in 1 yr
Body fat loss	Mild	Moderate	Mild	Severe	Mild	Severe
Muscle mass loss	Mild	Moderate	Mild	Severe	Mild	Severe
Fluid accumulation	Mild	Moderate to severe	Mild	Severe	Mild	Severe
Reduced grip strength	N/A	Measurable reduced	N/A	Measurably reduced	N/A	Measurably reduced

Abbreviation: Academy/ASPEN = Academy of Nutrition and Dietetics / American Society of Parenteral and Enteral Nutrition.

Source: Reprinted with permission from World Health Organization, *Management of SevereMalnutrition: A Manual for Physicians and Other Senior Health Workers* (Geneva, 1999).

The work group published a consensus statement in 2012 to provide a definition for malnutrition based on etiologies including social and environmental circumstances, chronic illness and acute illness.[24] A distinction between acute and chronic illness was provided explaining that chronic is a disease or condition that lasts three months or longer. Inflammation was once again acknowledged as a major factor in the development of malnutrition. However, the consensus statement did not propose any inflammatory markers for diagnostic purposes.

The consensus statement proposed a set of diagnostic characteristics and recommended the presence of two or more of the following six characteristics to diagnose malnutrition.[24]

- Insufficient energy intake
- Weight loss
- Loss of subcutaneous fat
- Loss of muscle mass
- Localized or generalized fluid accumulation that may sometimes mask weight loss
- Diminished functional status as measured by hand grip strength

A distinction was made between severe and non-severe malnutrition, but the consensus indicated that at the time there was insufficient evidence to make a distinction between mild and moderate forms of malnutrition (see Table 2.4).[24] Chapters 6 and 7, which describe the Nutrition Focused Physical Exam (NFPE), provide a more in-depth discussion of these characteristics in facilitating the diagnosis of malnutrition.

Visceral protein or hepatic protein laboratory data such as serum albumin and prealbumin have historically been used as markers of nutritional status. Investigators in the 1960s noted that plasma proteins, especially albumin, were reduced in cases of kwashiorkor.[8] The opinion at the time was that a decreased serum albumin would confirm the existence of severe protein depletion.[8] However, the Academy/ASPEN 2012 consensus statement emphasized that acute-phase proteins such as serum albumin and prealbumin reflect severity of the inflammatory response and should not be used as a marker of poor nutritional status.[24]

Since its publication, research has commenced to validate the Academy/ASPEN malnutrition consensus criteria. Studies published by Mogensen et al.[25] and Hiura et al.[26] have demonstrated that the criteria are able to effectively identify patients with malnutrition as well as an association with negative outcomes, such as an increased hospital length of stay, hospital readmissions and 90-day mortality.[25,26] More data regarding the validity of the criteria will become available as the results of clinical trials in progress are published.[27] In May of 2021, the Academy and ASPEN published the rationale and protocol of a large study involving 120 acute care hospitals across the United States. Its purpose is to assess the validity and reliability of the consensus criteria, and renamed Academy of Nutrition and Dietetics (Academy) / American Society for Parenteral and Enteral Nutrition indicators for the diagnosis of adult and pediatric malnutrition or AAIM.[28] The Academy/ASPEN consensus criteria or AAIM appear to be the most common diagnostic tool used by practitioners in the United States.[25]

TABLE 2.5
Two Alternate Ways to Diagnose Malnutrition[29]

Alternative 1	• BMI < 18.5 kg/m²
Alternative 2	• Weight loss (unintentional) > 10% indefinite of time, or > 5% over the last 3 months combined with **either**
	• BMI < 20 kg/m² if < 70 years of age, or < 22 kg/m² if ≥ 70 years of age **or**
	• FFMI < 15 and 17 kg/m² in women and men, respectively

Abbreviations: BMI = body mass index; FFMI = fat free mass index.

Note: Before the diagnosis of malnutrition, it is mandatory to fulfill criteria for being "at risk" of malnutrition by any validated risk-screening tool.

Source: Reprinted with permission from World Health Organization, *Management of SevereMalnutrition: A Manual for Physicians and Other Senior Health Workers* (Geneva, 1999).

E EUROPEAN SOCIETY FOR CLINICAL NUTRITION AND METABOLISM (ESPEN) CONSENSUS STATEMENT

In 2012, the ESPEN appointed a group of experts to provide a consensus on simple, clear diagnostic criteria for malnutrition.[29] Additionally, the group was charged with defining the relationship between the screening and the diagnostic process. The group determined that nutritional screening should be mandatory for patients in all clinical settings. Furthermore, it was agreed upon that a malnutrition diagnosis should be based on the outcome of a screening evaluation, thus diagnostic measures are only needed for patients who were identified as being at nutritional risk by a validated nutrition screening tool. No recommendations were made on which screening tool to use, only that the tool should be validated for the setting in which it is applied.[29] Chapter 4 provides more details on nutrition screening.

Three diagnostic variables were chosen by the group of experts to best reflect malnutrition: Percent of weight loss, low BMI and reduced fat-free mass index (FFMI).[29] Two ways in which a malnutrition diagnosis can be determined, as shown in Table 2.5, were suggested. The BMI criteria were based on the global acceptance of the WHO guideline of ≤ 18.5 kg/m², but due to the increasing BMI in some populations, additional values of < 20 and < 22 kg/m² were included for populations < 70 and ≥ 70 years, respectively.[29] Patients with these BMI levels must also experience unintentional weight loss in order to meet the criteria for malnutrition. The FFMI cut-offs were established based on a review of evidence.[29]

However, studies are needed to validate this method. It was acknowledged that at the time, various global initiatives were in the process of developing diagnostic criteria for malnutrition internationally and that achieving a global consensus is important.[29]

F GLOBAL LEADERSHIP INITIATIVE ON MALNUTRITION (GLIM)

In 2016, representatives from ASPEN, ESPEN, the Federacion Latinoamericana de Terapia Nutricional, Nutricion Clinica y Metabolismo (FELANPE) and Parenteral and Enteral Nutrition Society of Asia (PENSA) formed a leadership committee to create the Global Leadership Initiative on Malnutrition (GLIM).[30] The core leadership committee created a larger supporting work group to include members that could provide additional diversity and expertise in order to develop a global consensus on a standardized approach to diagnose malnutrition in clinical practice.[30]

The consensus report published in 2019 promotes a two-step model.[30] First, individuals at risk of malnutrition should be identified with the use of a validated nutrition screening tool, followed by a comprehensive assessment to determine the diagnosis and severity of malnutrition.[30] After completing a comprehensive review of potential malnutrition diagnostic criteria, the group chose the following criteria:

- Unintentional weight loss
- Low BMI
- Reduced muscle mass
- Reduced food intake or assimilation
- Disease burden/Inflammation

Due to robust literature and well-established validity, there was strong GLIM consensus for the inclusion of non-volitional weight loss as a malnutrition criterion. Percentage of weight loss thresholds were established for the diagnosis of malnutrition as well as the severity grading of malnutrition.[30] (See Tables 2.6 and 2.7.) The experts agreed that repeated measures are recommended to evaluate the rate of weight change or if weight loss has stabilized.[30]

The committee found substantial variation in the use of BMI.[30] In North America, low BMI is not typically used in malnutrition identification due to the higher prevalence of overweight and obesity as many adults would need to lose substantial amounts of weight before they would achieve a BMI low enough to meet the malnutrition guideline.[30] However, since it is applicable to assessing nutritional status in many regions of the world, the GLIM consensus report recommends using BMI. As BMI can be misleading when applied as a malnutrition diagnostic tool to the overweight/obese population, any healthcare facility in North America adopting GLIM should consider avoiding the use of BMI as a criterion.[31]

There was strong consensus for inclusion of reduced muscle mass; however, there was disagreement on how to best measure and define it.[30] GLIM recommends methods such as dual-energy X-ray absorptiometry (DEXA), bioelectrical impedance analysis (BIA), ultrasound, computed tomography (CT) or magnetic resonance imaging (MRI). However, recognizing that these technologies may not be available in most settings, they also suggest physical examination and measurement of calf/arm muscle circumference as alternate solutions. The GLIM group recommends assessing muscle function and functional status by using modalities such as hand grip strength, as supportive evidence.[30]

There was strong validation by studies of reduced food intake as a criterion. GLIM experts identified multiple causes as well as disease states which affect food intake and absorption.[30]

Finally, disease burden/inflammation was recognized as an underlying or contributing cause of malnutrition, similar to the previously published guidelines in the

TABLE 2.6
GLIM Phenotypic and Etiologic Criteria for the Diagnosis of Malnutrition[30]

Phenotypic criteria			Etiologic criteria	
Weight loss (%)	Low body mass index (kg/m²)	Reduced muscle mass	Reduced food intake or assimilation	Inflammation
> 5% within past 6 months, or > 10% beyond 6 months	< 20 if < 70 years < 22 if ≥ 70 years *Asia*: < 18.5 if < 70 years, or < 20 if ≥ 70 years	Reduced by validated body composition measuring techniques	≤ 50% of energy requirements > 1 week, or any reduction for > 2 weeks, or any chronic condition that adversely impacts food assimilation or absorption	Acute disease/ injury or chronic disease-related

Abbreviation: GLIM = Global Leadership Initiative on Malnutrition.

Source: Reprinted with permission from World Health Organization, *Management of SevereMalnutrition: A Manual for Physicians and Other Senior Health Workers* (Geneva, 1999).

United States and Europe. The GLIM committee proposed a simple acute (severe and sudden onset) or chronic (disease or condition that persists over time) approach to recognize inflammation.[30] Major infections and injuries such as burns and trauma are examples of acute or severe inflammation, whereas most chronic organ diseases such as congestive heart failure, cancer or rheumatoid arthritis are examples of chronic inflammation. Fever, negative nitrogen balance and elevated resting energy expenditure may also be indicators of inflammation. Serum C-reactive protein, albumin, or prealbumin can also be supportive proxy measures of inflammation.[30]

Criteria are classified as either phenotypic (observable clinical signs of malnutrition) or etiologic (causal factors to the development of malnutrition). These two categories were grouped together to identify the underlying factors promoting malnutrition. GLIM identified non-volitional weight loss, low BMI and reduced muscle mass as phenotypic criteria, whereas reduced food intake/assimilation and disease burden/inflammation are etiologic criteria. Malnutrition is diagnosed by the presence of at least one phenotypic and one etiologic criterion. [30] (See Table 2.6.)

The GLIM consensus report recommends using the phenotypic criteria to grade the severity of malnutrition as stage 1 — moderate and stage 2 — severe. [30] (See Table 2.7.)

GLIM endorses an etiology-based diagnosis classification such as that proposed by the International Consensus Guideline Committee, the Academy/ASPEN consensus statement and the ESPEN guidelines.[30] The group acknowledges that the GLIM criteria require validation testing and should be re-evaluated based on new evidence every three to five years.[30]

TABLE 2.7
GLIM Severity Grading of Malnutrition Based on Phenotypic Criteria[30]

	Weight loss (%)	Low body mass index (kg/m²)	Reduced muscle mass
Stage 1 / Moderate malnutrition (requires 1 phenotypic criterion that meets this grade)	5–10% within the past 6 mo, or 10–20% beyond 6 mo	< 20 if < 70 yr < 22 if ≥ 70 yr	Mild to moderate deficit (per validated assessment methods)
Stage 2 / Severe malnutrition (requires 1 phenotypic criterion that meets this grade)	> 10% within the past 6 mo, or > 20% beyond 6 mo	< 18.5 if < 70 yr < 20 if ≥ 70 yr	Severe deficit (per validated assessment methods)

Abbreviation: GLIM = Global Leadership Initiative on Malnutrition.

Source: Reprinted with permission from World Health Organization, *Management of SevereMalnutrition: A Manual for Physicians and Other Senior Health Workers* (Geneva, 1999).

The GLIM criteria are similar to the Academy/ASPEN consensus criteria and the two are not mutually exclusive. GLIM provides core variables that should be collected to obtain global data on the prevalence of malnutrition, effective interventions, and outcomes.

II OVERLAPPING CONDITIONS

To add a bit more complexity to the diagnostic process, clinical characteristics used to diagnose malnutrition can also be associated with other conditions such as cachexia, sarcopenia and frailty. These are medical conditions that are similar to malnutrition but also may have different etiologies.[29,30]

Cachexia develops due to the dysfunction of multiple metabolic pathways involving systemic inflammation that results in unintentional weight loss and muscle and fat wasting in the presence of a chronic illness.[32] Sarcopenia is defined by aging and normal loss of muscle mass and strength, although sarcopenia can be found in obese patients as body composition analyses have demonstrated significant muscle loss with maintenance of adipose tissue.[33-35] Frailty presents as overall functional decline, characterized by fatigue, illness and weight loss.[33]

No single tool can be used to screen for all these syndromes.[34,36] For example, while a measure of muscle mass can be performed using DEXA, BIA or L3 Total Psoas Index with CT measurement to diagnose sarcopenia, this would not necessarily diagnose cachexia, frailty or malnutrition. Similarly, global consensus criteria that differentiate and aid in the diagnosis of these syndromes do not yet exist.[36]

TABLE 2.8
Comparison of Criteria Used in SGA, Academy/ASPEN, and GLIM

Criteria	SGA	Academy/ASPEN	GLIM
Weight loss	√	√	√
Energy intake	√	√	√
Muscle mass	√	√	√
Body fat	√	√	
BMI			√
Fluid accumulation or ascites	√	√	
Reduced grip strength / Functional capacity	√	√	
Disease burden / Inflammation	√	*	√
Gastrointestinal symptoms	√		

Abbreviations: SGA = Subjective Global Assessment; Academy/ASPEN = Academy of Nutrition and Dietetics / American Society of Parenteral and Enteral Nutrition; GLIM = Global Leadership Initiative on Malnutrition.

*Metabolic stress or inflammation is considered as part of the etiology-based diagnosis of malnutrition.

III CONCLUSION

It is difficult to adopt global criteria for diagnosing malnutrition when the clinical presentation of malnutrition varies. The concepts of kwashiorkor and marasmus are seen in children suffering from famine; however, these conditions are rarely found in most parts of the world. In North America, the etiology of malnutrition stems from a combination of multiple factors involving the presence of acute or chronic illness, and the degree and recurrence of the inflammatory process that lead to reductions in oral intake, weight, and fat and lean body mass. While disease processes may influence the ability to consume, absorb and utilize nutrients, they may also increase physiological demand or nutrient utilization.[4] Malnutrition can also occur in the social or environmental context such as food insecurity or voluntary restriction.[2] The issue becomes even more complicated when other related conditions overlap with malnutrition.

The scientific community has made tremendous progress since 2010 to provide different tools to diagnose malnutrition. However, the availability of several sets of criteria may result in a failure to fully recognize malnutrition in clinical practice. For example, a clinician may diagnose malnutrition using one of the previously discussed criteria, while the insurance provider may disagree and deny payment if they define malnutrition using a different standard. Perhaps the focus should be on the criteria used in the diagnosis of malnutrition rather than the tool itself. It is clear from this perspective that many of these tools apply similar criteria which may facilitate the concurrence of opinions. (See Table 2.8.) However, a validated diagnostic method should be used to accurately diagnose and document malnutrition to better measure the efficacy of nutrition interventions. Further research in recognizing or standardizing the approach to detect malnutrition and to establish one global approach is ongoing.

REFERENCES

1. Soeters PB, Schols AMWJ. Advances in understanding and assessing malnutrition. *Curr Opin Clin Nutr Metab Care*. 2009;12(5):487–494.
2. Jensen GL, Bistrian B, Roubenoff R, Heimburger DC. Malnutrition syndromes: a conundrum vs continuum. *JPEN J Parenter Enter Nutr*. 2009;33:710–716.
3. Roubenoff R, Heymsfield SB, Kehayias JJ, Cannon JG, Rosenberg IH. Standardization of body composition in weight loss. *Am J Clin Nutr*. 1997;66(1):192–196.
4. Elia M. Defining, recognizing, and reporting malnutrition. *Int J Low Extrem Wounds*. 2017;16(4):230–237.
5. American Diabetes Association. Standards of Medical Care in Diabetes-2021. *Diabetes Care*. 2021;44(Supplement 1):S15–S33.
6. Whelton PK, Carey RM, Aronow WS, et al. ACC/AHA/AAPA/ABC/ACPM/AGS/APhA/ASH/ASPC/NMA/PCNA guideline for the prevention, detection, evaluation, and management of high blood pressure in adults: executive summary: a report of the American College of Cardiology/American Heart Association task force on clinical practice guidelines. *Hypertension*. 2018;71(6):1269–1324.
7. World Health Organization. Constitution of the World Health Organization. Geneva. 2005. Published April 7, 1948. Updated September 15, 2005. Accessed January 19, 2021. https://apps.who.int/gb/bd/PDF/bd47/EN/constitution-en.pdf?ua=1.
8. Jelliffe DB. The assessment of the nutritional status of the community. World Health Organization. Published 1966. Accessed May 23, 2021. https://apps.who.int/iris/bitstream/handle/10665/41780/WHO_MONO_53_%28part1%29.pdf?sequence=1&isAllowed=y.
9. World Health Organization. The treatment and management of severe protein-energy malnutrition. Published 1981. Accessed January 22, 2021. https://apps.who.int/iris/bitstream/handle/10665/38925/9241541598_eng.pdf?sequence=1&isAllowed=y.
10. Bailey KV, Ferro-Luzzi A. Use of body mass index of adults in assessing individual and community nutritional status. *Bull World Health Organ*. 1995;73(5):673–680.
11. World Health Organization. *Management of Severe Malnutrition: A Manual for Physicians and Other Senior Health Workers*. Geneva. Published 1999. Accessed January 22, 2021. www.who.int/nutrition/publications/en/manage_severe_malnutrition_eng.pdf.
12. Vicente MA, Barão K, Silva TD, Forones NM. What are the most effective methods for assessment of nutritional status in outpatients with gastric and colorectal cancer? *Nutr Hosp*. 2013;28(3):585–591.
13. van Bokhorst-de van der Schueren MAE, Realino Guaitoli P, Jansma EP, de Vet HCW. Nutrition screening tools: Does one size fit all? A systematic review of screening tools for the hospital setting. *Clin Nutr*. 2013;33(1):39–58.
14. Baker JP, Detsky AS, Wesson DE, et al. Nutritional assessment: a comparison of clinical judgment and objective measurements. *N Engl J Med*. 1982;306(16):969–972.
15. Detsky AS, Baker JP, Mendelson RA, Wolman SL, Wesson DE, Jeejeebhoy KN. Evaluating the accuracy of nutritional assessment techniques applied to hospitalized patients: methodology and comparisons. *JPEN J Parenter Enter Nutr*. 1984;8(2):153–159.
16. Detskey AS, McLaughlin JR, Baker JP, et al. What is subjective global assessment of nutritional status? *JPEN J Parenter Enter Nutr*. 1987;11(1):8–13.
17. Enia G, Sicuso C, Alati G, Zoccali C. Subjective global assessment of nutrition in dialysis patients. *Nephrol Dial Transplant*. 1993;8(10):1094–1098.

18. Lupo L, Pannarale O, Altomare D, Memeo V, Rubino M. Reliability of clinical judgment in evaluation of the nutritional status of surgical patients. *Brit J Surg.* 1993;80(12):1553–1556.

19. Ek AC, Unosson M, Larsson J, Ganowiak W, Bjurulf P. Interrater variability and validity in subjective nutritional assessment of elderly patients. *Scand J Caring Sci.* 1996;10(3):163–168.

20. Jones CH, Newstead CG, Will EJ, Smye SW, Davison AM. Assessment of nutritional status in CAPD patients: serum albumin is not a useful measure. *Nephrol Dial Transplant.* 1997;12(7):1406–1413.

21. Naber THJ, Schermer T, de Bree A, et al. Prevalence of malnutrition in nonsurgical hospitalized patients and its association with disease complications. *Am J Clin Nutr.* 1997;66(5):1232–1239.

22. Canadian Malnutrition Task Force. Subjective global assessment (SGA) – diagnosing malnutrition. Assessed February 4, 2021. https://nutritioncareincanada.ca/resources-and-tools/hospital-care-inpac/assessment-sga.

23. Jensen GL, Mirtallo J, Compher C, et al. Adult starvation and disease-related malnutrition: a proposal for etiology-based diagnosis in the clinical practice setting from the International Consensus Guideline Committee. *JPEN J Parenter Enter Nutr.* 2010;34(2):156–159.

24. White JV, Guenter P, Jensen G, et al. Consensus statement of the Academy of Nutrition and Dietetics/American Society of Parenteral and Enteral Nutrition: characteristics recommended for the identification and documentation of adult malnutrition (undernutrition). *J Acad Nutr Diet.* 2012;112(5):730–738.

25. Mogensen KM, Malone A, Becker P, et al. Academy of Nutrition and Dietetics/ American Society for Parenteral and Enteral Nutrition consensus malnutrition characteristics: usability and association with outcomes. *Nutr Clin Pract.* 2019;34(5):657–665.

26. Hiura G, Lebwohl B, Seres DS. Malnutrition diagnosis in critically ill patients using 2012 Academy of Nutrition and Dietetics/American Society for Parenteral and Enteral Nutrition standardized diagnostic characteristics is associated with longer hospital and intensive care unit length of stay and increased in-hospital mortality. *JPEN J Parenter Enter Nutr.* 2020;44(2):256–264.

27. Jensen GL, Malone A, Guenter P. The Academy of Nutrition and Dietetics/The American Society for Parenteral and Enteral Nutrition consensus malnutrition characteristics: usability and association with outcomes – a commentary. *Nutr Clin Pract.* 2019;34(5):655–656.

28. Yakes Jimenez E, Long JM, Lamers-Johnson E, et al. Academy of Nutrition and Dietetics Nutrition Research Network: rationale and protocol for a study to validate the Academy of Nutrition and Dietetics/American Society for Parenteral and Enteral Nutrition consensus-derived diagnostic indicators for adult and pediatric malnutrition and to determine optimal registered dietitian nutritionist staffing in acute care hospital settings. *J Acad Nutr Diet.* Published May 04, 2021. Accessed August 23, 2021. https://doi.org/10.1016/j.jand.2021.03.017.

29. Cederholm T, Bosaeus I, Barazzoni R, et al. Diagnostic criteria for malnutrition – an ESPEN consensus statement. *Clin Nutr.* 2015;34(3):335–340.

30. Jensen GL, Cederholm T, Correia MITD, et al. GLIM criteria for the diagnosis of malnutrition: a consensus report from the global clinical nutrition community. *JPEN J Parenter Enter Nutr.* 2019;43(1):32–40.

31. Phillips W, Doley J, Boi K. Malnutrition definitions in clinical practice: to be E43 or not to be? *Health Inf Manag J.* 2020;49(1):74–79.

32. Fearon K, Strasser F, Anker SD, et al. Definition and classification of cancer cachexia: an international consensus. *Lancet Oncol.* 2011;12(5):489–495.

33. Morley JE, Anker SD, von Haehling S. Prevalence, incidence, and clinical impact of sarcopenia: facts, numbers, and epidemiology-update. *J Cachexia Sarcopenia Muscle.* 2014;5(4):253–259.

34. Miller J, Wells L, Nwulu U, Currow D, Johnson MJ, Skipworth RJE. Validated screening tools for the assessment of cachexia, sarcopenia and malnutrition: a systematic review. *Am J Clin Nutr.* 2018;108(6):1196–1208.

35. Gallagher D, DeLegge M. Body composition (sarcopenia) in obese patients: implications for care in the intensive care unit. *JPEN J Parenter Enter Nutr.* 2011;35(5S):21S–28S.

36. Jensen GL, Cederholm T. The malnutrition overlap syndromes of cachexia and sarcopenia: a malnutrition conundrum. *Am J Clin Nutr.* 2018;108(6):1157–1158.

3 Prevalence and Risk Factors

Jennifer Doley

CONTENTS

I INTRODUCTION

Adult malnutrition is recognized as a common global health problem and has recently garnered increased focus, especially in the acute care setting. As a debilitating condition that increases mortality and healthcare costs, and worsens clinical outcomes, it is essential to understand malnutrition prevalence and risk factors for various populations so that effective identification and treatment strategies can be implemented.[1,2]

Researchers have studied the prevalence and risk of malnutrition in various healthcare settings worldwide. However, data are inconsistent and reported risk and prevalence rates vary widely. Several factors confound accurate interpretation of the scientific literature on malnutrition. Researchers have used a variety of definitions for malnutrition, including some previously accepted criteria that are not evidence-based, such as albumin and prealbumin levels.[3,4] Additionally, some study reports refer to malnutrition prevalence when only a screening tool, not a diagnostic tool, was used.[5] Data from these studies reflect prevalence of malnutrition *risk*, not prevalence of an actual malnutrition diagnosis. Some studies of adults of all ages used the Mini Nutritional Assessment tool,[6,7] which has only been validated in populations $\geq$ 65 years of age.[8]

DOI: 10.1201/9781003177586-3

Many malnutrition research studies focus on specific diagnoses or age groups, and some may not report data on certain demographic factors, such as subjects' race and ethnicity. It is therefore difficult to extrapolate these prevalence and risk data to all populations. Assessment of risk factors is especially challenging, as most studies only identify factors that are *associated* with malnutrition. As association does not signify causation, it is unclear if these factors cause or result from malnutrition, or both. While statistical analyses in some research may consider confounding variables, some do not. Lastly, some risk factors may influence or be related to others.[9]

II GEOGRAPHY

In 2019, Crichton et al. published a meta-analysis of studies on global malnutrition prevalence in the community setting.[10] The review included 111 studies that used validated diagnostic tools for malnutrition (Mini Nutritional Assessment or Subjective Global Assessment) with a total of 69,702 participants from 38 countries. The majority of the studies were conducted in Europe (45.9%) and Asia (34.2%), with other areas of the globe not well represented (North America (10.8%), Australia (6.3%), South America (3.6%) and Africa (1.8%)). Results were pooled by geographic location, with the lowest reported malnutrition prevalence in Northern Europe (2.5%) and the highest in Southeast Asia (24.6%). Study limitations include high heterogeneity of subjects between studies due to the types of participants enrolled, uneven geographic distribution, and low sample size for some regions. While these data should be interpreted with caution considering the study limitations, they do provide some insight into malnutrition prevalence based on geographic location.[10]

A systematic review of hospitalized adult patients from 12 countries in Latin America revealed a wide range of disease-related malnutrition prevalence (2.6 to 73.2%), although prevalence was in the range of 40–60% in many of the studies. While the total number of subjects was high (*n* = 29,474), several variables may have confounded the results. A significant limitation was the heterogeneity of subjects, including studies that focused only on specific disease states, such as critical illness and surgery, older adults only and geographic location, as a majority of the studies were conducted in Brazil. Further, although most studies used evidence-based malnutrition assessment tools, some used body mass index (BMI) only. The authors reported that malnutrition risk tended to be lower in the studies that used BMI only.[11]

III HEALTHCARE SETTING

Malnutrition risk and prevalence have been identified in a variety of healthcare settings, including acute care, long-term care, rehabilitation centers or units, and the community. Research studies may characterize "community" in a variety of ways; however, it can be broadly defined as any setting outside of an inpatient healthcare facility, including outpatient clinics, home healthcare, adult daycare and congregate meal sites, among others.[12] Reported prevalences for each setting vary widely due to factors including gender, ethnicity and geographic location, as well as study design

TABLE 3.1

Malnutrition Prevalence in the Acute Care / Hospital Setting

Study	Location	Number of subjects	Age (years)	Condition	Screen/ Assess tool	Prevalence/Risk	Factors associated with malnutrition
Ostrowska[19] 2021	Europe	10,863	≥ 60	—	MST ESPEN	Prevalence – 12.9% Risk – 29.9%	Taking > 5 medications, unable to walk without assist, self-reported poor health status
D'Almeida[20] 2020	Brazil	3061	> 65	Cancer	MNA-SF	Prevalence – 33.4% Risk – 39.3%	Female, increasing age
Fukui[21] 2020	Japan	300	≥ 75	Aortic stenosis	MNA-SF	Prevalence – 11.3% Risk – 42.3%	Severity of cardiac function, impaired IADLs, female
Van Vliet[16] 2020	Netherlands	584	Adult	—	PG-SGA	Prevalence (moderate and severe) – 31% at admission (n = 584) 56% on day 5 (n = 292) 66% on day 10 (n = 101) 79% on day ≥15 (n = 14) Of 91 pts assessed both at admit and before DC, 30% of well-nourished became malnourished, 82% of malnourished remained so	—
Chatindiara[22] 2018	New Zealand	234	≥ 65 ≥ 60 for Maori	—	MNA-SF	Prevalence – 26.9% Risk – 46.6%	Decline in cognition, dysphagia risk
Rinninella[23] 2018	Italy	300	Adult	—	NRS-2002, ESPEN	Prevalence – 38.7% Risk – 52.3%	Cirrhosis, upper GI disease
Alzahrani[24] 2017	Saudi Arabia	248	≥ 60	—	MNA-SF	Prevalence – 29% Risk – 47.6%	Living alone

(Continued)

TABLE 3.1 (Continued)
Malnutrition Prevalence in the Acute Care / Hospital Setting

Study	Location	Number of subjects	Age (years)	Condition	Screen/ Assess tool	Prevalence/Risk	Factors associated with malnutrition
Kim[25] 2016	Korea	102	> 20	PD	MNA	Prevalence – 25.5% Risk – 26.5%	Anxiety, duration of levodopa therapy, weight at onset of disease
Planas[26] 2016	Spain	401	Adult	Cancer	NRS-2002	*All* Risk on admit – 33.9% Risk on DC – 36.4% *> 70 yo* Risk on admit – 38.3% Risk on DC – 50%	Increasing age
Hernandez[17] 2015	Spain	352	Adult	Dysphagia	NRS-2002	*All:* 45.6% admit*, 42.2% DC^ ≥ 70 yo: 54.6% admit, 57.5% DC < 70 yo: 25.5% admit, 21.3% DC * w/in 48 h ^ at DC or day 28 if LOS > 28 days	Increasing age, reason for admission (urgent > scheduled)
Paris[27] 2013	Spain	1098 (35 hospitals)	≥ 65	DM	MNA	Prevalence – 21.2% Risk – 39.1%	Older age, female, DM complications
Lamb[28] 2009	United Kingdom	328	> 16	Medical, surgical, orthopedic, ICU	MUST	High risk – 32% Mod risk – 11.9%	Female, increasing age

						Prevalence	Risk factors
Pirlich[29] 2005	Germany	794	Adult	—	SGA	Prevalence – 22%	*All ages* Malignancy, multiple prescriptions, living alone, lower education, age ≥ 60 *Age < 60* Polypharmacy, malignancy *Age ≥ 60* Polypharmacy, living alone
Correia[30] 2003	Latin America	9348	Adult	—	SGA	Prevalence – 50.2% (11.2% severe)	Age > 60, cancer, infection, LOS

Abbreviations: MNA-SF = Mini Nutritional Assessment – Short Form; IADLs = independent activities of daily living; MST = Malnutrition Screening Tool; ESPEN = European Society for Clinical Nutrition and Metabolism; PG-SGA = Patient Generated Subjective Global Assessment; DC = discharge; NRS-2002 = Nutritional Risk Screening 2002; GI = gastrointestinal; PD = Parkinson's disease; MNA = Mini Nutritional Assessment; LOS = length of stay; DM = diabetes mellitus; ICU = intensive care unit; MUST = Malnutrition. Universal Screening Tool; SGA = Subjective Global Assessment.

TABLE 3.2
Malnutrition Prevalence in the Rehabilitation Setting

Study	Location	Number of subjects	Age (years)	Screen/ Assess tool	Prevalence/ Risk	Factors associated with malnutrition
Marshall[31] 2016	Australia	57	≥ 65	ICD-10-AM PG-SGA MNA	Prevalence ICD-10-AM – 46% PG-SGA – 53% MNA – 28%	—
Charlton[32] 2012	Australia	476	≥ 65	MNA	Prevalence – 30% Risk – 53%	Increasing age
Kaiser[14] 2010	12 countries	4507	Mean age 82.3	MNA	Prevalence – 50.5%	—

Abbreviations: ICD-10-AM = International Statistical Classification of Diseases and Related Health Problems, Australian Modification; PG-SGA = Patient Generated Subjective Global Assessment; MNA = Mini Nutritional Assessment.

elements such as the age of subjects and how each healthcare setting is defined. Malnutrition risk and prevalence are high in the acute care setting, and reportedly affect at least one-third of all inpatient stays in the United States.[1]

Research has also found a high prevalence of malnutrition in the rehabilitation setting. In a review of 17 studies conducted on older patients in rehabilitation facilities or units, malnutrition prevalence ranged from 0.1 to 68%, although prevalence reported in most of the studies was 25–50%.[13] Similarly, in a pooled analysis of 24 studies that included 4507 older adults, the highest incidence of malnutrition was 50.5% in the rehabilitation setting, followed by hospitals (38.7%), nursing homes (13.8%) and the community (5.8%).[14]

In another analysis of 240 studies with over 113,000 subjects, researchers also found the highest incidence of malnutrition in the rehabilitation setting (29.7%) and lowest in the community setting (3.1%).[15] The reported prevalence in other settings were long-term care (28.7%), hospital (22%), home care (8.7%) and outpatient (6%). Investigators in both analyses included only studies that used validated screening and assessment tools; however, both cited heterogeneity of subjects to be a significant study limitation.[15] Patients already nutritionally compromised on admission to an acute care hospital generally see further decline in nutrition status upon discharge.[16,17] As patients are generally admitted to rehabilitation units after prolonged hospital stays related to severe acute illness or exacerbation of chronic illness[18], it is not surprising that malnutrition prevalence is high in this population.

TABLE 3.3

Malnutrition Prevalence in the Community Setting

Study	Location	Number of subjects	Age (Years)	Condition	Screen / Assess Tool	Prevalence / Risk	Factors associated with malnutrition
Wojteczek[33] 2020	Poland	56	> 18	Scleroderma	Prevalence: ESPEN, GLIM Risk: SGA, SNAQ	Prevalence (ESPEN) – 17.9% Prevalence (GLIM) – moderate 50%, severe 12.5% Risk (SGA) – moderate 21.4%, severe 1.8% Risk (SNAQ) – moderate 0%, severe 16.1%	
Rodriguez-Sanchez[34] 2020	Spain	1660	≥ 65	—	Prevalence: GLIM (for those at risk using MNA-SF) Risk: MNA-SF	Prevalence – 12.6% Risk – 15%	Increasing age, frailty, depression, polypharmacy
Vandewoude[35] 2019	Belgium	819	≥ 70	—	MNA-SF	Prevalence – 7% Risk – 29%	Dementia, depression, cancer
Kuczmarski[7] 2019	United States	2177	Adult; Cohort ≥ 60	—	MNA-SF	Prevalence – 7.8% Risk – 63.7%	Lower income, less education, depression (symptoms or diagnosis), food insecurity, bipolar, anxiety, reduced functional status
Wei[36] 2018	China	6450	≥ 60	—	ESPEN	Prevalence – 12.6%	Increasing age, male, rural, lack health insurance
Damayanthi[37] 2018	Sri Lanka	999		—	MNA-SF	Prevalence – 12.5% Risk – 52.4%	Increasing age, alcohol abuse, hypertension, living alone

(Continued)

TABLE 3.3 (Continued)
Malnutrition Prevalence in the Community Setting

Study	Location	Number of subjects	Age (Years)	Condition	Screen / Assess Tool	Prevalence / Risk	Factors associated with malnutrition
Van den Broeke[38] 2018	Belgium	657	≥ 70	Cancer	MNA-SF	All Prevalence – 7% Risk – 30% Cancer ($n = 274$) – combined prevalence and risk – 66% No cancer ($n = 383$) – combined prevalence and risk – 16.7%	Depression, impaired IADLs (especially shopping, cooking and transport), distress, cancer
Shidfar[6] 2016	Iran	130	Adult	PD	MNA	Prevalence – 11.5% Risk – 58.5%	Increasing age, severity of disease
Wang[39] 2010	China	117	Adult	PD	MNA	Prevalence – 1.7% Risk – 19.7%	Constipation, depression

Abbreviations: ESPEN = European Society for Clinical Nutrition and Metabolism; SGA = Subjective Global Assessment; SNAQ = Simplified Nutritional Appetite Questionnaire; GLIM = Global Leadership Initiative on Malnutrition; MNA-SF = Mini Nutritional Assessment – Short Form; IADLs = independent activities of daily living; LTC = long-term care; PD = Parkinson's disease; MNA = Mini Nutritional Assessment.

TABLE 3.4
Malnutrition Prevalence in the Long-Term Care Setting

Study	Setting	Number of subjects	Age (years)	Screen/ Assess tool	Prevalence/Risk	Factors associated with malnutrition
Velazques-Alva[40] 2020	Mexico	262	≥ 65	MNA	Prevalence – 21.1% Risk – 59.9%	Increasing age, depression, decreasing functional status
Balci[41] 2019	Turkey	1224	≥ 65	MNA	Prevalence – 23.4% Risk – 45.7%	Dysphagia, poor cognition, dependence on ADLs
Vandewoude[35] 2019	Belgium	2480	≥ 70	MNA-SF	Prevalence – 14% Risk – 49%	Dementia, depression, cancer, PD, dependence on ADLs, number of comorbidities
Basibüyük[42] 2019	Turkey	773	≥ 60	MNA-SF	Prevalence – 8.4% Risk – 37%	Increasing age, dementia, depression, female, taking ≥ 3 medications per day
Madeira[43] 2018	Portugal	1186	≥ 65	MNA	Prevalence – 4.8% Risk – 38.7%	Increasing age, women, symptoms of depression, dependence on ADLs
Nazemi[44] 2015	Iran	263	> 60	MNA	Prevalence – 10.3% Risk – 68.8%	Independent variables – DM, poor/no teeth Associated with – sleep < 6 h per night, female
Papparotto[45] 2013	Italy	186	≥ 65	MNA	Prevalence – 36% Risk – 43%	Increasing age, female, dependence on ADLs, stroke, ≥ 4 illnesses

Abbreviations: LTC = long-term care; MNA = Mini Nutritional Assessment; ADLs = activities of daily living; MNA-SF = Mini Nutritional Assessment – Short Form; PD = Parkinson's disease; DM = diabetes mellitus.

TABLE 3.5

Malnutrition Prevalence in the Home-Based Care Setting

Study	Setting	Number of subjects	Age (years)	Screen/ Assess tool	Prevalence/ Risk	Factors associated with malnutrition
Berggren[46] 2020	Sweden	121	≥ 80	Prevalence: PG-SGA Risk: MNA	Prevalence – 7.4% Risk – 42%	Tiredness, anxiety, lower physical activity
Baz[47] 2019	Turkey	288	≥ 65	MNA	Prevalence – 15.6% Risk – 47.2%	Increasing age, lower education attainment, decreasing functional ability
Win[48] 2017	United States	2252	≥ 65	MNA-SF	Prevalence – 15% Risk – 40.3%	Not reported

Abbreviations: MNA = Mini Nutritional Assessment; MNA-SF = Mini Nutritional Assessment – Short Form; PG-SGA = Patient Generated Subjective Global Assessment.

Tables 3.1 to 3.5 review recent select studies that used validated screening and/or assessment tools to measure malnutrition risk and/or prevalence in several settings: hospitals (Table 3.1), rehabilitation (Table 3.2), community programs (Table 3.3), long-term care (Table 3.4) and home-based or palliative care (Table 3.5).

IV   ACUTE AND CHRONIC DISEASE

Acute disease or injury-related malnutrition is characterized by an acute and severe degree of inflammation, such as is seen in burns, trauma or major infections. Chronic disease-related malnutrition is generally recognized as having a duration longer than three months, and is associated with mild or moderate chronic inflammation, as seen in some cancers and liver or kidney failure.[49]

Prevalence and risk of malnutrition have been studied in multiple disease states and medical conditions. Research has shown a significantly higher risk of malnutrition in individuals with cancer, especially pancreatic, gastrointestinal and head/neck cancers,[50] in both the inpatient[20,26,29,30] and community settings.[25,35,38] Other diseases and conditions with reported higher rates of malnutrition risk and prevalence include dysphagia,[17,22,41] Parkinson's disease,[6,25,39,51] dementia or impaired cognition,[22,35,41,42,52] depression or anxiety,[34,35,38,39,43,46] stroke,[45] chronic obstructive pulmonary disease,[53,54] inflammatory bowel disease,[55,56] advanced liver disease,[57] acquired immune deficiency syndrome[58,59] and renal disease,[60] among others.

In addition to specific medical conditions, a greater number of overall comorbidities is also associated with higher nutrition risk.[27,45,52] Other factors related to comorbidities include the duration of a disease or its treatment,[25,51] duration of hospitalization,[16,26,30] disease severity,[6,21,54] and polypharmacy.[29,34,42]

Many factors can result in disease-related malnutrition, such as an array of symptoms that decrease intake, as well as alterations in nutrient absorption and metabolism. See Chapters 11 and 12 for more information on the causes and treatments for these conditions.

A REDUCED INTAKE

In acute or chronic illness, inadequate nutrient intake may result from symptoms such as poor appetite, difficulty chewing or swallowing, shortness of breath, altered level of consciousness or cognition, nausea, vomiting, constipation, diarrhea, taste changes, early satiety, fatigue and decreased mobility. These symptoms may be caused by the disease process itself, or its treatments, such as medications, surgeries and other procedures. Intentional restrictions of food may also occur with psychiatric conditions such as anorexia nervosa.

B INCREASED NUTRIENT NEEDS

A number of medical conditions increase nutrient needs. Acute illness or injury causing high levels of inflammation can increase energy expenditure and protein turnover. Chronic diseases such as obstructive pulmonary disease,[61] liver disease[62] and some types of cancer may also increase nutrient needs.[50] Additionally, nutrient needs may be heightened to facilitate healing of burns, pressure injuries, opened surgical incisions and other types of wounds.

C IMPAIRED NUTRIENT ABSORPTION AND UTILIZATION

Nutrient malabsorption can be a significant contributor to chronic disease-related malnutrition. Some malabsorptive conditions directly affect the surface or lining of the gastrointestinal tract, either by reduction of the total surface area available for absorption, or by damage to the mucosa. Such conditions include inflammatory bowel disease, short bowel syndrome, small bowel bacterial overgrowth, chronic pancreatitis and celiac disease, which can lead to a significant loss of the nutrients consumed.[63] Bariatric surgery is a unique circumstance, as some types of surgical interventions deliberately create malabsorption as a treatment for obesity; however, they can also lead to malnutrition and micronutrient deficiencies.[64]

Other diseases may cause insufficient production of enzymes required for digestion, such as pancreatic disease[65] and cystic fibrosis.[66] Hypochlorhydria, or reduced production of gastric acid, can impair breakdown of some nutrients and thus hinder absorption. Hypochlorhydria may be seen with increasing age, use of proton-pump inhibitor medications or gastric resections.[67]

Nutrient losses may also occur through other means besides a dysfunctional gastrointestinal tract. Poorly controlled diabetes mellitus (DM) causes hyperglycemia, which results in the loss of glucose in the urine. Liver disease can result in functional nutrient deficits, as the liver serves as a primary site for metabolism and storage of many nutrients, and produces proteins used for their transport.[62] Individuals with end stage renal disease can lose nutrients through blood filtration that occurs in the dialysis process.[68]

V   FUNCTIONAL STATUS

The US Centers for Disease Control and Prevention (CDC) defines disability as any condition or impairment of the body or mind that makes it more difficult for a person to do certain activities and interact with the world around them.[69] Conditions include those that impair various functions, including mobility, sensory (vision, hearing), cognitive (comprehension, learning, memory), mental health, communication, and social relationships. Disabilities or impairments may be present at birth (e.g. caused by genetic disorders or maternal exposure to infection or substances), develop during childhood (e.g. autism spectrum disorder), result from injury (e.g. traumatic brain injury) or result from chronic conditions (e.g. poorly controlled diabetes leading to impaired vision). Impairments may be progressive, such as muscular dystrophy, static, such as loss of a limb, or intermittent, such as some forms of multiple sclerosis.[69]

Disability or impaired functional status can result in reduced ability to obtain, prepare and eat food, especially in individuals without sufficient social or financial support to assist in these activities. Impaired functional status is strongly associated with malnutrition.[7,19,21,24,38,40,41,43,45,47,52] As with many other conditions, it is difficult to determine if declining functional status is a cause or effect of malnutrition, or both.[70]

Functional status can be assessed by factors such as independence in activities of daily living, as well as more specific measurement tools such as hand grip strength and the Short Physical Performance Battery test.[71] See Chapter 5 for additional information on assessing functional status.

VI   DEMOGRAPHICS

The more traditional term "demographics" may be better described as social determinants of health (SDOH). The World Health Organization (WHO) defines SDOH as "the conditions in which people are born, grow, live, work and age. These circumstances are shaped by the distribution of money, power and resources at global, national and local levels".[72] Social determinants of health include factors such as income, education and housing, among many others. Social determinants of health play a significant role in an individual's access to quality healthcare and healthy food, as well as health behaviors.[73] The following sections review select SDOH (and factors that impact SDOH) which can affect the prevalence and risk of malnutrition.

A   AGE

Many malnutrition studies conducted on older adults aged ≥ 60 or 65 years have found that as people age, the risk and prevalence of malnutrition increase. This relationship has been noted in a variety of settings, include acute and long-term care, and community and home care.[6,17,27–30,34,36,37,40,42] The contribution of age to malnutrition can also be multifactorial, as increasing age may be associated with an increase in the number and severity of acute and chronic diseases, social isolation, reduced income and impaired functional status.[74]

B GENDER

Gender may have an effect on malnutrition prevalence, although this appears to vary depending on the population and setting. Many studies have reported no statistically significant difference between sexes.[7,17,19,22–25,29,30,52,75] However, other studies have identified women at higher risk,[20,21,27,28,42,43,45] while very few have reported men at higher risk.[36] The meta-analysis conducted by Crichton et al. on malnutrition prevalence in the community reported that, based on 27 studies and 38,703 participants, women were 45% more likely to have malnutrition than men ($p < 0.00001$).[10] These data suggest that in circumstances where gender may influence malnutrition risk, such as increased needs in pregnancy and lactation, women are more likely to be negatively affected. Further, in some societies, when food is scarce, males are given priority at meals. Women are also less likely than men to have access to income and other financial support, which contributes to food insecurity.[76]

C RACE/ETHNICITY

There are significant limitations in evaluating research on malnutrition prevalence based on race or ethnicity. Race is often erroneously identified as a biological or physiological variable, but it is essentially a social construct. Race categories are generally applied to very large groups of the population, thus there is very wide genetic variability within any one group. It can be difficult to interpret some research studies, as the authors may not clarify how they identified race, although self-identification is now the method most commonly used. Even self-identification is not without its drawbacks, as individuals may identify their race based on appearance, language, country or region of origin, religion, customs, traditions or lifestyles. Furthermore, in many studies, classifications of race may be limited only to a few groups (most commonly Black, Hispanic and White); however, more individuals now identify as multiracial.[77]

In addition to the inherent difficulties of interpreting research as it relates to race or ethnicity, malnutrition risk and prevalence based on race have not been widely reported in adults, although there are numerous reports in children, for both general malnutrition and deficiency of specific nutrients. In a small study on older adults in an adult daycare setting in the United States, researchers used a validated tool to measure nutrition risk and found that 65% of Blacks were at high nutrition risk, compared to non-Hispanic Whites, Hispanics and Asians (40%, 33% and 29%, respectively).[78] In a study on 1001 community-dwelling adults ≥ 55 years of age, Sheean et al. found significantly higher nutrition risk in Blacks (47%) and Hispanics (30%) compared to Whites (23%).[79] Some studies have reported higher prevalence of malnutrition in indigenous compared to non-indigenous populations.[80–82]

Despite its challenges, race should not be eliminated from nutrition research, as racial discrimination and disparities affect many aspects of health, including access to food, income, opportunities for healthy behaviors, and other SDOH.[83,84] Health disparities based on ethnicity/race are a widely recognized problem in the United States.[77,84] Compared to non-Hispanic Whites, Blacks and Hispanics have higher rates of food insecurity[84,85] and specific disease states such as cancer[84,86] and a wide variety of issues associated with reduced quality of and access to healthcare.[84,87]

D Socioeconomic Factors

Malnutrition not related to acute or chronic disease is often caused by social and environmental factors which can negatively affect nutrient intake, in both the quantity and quality of food consumed. Income, residential environment, access to transportation and housing conditions, among others, may limit access to healthy food, as well as the ability to purchase, store and prepare it.[84] The following reviews malnutrition risk related to marital status, residence, income and education level. However, there are other factors that influence SDOH, which may affect nutrition risk, such as immigration status, employment, language and disability, among others.[84]

1 Marital Status

A meta-analysis conducted by Besora-Moreno et al. on subjects ≥ 60 years of age reported that marital status was significantly correlated with malnutrition risk. Of the 24 studies that investigated marital status and malnutrition, 13 did not find significant results; however, of the 11 studies that did, ten reported a greater malnutrition risk in subjects who were single, widowed or divorced. It is important to note that subjects in the non-married category are more likely to live alone, thus it is difficult to determine the degree to which marital status or living alone each contributed to a correlation with malnutrition.[88]

2 Residence

Location of residence may influence nutrition risk, although research on this determinant is somewhat limited. Besora-Moreno's meta-analysis reported only three studies that investigated the location of residence (rural vs. urban). Two did not find any correlation, and the third reported a higher nutrition risk in rural areas as compared to urban. The authors concluded that there was insufficient evidence to determine if location of residence affected malnutrition risk and that further research was needed.[88] However, Crichton et al. analyzed more research; 17 studies investigated malnutrition prevalence in rural and 69 studies in urban communities. The pooled data showed the prevalence of malnutrition was higher in rural (9.9%) vs. urban (5.7%) areas.[10] While this analysis does suggest a correlation between malnutrition risk and rural settings, this evidence must be interpreted with caution, as the heterogeneity of subjects was high, especially regarding geographic location.[10]

In addition to the location of residence, the number of people with whom one lives is also a risk factor. Living alone is a social factor that appears to correlate with higher malnutrition risk.[24,29,37,88] The Besora-Moreno analysis of subjects ≥ 60 years of age reported that of the 27 studies that analyzed subjects living alone vs. those living with others, all but two indicated either a correlation between malnutrition risk and living alone, or no statistical difference.[88] This suggests that in circumstances where living situation affects nutrition status, the older population is at higher risk when living alone. Reduced caloric intake has been reported in older adults who eat alone vs. those who eat with others, regardless of the number of people in residence, suggesting that the reason those who live alone have a higher prevalence of malnutrition may be partly because they are eating alone.[89]

3 Income

In their analysis, Besora-Moreno et al. found that of the 20 studies that investigated income level, 12 found a significant correlation between lower income level and higher malnutrition risk.[88] Similarly, in a longitudinal study of community dwelling adults, Kuczmarski reported that malnutrition prevalence was associated with lower income levels, defined as < 125% of the US poverty level, in those ≥ 60 years of age.[7] In relation to income levels, more food insecurity is also associated with increased malnutrition prevalence and risk.[7,90]

4 Education Level

Some studies have shown that malnutrition is associated with a lower education level,[7,29,47] while others have not.[91] In the review and meta-analysis by Besora-Moreno et al., the authors analyzed 40 observational studies of participants ≥ 60 years of age, excluding those on subjects with specific disease states or conditions. Of the 31 studies that evaluated education level, 11 revealed a higher risk of malnutrition at lower education levels, four found lower risk, and 16 did not find that education level had a statistically significant effect on malnutrition.[88] It appears lower education level may increase risk of malnutrition in some settings in older populations, although further research is needed.

VII CONCLUSION

A number of acute and chronic illnesses as well as social, behavioral and environmental factors can contribute to malnutrition. Malnutrition research results can be challenging to interpret given the heterogeneity of subjects and varying definitions of malnutrition; however, it is clear that there are a number of factors related to malnutrition risk, including healthcare setting, demographics and socioeconomic considerations. It is important to understand the common etiologies and risk factors of malnutrition so that health professionals can effectively screen for high-risk patients, and implement nutrition treatment and monitoring plans in a timely manner.

REFERENCES

1. Tappenden KA, Quatrara B, Parkhurst ML, Malone A, Fanjiang G, Ziegler TR. Critical role of nutrition in improving quality of care: an interdisciplinary call to action to address adult hospital malnutrition. *JPEN J Parenter Enteral Nutr.* 2013;37(4):482–497.

2. White JV, Guenter P, Jensen G, Malone A, Schofield M, the Academy Malnutrition Workgroup, the ASPEN Malnutrition Task Force. Consensus statement of the Academy of Nutrition and Dietetics / American Society of Parenteral and Enteral Nutrition: characteristics recommended for the identification and documentation of adult malnutrition (undernutrition). *JPEN J Parenter Enteral Nutr.* 2012;36(3):275–283.

3. Evans DC, Corkins MR, Malone A, et al. The use of visceral proteins as nutrition markers: an ASPEN position paper. *Nutr Clin Pract.* 2021;36(1):22–28.

4. Scrutinio D, Lanzillo B, Guida P, Passantino A, Spaccavento S, Battista P. Association between malnutrition and outcomes in patients with severe ischemic stroke undergoing rehabilitation. *Arch Phys Med Rehabil.* 2020;101(5):852–860.

5. Koifman E, Mashiach T, Papier I, Karban A, Eliakim R, Chermesh I. Proactive screening in Israel identifies alarming prevalence of malnutrition among hospitalized patients – action is needed. *Nutrition.* 2012;28(5):515–519.

6. Shidfar F, Darabkhani PB, Yazdanpanah L, Karkheiran S, Noorollahi-Moghaddam H, Haghani H. Assessment of nutritional status in patients with Parkinson's disease and its relationship with severity of the disease. *Med J Islam Repub Iran.* 2016;30:454.

7. Kuczmarski MF, Shupe ES, Pohlig RT, Rawal R, Zonderman AB, Evans MK. A longitudinal analysis of diet quality and risks associated with malnutrition in socioeconomic and racially diverse adults. *Nutrients.* 2019;11(9):2046.

8. van Bokhorst-de van der Schueren MA, Guaitoli PR, Jansma EP, et al. Nutrition screening tools: does one size fit all? A systematic review of screening tools for the hospital setting. *Clin Nutr.* 2014;33(1):39–58.

9. Boushey CJ, Harris J, Bruemmer B, Archer SL. Publishing nutrition research: a review of study design, statistical analyses and other key elements of manuscript preparation, part 1. *J Am Diet Assoc.* 2006;106(1):89–96.

10. Crichton M, Craven D, Mackay H, Marx W, Van Der Schueren M, Marshall S. A systematic review, meta-analysis and meta-regression of the prevalence of protein-energy malnutrition: associates with geographical region and sex. *Age Ageing.* 2019;48(1):38–48.

11. Correia MITD, Perman MI, Waitzberg DL. Hospital malnutrition in Latin America: a systematic review. *Clin Nutr.* 2017;36(4):958–967.

12. Centers for Medicare & Medicaid Services. Medicaid Program; State Plan Home and Community-Based Services, 5-Year Period for Waivers, Provider Payment Reassignment, and Home and Community-Based Setting Requirements for Community First Choice and Home and Community-Based Services (HCBS) Waivers. Federal Register, January 2014. Accessed May 3, 2021. www.federalregister.gov/documents/2014/01/16/2014-00487/medicaid-program-state-plan-home-and-community-based-services-5-year-period-for-waivers-provider.

13. Marshall S. Protein-energy malnutrition in the rehabilitation setting: Evidence to improve identification. *Maturitas.* 2016;86:77-85.

14. Kaiser MJ, Bauer JM, Rämsch C, et al. Frequency of malnutrition in older adults: a multinational perspective using the Mini Nutritional Assessment. *J Am Geriatr Soc.* 2010;58(9):1734.

15. Cereda E, Pedrolli C, Klersy C, et al. Nutritional status in older persons according to healthcare setting: A systematic review and meta-analysis of prevalence data using MNA®. *Clin Nutr.* 2016;35(6):1282–1290.

16. Van Vliet IMY, Gomes-Neto AW, de Jong MFC, Jager-Wittenaar H, Navis GJ. High prevalence of malnutrition both on hospital admission and predischarge. *Nutrition.* 2020;77.

17. Hernandez JA, Sanz ML, Vila MP, Arujo K, Garcia de Lorenzo A, Perez SC. Prevalence and costs of malnutrition in hospitalized dysphagic patients: a subanalysis of the PREDyCES study. *Nutr Hosp.* 2015;32(4):1830–1836.

18. Medicare Interactive. Inpatient rehabilitation hospital care. Available at www.medi careinteractive.org/get-answers/medicare-covered-services/inpatient-hospital-servi ces/inpatient-rehabilitation-hospital-care. Accessed May 31, 2021.

19. Ostrowska J, Suz I, Tarantino S, Hiesmayr M, Szostak-Wegierek D. Hospital malnutrition, nutritional risk factors, and elements of nutritional care in Europe: comparison of Polish results with all European countries participating in nDay Survey. *Nutrients.* 2021;13(1):263.

20. D'Almeida CA, Peres WAF, De Pinho DE, Martucci RB, Rodrigues VD, Ramalho A. Prevalence of malnutrition in older hospitalized cancer patients: a multicenter and multiregional study. *J Nutr Health Aging.* 2020;24(2):166–171.

21. Fukui S, Kawakami M, Otaka Y, et al. Malnutrition among elderly patients with severe aortic stenosis. *Aging Clin Exp Res.* 2020;32(3):373–379.

22. Chatindiara I, Allen J, Popman A, et al. Dysphagia risk, low muscle strength and poor cognition predict malnutrition risk in older adults at hospital admission. *BMC Geriatrics.* 2018;18(1):78.

23. Rinninella E, Intoni M, De Lorenzo A, et al. Risk, prevalence and impact of hospital malnutrition in a tertiary care referral university hospital: a cross-sectional study. *Intern Emerg Med.* 2018;13(5):689–697.

24. Alzahrani SH, Alamari SH. Prevalence of malnutrition and associated factors among hospitalized elderly patients in King Abdulaziz University Hospital, Jeddah, Saudi Arabia. *BMC Geriatrics.* 2017;17:136.

25. Kim SR, Chung SJ, Yoo S-H. Factors contributing to malnutrition in patients with Parkinson's disease. *Int J Nurs Pract.* 2016;22(2):129–137.

26. Planas M, Alvarez-Hernandez J, Leon-Sanz M, Celaya-Perez S, Araujo K, Garcia de Lorenzo A. Prevalence of hospital malnutrition in cancer patients: a sub-analysis of the PREDyCES study. *Support Care Cancer.* 2016;24(1):429–435.

27. Paris AS, Garcia JM, Gomez-Candela C, et al. Malnutrition prevalence in hospitalized elderly diabetic patients. *Nutr Hosp.* 2013;28(3):592–599.

28. Lamb CA, Parr J, Lamb EIM, Warren MD. Adult malnutrition screening, prevalence and management in a United Kingdom hospital: cross-sectional study. *Br J Nutr.* 2009;102(4):571–575.

29. Pirlich M, Schutz T, Kemps M, et al. Social risk factors for hospital malnutrition. *Nutrition.* 2005;21(3):295–300.

30. Correia MITD, Campos ACL. Prevalence of hospital malnutrition in Latin America: the multicenter ELAN study. *Nutrition.* 2003;19(10):823–825.

31. Marshall S, Young A, Bauer J, Isenring E. Malnutrition in geriatric rehabilitation: prevalence, patient outcomes, and criterion validity of the scored Patient-Generated Subjective Global Assessment and the Mini Nutritional Assessment. *J Acad Nutr Diet.* 2016;116(5):785–94.

32. Charlton K, Nichols C, Bowden S, et al. Poor nutritional status of older subacute patients predicts clinical outcomes and mortality at 18 months of follow-up. *Eur J Clin Nutr.* 2012;66(11):1224–1228.

33. Wojteczek A, Dardzinska JA, Malgorzewicz S, Gruszecka A, Zdrojewski Z. Prevalence of malnutrition in systemic sclerosis patients assessed with different diagnostic tools. *Clin Rheumatol.* 2020;39(1):227–232.

34. Rodriguez-Sanchez B, Sulo S, Carnicero JA, Rueda R, Rodriguez-Manas L. Malnutrition prevalence and burden on healthcare resource use among Spanish

community-living older adults: results of a longitudinal analysis. *ClinicoEcon Outcomes Res.* 2012;12:355–367.

35. Vandewoude MFJ, van Wijngaarden JP, De Maesschalck L, Luiking YC, Van Gossum A. The prevalence and health burden of malnutrition in Belgian older people in the community or residing in nursing homes: results of the NutriAction II study. *Aging Clin Exp Res.* 2019;31(2):175–183.

36. Wei J-M, Li S, Claytor L, Partridge J, Goates S. Prevalence and predictors of malnutrition in elderly Chinese adults: results from the China Health and Retirement Longitudinal Study. *Public Health Nutr.* 2018;21(17):3129–3134.

37. Damayanthi HDWT, Moy FM, Dharmaratne SD. Prevalence of malnutrition and associated factors among community-dwelling older persons in Sri Lanka: a cross-sectional study. *BMC Geriatrics.* 2018;18(1):1990

38. Van Den Broeke C, De Burghgraeve T, Ummels M, et al. Occurrence of malnutrition and associated factors in community-dwelling older adults: those with a recent diagnosis of cancer are at higher risk. *J Nutr Health Aging.* 2018;22(2):191–198.

39. Wang G, Wan Y, Cheng Q, Wang X-J, Zhou H-Y, Chen S-D. Malnutrition and associated factors in Chinese patients with Parkinson's disease: results from a pilot investigation. *Parkinsonism Relat Disord.* 2010;16(2):119–123.

40. Velazquez-Alva MC, Irigoyen-Camacho ME, Cabrer-Rosales MF, et al. Prevalence of malnutrition and depression in older adults living in nursing homes in Mexico City. *Nutrients.* 2020;12(8):2429.

41. Balci C, Ulger Z, Halil MG, et al. Malnutrition and associated risk factors in nursing home residents in Turkey. *Clin Sci Nutr.* 2019;1(3):129–133.

42. Özgün Başibüyüka G, Ayremloub P, Nouri Saeidlouc S, et al. Evaluation of malnutrition among elderly people living in nursing homes by Mini Nutritional Assessment Short Form (MNA-SF) in Turkey. *MAEDICA – A Journal of Clinical Nutrition.* 2019;14(1):38–44.

43. Madeira T, Peixoto-Plácido C, Sousa-Santos N, et al. Malnutrition among older adults living in Portuguese nursing homes: the PEN-3S study. *Pub Health Nutr.* 2019;22(3):486–497.

44. Nazemi L, Skoog I, Karlsson I, et al. Malnutrition, prevalence and relation to some risk factors among elderly residents in nursing homes in Tehran, Iran. *Iran J Public Health.* 2015;44(2):218–227.

45. Papparotto C, Bidoli E, Palese A. Risk factors associated with malnutrition in older adults living in Italian nursing homes: a cross-sectional study. *Res Gerontol Nurs.* 2013;6(3):187–197.

46. Berggren E, Strang P, Orrevall Y, Olin AO, Tornkvist L. Symptom burden in patients with home care who are at risk for malnutrition: a cross-sectional study. *J Palliat Care.* 2020;35(2):103–109.

47. Baz S, Ardahan M. Relationship between malnutrition risks and functional abilities of the elderly in home care services. *Int J Caring Sci.* 2019;12(2):603–610.

48. Win AZ, Ceresa C, Arnold K, Allison TA. High prevalence of malnutrition among elderly veterans in home based primary care. *J Nutr Health Aging.* 2017;21(6):610–613.

49. Jensen GL, Mirtallo J, Compher C, et al. Adult starvation and disease-related malnutrition: A proposal for etiology-based diagnosis in the clinical practice setting from the International Consensus Guideline Committee. *JPEN J Parenter Enteral Nutr.* 2010;34(2):156–159.

50. Gangadharan A, Choi SE, Hassan A, et al. Protein calorie malnutrition, nutritional intervention and personalized cancer care. *Oncotarget.* 2017; 8: 24009–24030.

51. Barichella M, Villa MC, Massarotto A, et al. Mini Nutritional Assessment in patients with Parkinson's disease: correlation between worsening of the malnutrition and increasing number of disease-years. *Nutr Neurosci*. 2008;11(3):128–134.

52. Drevet S, Bioteau C, Maziere S, et al. Prevalence of protein-energy malnutrition in hospital patients over 75 years of age admitted for hip fracture. *Orthop Traumatol-Surg*. 2014;100(6):669–674.

53. Bellini LM. Malnutrition in advanced lung disease. UpToDate. October 8, 2020. Accessed April 15, 2021.

54. Mete B, Pehlivan E, Gulbas G, Gunen H. Prevalence of malnutrition in COPD and its relationship with the parameters related to disease severity. *Int J Chron Obstruct Pulmon Dis*. 2018; 11;13:3307–3312.

55. Casanova MJ, Chaparro M, Molina B, et al. Prevalence of malnutrition and nutritional characteristics of patients with inflammatory bowel disease. *Crohns Colitis*. 2017;11(12):1430–1439.

56. Balestrieri P, Ribolsi M, Guarino MPL, Emerenziani S, Altomare A, Cicala M. Nutritional aspects in inflammatory bowel diseases. *Nutrients*. 2020;12(2):372.

57. Cheung K, Lee SS, Raman M. Prevalence and mechanisms of malnutrition in patients with advanced liver disease, and nutrition management strategies. *Clin Gastroenterol Hepatol*. 2012;10(2):17–125.

58. Teklu T, Chauhan NM, Lemessa F, Teshome G. Assessment of prevalence of malnutrition and its associated factors among AIDS patients form Asella, Oromia, Ethiopia. *Biomed Res Int*. 2020; doi:10.1155/2020/7360190.

59. Mulu H, Hamza L, Alemseged F. Prevalence of malnutrition and associated factors among hospitalized patients with acquired immunodeficiency syndrome in Jimma University Specialized Hospital, Ethiopia. *Ethiop J Health Sci*. 2016;26(3):217–26.

60. Carrero JJ, Thomas F, Nagy K, et al. Global prevalence of protein-energy wasting in kidney disease: a meta-analysis of contemporary observational studies from the International Society of Renal Nutrition and Metabolism. *J Ren Nutr*. 2018;28(6):380–392.

61. Itoh M, Tsuji T, Nemoto K, Nakamura H, Aoshiba K. Undernutrition in patients with COPD and its treatment. *Nutrients*. 2013;5(4):1316–1335.

62. Ghufran A. Nutrition in chronic liver disease: a point-of-care review. *Nutr Clin Pract*. 2020;35(2):211–217.

63. Schiller LR. Nutrition management of chronic diarrhea and malabsorption. *Nutr Clin Pract*. 2006;21(1)34–39.

64. Dagan SS, Goldenshluger A, Globus I, et al. Nutritional recommendations for adult bariatric surgery patients: clinical practice. *Adv Nutr*. 2017;8(2):382–394.

65. Duggan SN, Conlon K. A practical guide to the nutritional management of chronic pancreatitis. *Practical Gastroenterology*. 2013;118(June):24–32.

66. Rogers CL. Nutritional management of the adult with cystic fibrosis – part 1. *Practical Gastroenterology*. January 2013. Available at https://med.virginia.edu/ginutrition/wp-content/uploads/sites/199/2014/06/Parrish_Jan_13_Part_1__CF.pdf. Accessed May 31, 2021.

67. Schubert ML, Peura DA. Control of gastric acid secretion in health and disease. *Gastroenterology*. 2008;134(7):1842–1860.

68. Kalantar-Zateh K, Fouque D. Nutritional management of chronic kidney disease. *N Engl J Med*. 2017;377(17):1765–1776.

69. Centers for Disease Control and Prevention (CDC). *Disability and health*. Available at www.cdc.gov/ncbddd/disabilityandhealth/disability.html. Accessed July 1, 2021.

70. Groce N, Challenger E, Berman-Bieler R, Farkas A, Yilmaz N, Schultink W, et al. Malnutrition and disability: unexplored opportunities for collaboration. *Paediatr Int Child Health.* 2014;34(4):308–314.

71. Pavasini R, Guralnik J, Brown JC, et al. Short Physical Performance Battery and all-cause mortality: systematic review and meta-analysis. *BMC Med.* 2016;14(1):215.

72. World Health Organization. 2012. *What are the social determinants of health?* Available at: www.who.int/health-topics/social-determinants-of-health#tab=tab_1/. Accessed May 25, 2021.

73. Mangan S. Social determinants of health 101 for health care: five plus five. *National Academy of Medicine.* Published October 9, 2017. Available at https://nam.edu/social-determinants-of-health-101-for-health-care-five-plus-five/. Accessed May 25, 2021.

74. Guyonnet S, Rolland Y. Screening for malnutrition in older people. *Clin Geriatr Med.* 2015;31(3):429–437.

75. Griffin A, O'Neill A, O'Connor M, Ryan D, Tierney A, Galvin R. The prevalence of malnutrition and impact on patient outcomes among older adults presenting at an Irish emergency department: a secondary analysis of the OPTI-MEND trial. *BMC Geriatrics.* 2020;20:455.

76. Food and Agriculture Organization (FAO) of the United Nations. *Gender and nutrition.* Available at www.fao.org/3/al184e/al184e00.pdf. Accessed May 31, 2021.

77. Duggan C, Kurpad A, Stanford F, Sunguya B, Wells JC. Race, ethnicity, and racism in the nutrition literature: an update for 2020. *Am J Clin Nutr.* 2020;112(6):1409–1414.

78. Sadarangani TR, Missaelides L, Yu G, Trinh-Shevrin C, Brody A. Racial disparities in nutritional risk among community dwelling older adults in adult day health care. *J Nutr Gerontol Geriatr.* 2019:38(4):345–360.

79. Sheean P, Farrar IC, Sulo S, Partridge J, Schiffer L, Fitzgibbon M. Nutrition risk among an ethnically diverse sample of community-dwelling older adults. *Public Health Nutr.* 2019;22(5):894–902.

80. Sauer J, Berrang- Ford L, Patterson K, et al. An analysis of the nutrition status of neighboring Indigenous and non-Indigenous populations in Kanungu District, south-western Uganda: Close proximity, distant health realities. *Soc Sci Med.* 2018;217:55–64.

81. Morris NF, Stewart S, Riley MD, Maguire GP. The burden and nature of malnutrition among patients in regional hospital settings: A cross-sectional survey. *Clin Nutr ESPEN.* 2018;23:1–9.

82. Batis C, Mazariegos M, Martorell R, Gil A, Rivera JA. Malnutrition in all its forms by wealth, education and ethnicity in Latin America: Who are more affected? *Public Health Nutr.* 2020;23(S1):S1–S12.

83. Walker RJ, Strom Williams J, Egede LE. Influence of race, ethnicity and social determinants of health on diabetes outcomes. *Am J Med Sci.* 2016;351(4):366–373.

84. Satia JA. Diet-related disparities: understanding the problem and accelerating solutions. *J Am Diet Assoc.* 2009;109(4):610–615.

85. US Department of Agriculture, Economic Research Service. Food insecurity – key statistics and graphs (2019). Accessed May 4, 2021 at www.ers.usda.gov/topics/food-nutrition-assistance/food-security-in-the-us/key-statistics-graphics.aspx/.

86. Nesbitt S, Palomarez RE. Review: increasing awareness and education on health disparities for health care providers. *Ethn Dis.* 2016;26(2):181–190.

87. Agency for Healthcare Research and Quality. 2019 National Healthcare Quality & Disparities Report. 2019. Accessed April 11, 2021 at www.ahrq.gov/sites/default/files/wysiwyg/research/findings/nhqrdr/2019qdr.pdf.

88. Besora-Moreno M, Llaurado E, Tarro L, Sola R. Social and economic factors and malnutrition or the risk of malnutrition in the elderly: a systematic review and meta-analysis of observational studies. *Nutrients.* 2020;12(3):737.

89. Locher JL, Robinson CO, Roth DL, Ritchie CS, Burgio KL. The effect of the presence of others on caloric intake in homebound older adults. *J Gerontol A Biol Sci Med Sci.* 2005;60(11):1475–1478.

90. Grammatikopoulou MG, Gkiouras K, Theodoridis X, et al. Food insecurity increases the risk of malnutrition among community-dwelling older adults. *Maturitas.* 2019;119:8–13.

91. Hoogendijk EO, Flores Ruano T, Martínez-Reig M, et al. Socioeconomic position and malnutrition among older adults: results from the FRADEA Study. *J Nutr Health Aging.* 2018;22(9):1086–1091.

4 Screening

Maureen Janowski

CONTENTS

I INTRODUCTION

Identifying patients at risk of or with malnutrition is a priority in all care settings to help the nutrition professional determine which patients would benefit from medical nutrition therapy (MNT). Healthcare providers should develop protocols to identify patients at nutrition risk and implement a process to refer those patients to the Registered Dietitian Nutritionist (RDN) for nutrition care. This is most often accomplished by using a validated nutrition risk screening tool. The Academy of Nutrition and Dietetics (Academy) defines nutrition screening as "the process of identifying patients, clients, or groups who may have a nutrition diagnosis and benefit from nutrition assessment and intervention by an RDN".[1] It is important to remember that nutrition screening is not the same as nutrition assessment. Screening occurs prior to the start of the Nutrition Care Process and does not need to be completed by an RDN, whereas only the RDN conducts a nutrition assessment. This chapter reviews the characteristics to consider when choosing a nutrition screening tool, and describes commonly used tools in acute care, long-term care (LTC) and community settings.

DOI: 10.1201/9781003177586-4

II SCREENING TOOL CHARACTERISTICS

A systematic review conducted in 2014 by van Bokhorst-de van der Schueren et al.[2] found that at least 33 different nutrition screening tools exist.[2] Selecting the appropriate tool can be daunting, but clinicians should carefully evaluate the options to ensure they choose the best tool. See Table 4.1 for characteristics to consider when selecting a nutrition screening tool.

The tool should require minimal training given the variety of individuals who may be responsible for completing the screen, including nutrition and dietetics technicians registered (NDTR), nursing, and medical assistants, among others. In some care settings, such as the community, the nutrition screen may be completed by individuals with little or no healthcare knowledge. Conversely, some screening tools may be completed by the patient, and the results evaluated by an RDN or other healthcare professional. Use of a nutrition screening tool that hasn't been validated increases the risk that patients who most need nutrition assessment and interventions may be missed. According to the American Society of Parenteral and Enteral Nutrition (ASPEN), in the United States approximately 15,000 hospitalized patients with malnutrition go undiagnosed daily.[3]

Screening tools should be validated for the patient populations and settings in which they will be used. For example, a screening tool validated for pediatric patients would not be accurate and reliable to screen older adults. Reliability means the tool will provide consistent results. Sensitivity (measuring "true positive") and specificity (measuring "true negative") should also be considered when choosing the screening tool. See Table 4.2 for explanations of common terminology used in the development and validation process.

Some screening tools may have a fee, licensing or copyright requirements, or other conditions for use. Prior to utilizing a screening tool, the organization should obtain all required permissions.

TABLE 4.1

Recommended Characteristics of a Malnutrition Screening Tool[10]

Characteristic	Explanation
Quick	No more than 5–10 minutes to administer
Reliable and valid	As indicated by research
Inexpensive	None or minimal cost to the facility to use
Non-invasive	Does not require invasive screening
Acceptable to the general population	Tool questions will not be offensive, the time to complete will not be lengthy, etc.
Collects dynamic information	Examples include recent weight loss, current BMI, current food intake versus asking static questions
Easy to use	Requires minimal training to administer

TABLE 4.2
Definitions of Research Terminology[11,12]

Term	Definition
Validity	Validity measures accuracy. Validity describes the extent to which the results measure what they are supposed to measure. A valid measurement is generally reliable. If the research produces accurate results, they should be reproducible.
Reliability	Reliability measures consistency. It describes the extent to which the same results will occur when the research is repeated under the same conditions. A reliable measurement is not always valid. The same results may occur but that doesn't mean they are necessarily correct.
Sensitivity	Sensitivity measures how often a test correctly generates a positive result for people who have the condition being tested. This is also known as a "true positive" rate. *Example*: 90% sensitivity means it will correctly return a positive result 90% of the time.
Specificity	Specificity measures how often the test correctly generates a negative result for people who don't have the condition being tested. This is also known as a "true negative" rate. *Example*: 90% specificity will correctly return a negative result 90% of the time.
Positive predictive value	The probability that the person with a positive screening result really has the condition.
Negative predictive value	The probability that a person with a negative screening result really does not have the condition.
Intra-rater reliability	The degree of agreement from repeated testing performed by a single person or "rater".
Inter-rater reliability	The degree of agreement from repeated testing performed by different people or "raters".
Evidence Analysis Library	The Academy of Nutrition and Dietetics' Evidence Analysis Library (EAL) provides an evidence strength/grade based on an analysis of the available literature. The EAL uses I–Good, II–Fair, III–Limited, IV–Expert Opinion, V–Not assignable.

III ACUTE CARE

It is estimated that 15–60% of patients in the hospital are either malnourished or at risk of malnutrition.[4] The objective of nutrition screening in the acute care environment is to identify which patients would more likely benefit from a nutrition assessment so that timely MNT can be implemented. In 1995, The Joint Commission (TJC) mandated that patients be screened for nutrition risk within 24 hours of hospital admission by a trained healthcare practitioner, followed by a full nutrition assessment completed by an RDN or a qualified nutrition professional, if the screen indicated the patient was at risk.[5] More recently, TJC has modified this requirement by allowing the hospital to define the timeframe for screening. Although it is no longer mandated that a nutrition screen be completed within 24 hours of admission, it is still recommended.[6]

Screening for nutrition risk is usually a part of the admission process and completed by nursing for all patients admitted to the hospital, regardless of the reason for admission. Patients on some units are more likely to be malnourished or at risk of malnutrition (e.g. oncology); however, nutrition screening should be completed for all patients admitted, even though some populations are less likely to be malnourished (e.g. maternity). In 2018, TJC updated standard CTS.02.01.11 for behavioral healthcare organizations or behavioral healthcare programs within a hospital surveyed under the TJC's Behavioral Healthcare standards.[6] The standard states "the organization screens all individuals served to identify those for whom a nutrition assessment is indicated".[7] At a minimum, the screening includes questions about the following: food allergies, weight loss or gain of ten pounds or more in the last three months, decrease in food intake and/or appetite, dental problems, and eating habits or behaviors that may be indicators of an eating disorder, such as binging or induced vomiting.[7]

The most common validated nutrition screening tools used in the acute care environment include the Malnutrition Screening Tool (MST), the Malnutrition Universal Screening Tool (MUST), the Nutritional Risk Screening (NRS 2002) and the NUTrition Risk in the Critically Ill (NUTRIC). The Subjective Global Assessment (SGA) is technically an assessment tool but is occasionally used as a screening tool. See Chapter 2 for more information on the SGA.

A   MALNUTRITION SCREENING TOOL (MST)

The MST was developed by Ferguson and colleagues in 1999 to detect malnutrition risk.[8] This tool has been validated in multiple countries and in a variety of settings including acute and LTC, rehabilitation, ambulatory care and oncology clinics. In these studies the MST exhibited a moderate degree of validity, agreement and inter-rater reliability in identifying malnutrition risk in adults.[8] Moreover, a systematic review by the Academy assigned the MST a Grade I, reflecting good/strong evidence, with consistency of results across studies, quantity of studies and number of subjects, clinical impact of outcomes with good generalizability.[1] In 2020, in a position paper published by the Academy called the *Malnutrition (Undernutrition) Screening Tools for All Adults*, the authors concluded "It is the position of the Academy of Nutrition and Dietetics that, based upon current evidence, the Malnutrition Screening Tool should be used to screen adults for malnutrition (undernutrition) regardless of their age, medical history, or setting".[1] This concurs with the conclusion reached by the Academy's systematic review on screening tools.[1] The MST is very easy to use, can be administered by anyone regardless of training or a healthcare background, and has two simple questions about weight loss and appetite (see Table 4.3).

B   MALNUTRITION UNIVERSAL SCREENING TOOL (MUST)

The MUST is a five-step process used to identify adults at risk of malnutrition, and was developed by the Malnutrition Advisory Group, A Standing Committee of British Association for Parenteral and Enteral Nutrition in 2003.[9] The first three steps pertain to body mass index (BMI), unplanned weight loss and lack of intake. Step 4 determines the overall risk of malnutrition by adding the results from steps 1 through 3. Step 5 includes management guidelines for each risk level. For example, if the overall score

TABLE 4.3
Malnutrition Screening Tool (MST) Questions[13]

Questions	Answer Choices	
1) Have you recently lost weight without trying?	0 points	= No
	2 points	= Unsure
	Yes:	
	1 point	= 2–13 lb
	2 points	= 14–23 lb
	3 points	= 24–33 lb
	4 points	= 34 lb or more
	2 points	= Unsure
2) Have you been eating poorly because of a decreased appetite?	0 points	= No
	1 point	= Yes

Scoring:
- 0–1: Not at risk. Eating well with little or no weight loss. If length of stay exceeds 7 days, then rescreen, repeating weekly as needed.
- 2 or more = At risk. Eating poorly and/or recent weight loss. Rapidly implement nutrition interventions. Perform nutrition assessment within 24–72 hours, depending on risk.

TABLE 4.4
Malnutrition Universal Screening Tool (MUST)[9]

Steps	Answer choices	
Step 1 – Measure height and weight to determine BMI	0 points	= > 20 (> 30 obese)
	1 point	= 18.5–20
	2 points	= < 18.5
Step 2 – Note percentage unplanned weight loss using scoring tables provided	0 points	= < 5%
	1 point	= 5–10%
	2 points	= > 10%
Step 3 – Establish acute disease effect and score	2 points	= If acutely ill and there has been or is likely to be no nutrition intake for > 5 days.
Step 4 – Add scores from steps 1, 2, and 3 to obtain overall risk of malnutrition	*Total of Steps 1, 2, 3:*	
	0 points	= low risk
	1 point	= medium risk
	2 points or more	= high risk

Use management guidelines and/or local policy to develop care plan.

Abbreviation: BMI = body mass index.

is 2 or higher, the guidelines state the patient should be referred to an RDN, who will set goals to improve nutrition intake and review the care plan on an established schedule. Comprehensive information on all five steps is detailed in a six-page guide, which contains a flow chart depicting the five steps, BMI chart, weight loss tables and alternative measurements when BMI cannot be obtained (see Table 4.4). Although the MUST was first developed for use in community settings such as physicians' offices, it was subsequently validated for use in other healthcare settings, including hospitals. The MUST has excellent inter-rater reliability, concurrent validity with other tools, and a predictive validity for length of hospital stay and mortality in elderly wards.[10]

C   Nutritional Risk Screening – 2002 (NRS-2002)

The NRS-2002 was published by the European Society of Clinical Nutrition and Metabolism.[9] This tool incorporates nutrition components similar to the MUST, including BMI, unplanned weight loss and decreased intake, but also includes grading for severity of disease. This tool was developed based on a review of 128 randomized clinical trials in which the authors reported that patients identified as at-risk by the NRS-2002 were more likely to have positive clinical outcomes after receiving nutritional support than low-risk patients.[10] The NRS-2002 is a well-validated tool consisting of two steps; the first step includes four prescreening questions related to low BMI, weight loss, decreased intake, and if the patient is severely ill. If the answer is "yes" to any of the first four questions, then the second step is performed, in which a score is assigned based on the amount of weight loss, current intake compared to normal intake, severity of disease and age over 70 years. See Table 4.5 for an outline of both steps. The NRS-2002 has a moderate overall validity and moderate agreement when compared to the SGA.[1]

TABLE 4.5
Nutritional Risk Screening (NRS-2002)[10]

Questions	Answer choices
Is BMI > 20.5?	Yes / No
Has the patient lost weight within the last 3 months?	Yes / No
Has the patient had a reduced dietary intake in the last week?	Yes / No
Is the patient severely ill? (e.g. in intensive therapy?)	Yes / No
If answer Yes to any of these questions move to Final Screening	
Final Screening – Impaired Nutrition Status Section	
Weight loss > 5% in 2 months or food intake below 50–75% in preceding week.	Score 1 (mild)
Weight loss > 5% in 2 months or BMI 18.5–20.5 plus impaired general condition or food intake 25–60% in preceding week.	Score 2 (moderate)
Weight loss > 5% in 1 month (>15% in 3 months) or BMI < 18.5 plus impaired general condition or food intake 0–25% in preceding week.	Score 3 (severe)
Final Screening – Severity of Disease Section	
Hip fracture, chronic patients, in particular with acute complications: cirrhosis, COPD, chronic hemodialysis, diabetes, oncology.	Score 1 (mild)
Major abdominal surgery, stroke, severe pneumonia, hematologic malignancy.	Score 2 (moderate)

TABLE 4.5 (Continued)
Nutritional Risk Screening (NRS-2002)[10]

Questions	Answer choices
Head injury, bone marrow transplantation, intensive care patients (APACHE II > 10)	Score 3 (severe)

- Add impaired nutrition status section score to severity of disease section to equal total score. If ≥ 70 years of age add 1 to the total score.
  - Score ≥ 3: patient is nutritionally at risk.
  - Score < 3: weekly rescreening of the patient.

Abbreviations: BMI = body mass index; COPD = chronic obstructive pulmonary disease; APACHE = Acute Physiologic Assessment and Chronic Health Evaluation II.

D   NUTRITION RISK IN THE CRITICALLY ILL (NUTRIC SCORE)

The NUTRIC Score, the first tool developed and validated specifically for intensive care unit (ICU) patients, helps identify which ICU patients may benefit from aggressive nutrition intervention.[14] This tool uses easily obtained data such as age and health conditions related to the patient's current clinical status instead of food intake and weight loss, as these patients are often unable to provide this information due to mechanical ventilation and sedation. Scoring is based on age, Acute Physiology and Chronic Health Evaluation score (APACHE II), Sequential Organ Failure Assessment (SOFA) score, number of comorbidities, days from hospital to ICU admission and interleukin 6 (IL-6).[15] There are two different scoring tables, depending on if IL-6 is available. See Table 4.6 for scoring variables. In a 2019 systematic review of 12 studies, all chose not to use IL-6. The review indicated that a high NUTRIC score was significantly associated with mechanical ventilation in four studies, with ICU or hospital length of stay in three studies, and with mortality in seven studies, thereby indicating that these patients are most likely to benefit from aggressive nutrition therapy.[16]

IV   LONG-TERM CARE (LTC)

The terms LTC, Skilled Nursing Facility (SNF) and Nursing Home are often used interchangeably and refer to a facility or patient care unit that provides ongoing skilled nursing care to residents in need of assistance with activities of daily living. Many LTC facilities also have rehab units, often called sub-acute units, which provide rehabilitation services for short-stay patients. These facilities and units fall under the Centers for Medicare & Medicaid Services (CMS) regulations titled 42 CFR Subpart B – Requirements for Long Term Care Facilities. LTC federal regulations specify that an initial nutrition assessment and regular reassessments (required minimally every three months) must be completed by an RDN or qualified professional on all patients/residents.[17] This is in contrast to the acute care setting in which the RDN does not have to assess every patient admitted to the hospital. Since the purpose of a nutrition screen is to identify which patients should be seen by the RDN, the fact that RDNs assess all patients/residents in LTC mitigated the need for completing a

TABLE 4.6
Nutrition Risk in the Critically Ill (NUTRIC Score)[15]

Variable	Scoring		
Age	0 points	=	< 50
	1 point	=	50–74
	2 points	=	≥ 75
APACHE II	0 points	=	< 15
	1 point	=	15–19
	2 points	=	20–28
	3 points	=	> 28
SOFA	0 points	=	< 6
	1 point	=	6–9
	2 points	=	≥ 10
Number of comorbidities	0 points	=	0–1
	1 point	=	≥ 2
Days from hospital to ICU admission	0 points	=	0 – < 1
	1 point	=	≥ 1
IL-6	0 points	=	0 – < 400
	1 point	=	≥ 400

Scoring If IL-6 Available

- High score: Associated with worse clinical outcomes. These patients are most likely to benefit from aggressive nutrition therapy — 6–10 points
- Low score: These patients have a low malnutrition risk — 0–5 points

Scoring If IL-6 Is Not Available

- High score: Associated with worse clinical outcomes. These patients are most likely to benefit from aggressive nutrition therapy — 5–9 points
- Low score: These patients have a low malnutrition risk — 0–4 points

Abbreviations: APACHE = Acute Physiologic Assessment and Chronic Health Evaluation II; SOFA = Sequential Organ Failure Assessment; ICU = intensive care unit; IL-6 = interleukin 6.

nutrition screen in this setting. Some LTC facilities utilize Certified Dietary Managers (CDMs) or NDTRs to work with a consulting RDN to provide nutritional care instead of employing full-time or part-time RDNs. In these cases, since the RDN usually only visits the facility weekly or as little as monthly, the CDM or NDTR may complete a nutrition screen to identify which patients/residents the RDN should prioritize for assessment during their visit.

Effective October 1, 2019, the payment model for SNFs changed to the Patient Driven Payment Model (PDPM) for all patients/residents covered by Medicare Part A.[18] This new model consists of five case-mix adjusted components including Physical Therapy, Occupational Therapy, Speech Language Pathology, Nursing and Non-Therapy Ancillary (NTA).[18] The NTA classification uses a scoring system and is based on the presence of specific comorbidities or the use of certain extensive services.

Certain nutrition-related diagnoses, including malnutrition and risk of malnutrition, when coded in the Five-day Scheduled MDS (Minimum Data Set) Assessment, increase the NTA score and therefore could potentially increase reimbursement. The five-day MDS is the driver for the reimbursement for the entire Medicare Part A stay. This new payment model has increased the demand for the RDN to complete a full nutrition assessment within five days of admission. Due to the PDPM change, many LTC facilities have implemented nutrition screening to ensure that the RDN identifies and assesses the patients who are malnourished or at risk of malnutrition before the five-day MDS is submitted.

Nursing, a CDM or an NDTR may complete the nutrition screen. The most commonly used screening tools in LTC are the Mini Nutrition Assessment (MNA), and the Short Nutritional Assessment Questionnaire (SNAQ). While the MST is not commonly used in the LTC environment, its use may increase due to the 2019 Position Statement of the Academy of Nutrition and Dietetics, which states "It is the position of the Academy of Nutrition and Dietetics that, based upon current evidence, the Malnutrition Screening Tool should be used to screen adults for malnutrition (undernutrition) regardless of their age, medical history, *or setting*".[1]

A   MINI NUTRITIONAL ASSESSMENT (MNA)

The MNA, a validated nutrition screening and assessment tool that was developed to identify malnutrition or risk of malnutrition in patients 65 years and older, was created and copyrighted by the Nestlé Nutrition Institute in 2001.[19] Originally composed of 18 questions, the MNA has been shortened to six questions (MNA Short Form, or MNA-SF) to streamline the screening process and has been found to retain the validity and accuracy of the original 18-question form.[20] Unlike other screening tools, the MNA and MNA-SF have also been validated as nutrition assessment tools for older adults and are commonly used in LTC for both purposes. The questions relate to food intake, weight loss, mobility, psychological stress, acute disease, neuropsychological problems (dementia, depression) and BMI (see Table 4.7).

B   SHORT NUTRITIONAL ASSESSMENT QUESTIONNAIRE (SNAQ)

The SNAQ was developed in 2005 by Kruizenga et al.[21] in the Netherlands with the philosophy that nutrition screening should be as easy as possible.[18] The tool can be used by untrained personnel, does not require equipment or calculations, takes less than five minutes to complete and has been validated for older adults. The SNAQ contains three questions that address unintentional weight loss, decreased appetite and utilization of supplements or tube feeding over the last month. Dots are used for scoring (1, 2, or 3 dots) and upon completion of the form the dots are added up.

In 2009, SNAQ[RC] was developed specifically for individuals in residential care, and in 2010 SNAQ [65+] was developed for community-dwelling older men and women. While these newer versions have been validated, they are more commonly used in Europe. See Table 4.8 for details on SNAQ.

TABLE 4.7
Mini Nutritional Assessment (MNA) Questions[22]

Questions	Points
A) Has food intake declined over the past 3 months due to loss of appetite, digestive problems, chewing or swallowing difficulties?	0 = severe decrease in food intake 1 = moderate decrease in food intake 2 = no decrease in food intake
B) Weight loss during the last 3 months	0 = weight loss greater than 3 kg (6.6 lbs) 1 = does not know 2 = weight loss between 1 and 3 kg (2.2 and 6.6 lbs) 3 = no weight loss
C) Mobility	0 = bed- or chair-bound 1 = able to get out of bed/chair but does not go out 2 = goes out
D) Has suffered psychological stress or acute disease in the past 3 months?	0 = yes 2 = no
E) Neuropsychological problems	0 = severe dementia or depression 1 = mild dementia 2 = no psychological problems
F1) Body mass index (BMI) If BMI is not available replace F1 with F2:	0 = BMI less than 19 1 = BMI 19 to less than 21 2 = BMI 21 to less than 23 3 = BMI 23 or greater
F2) Calf circumference (CC) in centimeters	0 = CC less than 31 3 = CC 31 or greater

Scoring:
- 12–14 points: normal nutrition status
- 8–11 points: at risk of malnutrition
- 0–7 points: malnourished

TABLE 4.8
Short Nutritional Assessment Questionnaire (SNAQ)[21]

Questions	Scoring	
Did you lose weight unintentionally?	3 dots =	more than 6 kg in the last 6 months
	2 dots =	more than 3 kg in the last month
Did you experience a decreased appetite over the last month?	1 dot =	Yes
Did you use supplemental drinks or tube feeding over the last month?	1 dot =	Yes

Scoring:
- 1 dot = no intervention
- 2 dots = moderately malnourished; nutritional intervention
- 3 dots = severely malnourished; nutrition intervention and treatment from dietitian

V COMMUNITY

Nutrition screening, assessment and education that are completed outside of the acute care hospital or LTC facility are often referred to as community nutrition. Nutrition screening in the community can be completed in multiple different settings such as physician offices, outpatient medical clinics, congregate meal sites, the home care environment, and independent or assisted living facilities.[23]

Screening in the community setting is important for early identification of nutritional risk to facilitate referral to the appropriate services. Up to one out of two older adults are at risk of malnutrition[24], which is often attributed to long-standing inadequate intake.[25] Unfortunately, screening for malnutrition in the community is not as routine as it is in acute and LTC settings, although strides have been made in this area. When choosing a nutrition screening tool for the community setting, it is important to ensure that the tool is appropriate for the population on which it is used, but equally important is consideration of the person completing the screen. For example, in physicians' offices, outpatient clinics, independent or assisted living facilities, a physician, nurse or nurse aide may complete the screening, but in the home care environment, a case manager (with little or no medical background) or even a driver for a home-delivered meal program may complete the screen.[23]

The most common validated screening tools used in the community setting are the DETERMINE Checklist Nutrition Screening Initiative (NSI), the MNA-SF, and Seniors in the Community: Risk Evaluation for Eating and Nutrition (SCREEN II©). The Patient-Generated Subjective Global Assessment (PG-SGA©) may be used for screening although it is actually an assessment tool (see Chapter 2). Refer to the LTC section for more information on the MNA-SF.

A Determine Checklist

The DETERMINE Checklist was developed by the American Academy of Family Physicians and the American Dietetic Association (now the Academy of Nutrition and Dietetics) as part of the Nutrition Screening Initiative (NSI) in the United States in 1991.[26] Participants of the Older American's Act (OAA) Congregate Nutrition Services (Title III C1), Home-Delivered Nutrition Services (Title III C2) or Nutrition Services Incentive Program (NSIP) are screened for malnutrition risk based on the NSI's DETERMINE Checklist.[23] The DETERMINE scores can also be used to reassess an individual's improvement or decline in nutritional risk over time.

The acronym DETERMINE is derived from: **D**isease, **E**ating poorly, **T**ooth loss, **E**conomic hardship, **R**educed social contact, **M**ultiple medications, **I**nvoluntary weight loss/gain, **N**eeds assistance in self-care, and **E**lder years.[26] There are ten questions in the DETERMINE checklist relating to the conditions outlined by the DETERMINE acronym (see Table 4.9).

B Seniors in the Community: Risk Evaluation for Eating and Nutrition (SCREEN)

Seniors in the Community: **R**isk **E**valuation for **E**ating and **N**utrition (SCREEN) was originally developed in 2001 for epidemiological research using self- or telephone administration in cognitively intact community-living seniors.[27] The SCREEN© tools,

TABLE 4.9
DETERMINE Your Nutritional Health Questions[26]

Questions	Points
I have an illness or condition that made me change the kind and/or amount of food I eat.	2
I eat fewer than two meals a day.	3
I eat few fruits or vegetables, or milk products.	2
I have three or more drinks of beer, liquor or wine almost every day.	2
I have tooth or mouth problems that make it hard for me to eat.	2
I don't always have enough money to buy the food I need.	4
I eat alone most of the time.	1
I take three or more different prescribed or over-the-counter drugs a day.	1
Without wanting to, I have lost or gained ten pounds in the last six months.	2
I am not always physically able to shop, cook and/or feed myself.	2

Scoring:
- 0–2 = good
- 3–5 = moderate nutritional risk
- 6 or more = high nutrition risk

Abbreviation: DETERMINE = Disease, Eating poorly, Tooth loss/mouth pain, Economic hardship, Reduced social contact, Multiple medicines, Involuntary weight loss/gain, Needs assistance with self-care, Elder years above age 80.

previously titled SCREEN-II, SCREEN-II-AB and SCREEN-III, were rebranded in 2020 to SCREEN-14, SCREEN-8 and SCREEN-3. The updated names reflect the number of questions that are asked during the screening process.[28]

The SCREEN-14 and SCREEN-8 tools include questions about weight changes, intake and appetite, signs of aspiration, fluid intake, meal companions and meal preparation. SCREEN-14 also asks about difficulty chewing, use of supplements, meals and problems getting groceries. SCREEN-14 and SCREEN-8 were validated against an RDN's nutritional assessment, which included information on diet, anthropometrics, function and clinical risk identification such as swallowing problems. The SCREEN-3 is a shortened version; however, it has not been validated.[27–29] See Table 4.10 for details on SCREEN-14.

VI CONCLUSION

Nutrition risk screening should occur in all care settings (acute, LTC and community) and is a vital step in identifying patients who are malnourished or at risk of malnutrition. Choosing the most appropriate screening tool is equally important. It should be validated for the population that will be screened and consideration should be given for the skill set of the person who will be administering the screen. See Table 4.11 for a detailed list of the commonly used screening tools. The screening process plays an important role in the identification and treatment of patients with malnutrition.

TABLE 4.10

Seniors in the Community: Risk Evaluation for Eating and Nutrition (SCREEN-14)[28]

Question	Scoring
Has your weight changed in the past 6 months?	• Yes, I gained more than 10 pounds (0 points) • Yes, I gained 6 to 10 pounds (1 point) • Yes, I gained about 5 pounds (2 points) • No, my weight stayed within a few pounds (4 points) • Yes, I lost about 5 pounds (2 points) • Yes, I lost 6 to 10 pounds (1 point) • Yes, I lost more than 10 pounds (0 points) • I don't know how much I weigh or if my weight has changed (0 points)
Have you been trying to change your weight in the past 6 months?	• Yes (4 points) • No (4 points) • No, but it changed anyway (0 points)
Do you think your weight is …?	• More than it should be (0 points) • Just right (4 points) • Less than it should be (0 points)
Do you skip meals?	• Never or rarely (4 points) • Sometimes (2 points) • Often (1 point) • Almost every day (0 points)
Do you limit or avoid certain foods?	• I eat most foods (4 points) • I limit some foods and I am managing fine (2 points) • I limit some foods and I am finding it difficult to manage (0 points)
How would you describe your appetite?	• Very good (4 points) • Good (3 points) • Fair (2 points) • Poor (0 points)
How many pieces or servings of vegetables and fruits do you eat a day?	• Five or more (4 points) • Four (3 points) • Three (2 points) • Two (1 point) • Less than two (0 points)
How often do you eat meat, eggs, fish, poultry, tofu, dried peas, beans, lentils, nuts or nut butters?	• Two or more times a day (4 points) • One to two times a day (3 points) • Once a day (1 point) • Less than once a day (0 points)
How often do you have milk, soy beverages, or milk products such as cheese, yogurt, or kefir?	• Three or more times a day (4 points) • Two or three times a day (3 points) • One or two times a day (2 points) • Usually once a day (1 point) • Less than once a day (0 pints)

(Continued)

TABLE 4.10 (Continued)
Seniors in the Community: Risk Evaluation for Eating and Nutrition (SCREEN-14)[28]

Question	Scoring
How much fluid do you drink in a day?	• Eight or more cups (4 points) • Five to seven cups (3 points) • Three to four cups (2 points) • Above two cups (1 point) • Less than two cups (0 points)
Do you cough, choke, or have pain when swallowing food or fluids?	• Never (4 points) • Rarely (3 points) • Sometimes (1 point) • Often or always (0 points)
Is biting or chewing food difficult for you?	• Never (4 points) • Rarely (3 points) • Sometimes (2 points) • Often or always (0 points)
Do you use commercial meal replacements or supplements?	• Never or rarely (4 points) • Sometimes (2 points) • Often or always (0 points)
Do you eat one or more meals a day with someone?	• Never or rarely (0 points) • Sometimes (2 points) • Often (3 points) • Almost always (4 points)
Who usually prepares your meals?	• *These do not have points assigned to them* • I do • I share my cooking with someone else • Someone else cooks most of my meals
Which statement best describes meal preparation for you?	• I enjoy cooking most of my meals (4 points) • I sometimes find cooking a chore (2 points) • I usually find cooking a chore (0 points) • I'm satisfied with the quality of food prepared by others (4 points) • I'm not satisfied with the quality of food prepared by others (0 points)
Do you have problems getting your groceries?	• Never or rarely (4 points) • Sometimes (2 points) • Often (1 point) • Always (0 points)

Scoring – Scores can range from 0 to 64; the lower the score, the greater the nutritional risk. A score of 54–64 indicates low risk, 50–53 indicates medium risk and less than 50 is considered high nutrition risk.

TABLE 4.11
List of Commonly Used Nutrition Risk Screening Tools[1,3,14,29]

Name and basic information	Patient population	Nutrition screening parameters included	Criteria used to identify risk of malnutrition	Administration of screening tool	Validity
Malnutrition Screening Tool (MST)[8] Australia	Adults (including elderly) in hospital and outpatient Residential aged care facility	• Recent weight loss • Recent poor intake	Recent intake: score 0–1 Recent weight loss: score 0–4 Total score: ≥ 2 indicates at risk for malnutrition	Can be administrated by a person without clinical skills Can be self-administered	Overall validity – Moderate[1] Evidence grade, Strength – Good/strong[1]
Malnutrition Universal Screening Tool (MUST)[9] United Kingdom	Adults in hospital and community	Five-step screening: • BMI • Weight loss (%) • Acute disease • Total the scores from first three steps • Develop care plan	Each parameter: score 0–3 Total score: • ≥ 2 = high risk • 1 = medium risk • 0 = low risk	Care workers in hospitals, community and other care settings	Overall validity – High[1] Evidence grade, Strength – fair[1]
Nutritional Risk Screening (NRS 2002)[10] Denmark	Adults in hospital	• Recent weight loss (%) • Recent poor intake (%) • BMI • Severity of disease • Elderly	Each parameter: score 0–3 Total score: • ≥ 3 = start nutritional interventions	Care workers in hospitals, community and other care settings	Overall validity – Moderate[1] Evidence grade, Strength – fair[1]

(Continued)

TABLE 4.11 (Continued)
List of Commonly Used Nutrition Risk Screening Tools[1,3,14,29]

Name and basic information	Patient population	Nutrition screening parameters included	Criteria used to identify risk of malnutrition	Administration of screening tool	Validity
NUTrition Risk in the Critically ill (NUTRIC Score)[11]	Critical care	• Age • APACHE II (Acute Physiology and Chronic Health Evaluation II score) • SOFA (Sequential Organ Failure Assessment) • Number of comorbidities • Days from hospital to ICU admission • Interleukin 6 (IL-6)	Two scoring systems depending on if IL-6 is available. The resulting score indicates either low malnutrition risk or a high score, in which the patient will most likely benefit from aggressive nutrition therapy	Medical professional	NUTRIC has been found to have a statistically significant association with mortality
*Mini Nutritional Assessment – Short Form (MNA-SF®)[16] United States	Elderly May be used in community, sub-acute, LTC or other residential care facilities for older adults	• Recent intake • Recent weight loss • Mobility • Psychological stress or acute disease • Neuropsychological problems • BMI	Parameters have different possible points Total score: • 12–14 = normal nutritional status • 8–11 = at risk for malnutrition • 0–7 = malnourished	Care workers in hospitals, community and other care settings Can be self-administered	Overall validity – High[1] Evidence grade, Strength – fair[1] Sensitivity = 97.9% Specificity = 100% Diagnostic accuracy = 98.7% Compared with SGA in older inpatients: Sensitivity = 100% Specificity = 52%[29]
Short Nutritional Assessment Questionnaire (SNAQ)[18] Netherlands	Most often used for older adults in community dwelling settings	• Weight loss • Decreased appetite • Use of supplemental drinks or tube feeding in last month	Parameters have different possible points • 1 = no intervention • 2 = moderately malnourished • 3 = severely malnourished	Can be used by untrained personnel	Overall validity – High[1] Evidence grade, Strength – fair[1]

| DETERMINE Your Nutrition Health Checklist[22] United States | Community Used to evaluate those asking for services from the Older Americans Act Nutrition Program (OAANP) | • Disease
• Eating poorly
• Tooth loss
• Economic hardship
• Reduced social contact
• Multiple medications
• Involuntary weight loss/gain
• Needs assistance in self-care
• Elder years | Parameters have different possible points
• 0–2 = good nutritional status
• 3–5 moderate risk
• ≥ 6 = high risk | Can be used by professionals or untrained staff
Can be self-administered | Was not developed to be a stand-alone screening tool and has not been independently validated
It is not meant to be a diagnostic tool, but should predict overall perceived health status and identify persons whose estimated nutrient intakes fall below the Recommended Dietary Allowances |
| SCREEN© Seniors in the Community: Risk Evaluation for Eating and Nutrition SCREEN-3, SCREEN-8, SCREEN-14[23] | Community-living older adults | 3, 8, or 14 questions (depending on the tool selected) on these focus areas: weight change, perception of weight, food intake and appetite, swallowing/chewing difficulty, function (preparing food, shopping) | SCREEN 14: Total score ranges 0–64
• ≥ 54 = low risk
• 50–53 = medium risk
• < 50 = high risk | Can be used by professionals and untrained staff
Can be self-administered | SCREEN-14 was validated against Dietitian Nutrition Risk Rating = 85%
Sensitivity = 85%
Specificity = 62%[24] |

Abbreviations: BMI = body mass index; ICU = intensive care unit; LTC = long-term care; SGA = Subjective Global Assessment.

REFERENCES

1. Skipper A, Coltman A, Tomesko J, et al. Position of the Academy of Nutrition and Dietetics: Malnutrition (Undernutrition) screening tools for all adults. *J Acad Nutr Diet*. 2020;120(4):709–713.
2. van Bokhorst-de van der Schueren MA, Guaitoli PR, Jansma EP, de Vet HCW. Nutrition screening tools: does one size fit all? A systematic review of screening tools for the hospital setting. *Clin Nutr*. 2014;33(1):39–58.
3. American Society for Parenteral and Enteral Nutrition. 2020. ASPEN Malnutrition Solution Center. Accessed January 20, 2021. www.nutritioncare.org/Guidelines_and_ Clinical_Resources/Malnutrition_Solution_Center/.
4. White J, Guenter P, Jenson G, Malone A, Schofield M. Consensus statement of the Academy of Nutrition and Dietetics/American Society for Parenteral and Enteral Nutrition: Characteristics recommended for the identification and documentation of adult malnutrition (undernutrition). *J Acad Nutr Diet*. 2012;112(5):730–738.
5. The National Resource Center on Nutrition & Aging. Nutrition Screening and Assessment in Hospital Patients: A Survey of Current Practice in the United States. Updated July 25, 2021. Accessed August 22, 2021. https://nutritionandaging.org/nutrit ion-screening-and-assessment-in-hospital-patients-a-survey-of-current-practice-in-the-united-states/#wbounce-modal.
6. Malnutrition Quality Improvement Initiative. Academy of Nutrition and Dietetics and Avalere Health. Published 2018. Accessed May 16, 2021. https://malnutritionquality. org/wp-content/uploads/complete-mqii-toolkit-1.pdf.
7. Joint Commission Nutrition Screening Requirements for Behavioral Healthcare Programs. Barrins & Associates. Published August 22, 2018. Accessed January 24, 2021. https://barrins-assoc.com/tjc-cms-blog/behavioral-health/joint-commission-nutrition-screening-requirements-for-behavioral-healthcare-programs/.
8. Ferguson M, Capra S, Bauer J, Banks M. Development of a valid and reliable malnutrition screening tool for adult acute hospital patients. *Nutrition*. 1999;15(6): 458–64.
9. Malnutrition Advisory Group (MAG): A Standing Committee of the British Association for Parenteral and Enteral Nutrition (BAPEN). The 'MUST' Explanatory Booklet. A Guide to the 'Malnutrition Universal Screening Tool' ('MUST') for Adults: BAPEN; 2003.
10. Kondrup J, Allison SP, Elia M, Vellas B, Plauth M. ESPEN guidelines for nutrition screening 2002. *Clin Nutr*. 2003;22(4):415–421.
11. Understanding medical tests: Sensitivity, specificity, and positive predictive value. Health News Review.org. Accessed April 18, 2021. www.healthnewsreview.org/tool kit/tips-for-understanding-studies/understanding-medical-tests-sensitivity-specificity-and-positive-predictive-value/.
12. Middleton F. Reliability vs validity: what's the difference? Published July 3, 2019. Updated July 16, 2021. Accessed August 22, 2021. www.scribbr.com/methodology/ reliability-vs-validity/.
13. Alliance to Advance Patient Nutrition. Malnutrition Screening Tool (MST). Published February, 2014. Accessed August 22, 2021. http://static.abbottnutrition.com/cms-prod/malnutrition.com/img/Alliance_Malnutrition_Screening_Tool_2014_v1.pdf.
14. Heyland DK, Dhaliwal R, Jiang X, Day AG. Identifying critically ill patients who benefit the most from nutrition therapy: the development and initial validation of a novel risk assessment tool. *Crit Care*. 2011;15(6):R268.
15. NUTRIC Score. Critical Care Nutrition. Published December 16, 2015. Accessed April 18, 2021. www.criticalcarenutrition.com/resources/nutric-score.

16. Reis AMD, Fructhenicht AVG, Moreira LF. NUTRIC score use around the world: a systematic review. *Rev Bras Ter Intensiva*. 2019;31(3):379–385.

17. State Operations Manual Appendix PP – Guidance to Surveyors for Long Term Care Facilities. Centers for Medicare & Medicaid Services. Updated November 22, 2017. Accessed April 18, 2021. www.cms.gov/medicare/provider-enrollment-and-certificat ion/guidanceforlawsandregulations/downloads/appendix-pp-state-operations-man ual.pdf.

18. Centers for Medicare & Medicaid Services. Patient Driven Payment Model. Updated August 2, 2021. Accessed August 22, 2021. www.cms.gov/Medicare/Medicare-Fee-for-Service-Payment/SNFPPS/PDPM.

19. Rubenstein LZ, Harker JO, Salva A, Guigoz Y, Vellas B. Screening for undernutrition in geriatric practice: developing the short-form Mini Nutritional Assessment (MNA-SF). *J Gerontol A Biol Sci Med Sci*. 2001;56(6):M366–M372.

20. Nestlé Nutrition Institute. MNA® Mini Nutritional Assessment. Published 1994. Updated 2009. Accessed February 13, 2021. www.mna-elderly.com/forms/mini/mna_ mini_english.pdf.

21. Kruizenga HM, Seidell JC, de Vet HC, Wierdsma NJ, van Bokhorst-de van der Schueren MA. Development and validation of a hospital screening tool for malnutrition: the Short Nutritional Assessment Questionnaire (SNAQ). *Clin Nutr*. 2005;24(1):75–82.

22. Mini Nutritional Assessment MNA. Nestle Nutrition Institute. Accessed August 22, 2021. www.mna-elderly.com/forms/mna_guide_english_sf.pdf.

23. Niedert K, Carlson M. *Nutrition Care of the Older Adult: A Handbook of Nutrition Throughout the Continuum of Care*, 3rd ed. Academy of Nutrition and Dietetics; 2016.

24. Kaiser MJ, Bauer JM, Rämsch C, et al. Frequency of malnutrition in older adults: a multinational perspective using the Mini Nutritional Assessment. *J Am Geriatr Soc*. 2010;58(9):1734–8.

25. Laur C, Keller H. Making the Case for Nutrition Screening in Older Adults in Primary Care. Lippincott Nursing Center. Accessed February 13, 2021. www.nursingcenter. com/ce_articleprint?an=00017285-201705000-00004.

26. Texas Department of Aging and Disability Services Access & Intake / Area Agencies on Aging. Instructions for completing the Nutrition Risk Assessment (NRA) DETERMINE Your Nutrition Health Nutrition Screening Initiative (NSI). Published May 7, 2010. Accessed August 22, 2021. www.hhs.texas.gov/sites/default/files/ documents/doing-business-with-hhs/providers/health/nra.pdf.

27. Keller HH, Goy R, Kane S-L. Validity and reliability of SCREEN II (Seniors in the Community: Risk evaluation for eating and nutrition, Version II). *Eur J Clin Nutr*. 2005;59(10):1149–1157.

28. Older Adult Nutrition Screening. Using and Scoring SCREEN. Accessed April 18, 2021. https://olderadultnutritionscreening.com/faq/#SCREEN.

29. *NSCR: Adult Nutrition Screening Tool Comparison*. Evidence Analysis Library, Academy of Nutrition and Dietetics; 2009.

5 Assessment – Anthropometrics and Functional Status

Terese Scollard

CONTENTS

I INTRODUCTION

Since the early 1990s, significant improvements have been made in the science underpinning anthropometric and functional measurement tools, and examination methods utilized to assess and diagnose adult protein-energy malnutrition (PEM), sarcopenia, and frailty.[1] The impact of acute and chronic diseases, related metabolic derangements, and their consequences to muscle and fat tissue are now better understood. Terminology, clinical characteristics, and established standards are becoming more aligned internationally.

While this new information drives improvements in clinical practice, significant challenges remain which may hinder routine application, including the availability

DOI: 10.1201/9781003177586-5

of testing, insurance coverage, costs, and other business factors. Moreover, there is a new large body of information that clinicians need to learn to fully optimize routine application of anthropometric measurements and functional exams. Clinicians must choose the most appropriate measure, use the correct exam methodology, apply appropriate standardized comparison tables, accurately analyze results, interpret the implications for the patient, and communicate and document results succinctly and meaningfully.

This chapter outlines anthropometric measurements and functional examinations, with an emphasis on those that are most within the control of, and available to, the practicing clinician who does not work in a research setting.

II   PATIENT INTERACTION AND EXAM CONSIDERATIONS

There are many factors to consider both before and during a physical examination, including patient safety, privacy and consent, as well as cultural factors. See Chapter 6 for additional information relating to patient interactions.

A   PRESENTATION AND INTERVIEW

After review of the patient's medical record, performance of functional and anthropometric examination begins before entering the patient's room. Clinicians must be prepared, professional, and wear appropriate personal protective equipment (PPE), if needed, as their presentation may influence the willingness of the patient to communicate or allow the clinician to proceed with the examination. Respectfulness, terms of greeting, self-introduction, speed and tone of speaking, avoidance of terminology unfamiliar to the patient, listening skills, and attentiveness will help foster trust and successful patient interactions.

The patient's presentation and their environment can convey significant information for the clinician. For example, the presence or absence of walking equipment, slippers, meal service items, breathing devices, as well as the patient's ability to manage their position in the chair or bed, all communicate their capability to partner with the clinician to safely perform functional and anthropometric examinations. Presence of get well cards, flowers, and visitors may also provide clues regarding the patient's social support systems.

B   SAFETY

Precautions for patient and clinician safety are critical during an examination. In the acute care setting, for example, before interacting with the patient, it may be prudent to clarify with nursing staff the ideal timing for the examination, or the patient's capacity to cooperate. Can the patient safely sit on the side of the bed or walk to a chair? Are there obstructions that could cause the patient to become unbalanced when moving between the bed and chair? Obtaining assistance from a nurse or other caregiver, or delaying and rescheduling an examination may be necessary. In ambulatory settings, use of wheelchairs or walking devices may also require assistance from another caregiver. The patient can also share their mobility limitations with the clinician if they are alert and communicative.

Safety related to infection prevention is also critical. Practices such as hand washing and use of appropriate PPE should be visible to the patient upon entry to the room.

C PRIVACY

Privacy is essential and may vary based on each patient's level of comfort. The clinician should always ensure patient privacy to the fullest extent allowed by the environment, and in accordance with the patient's preferences. Privacy curtains should be used in rooms with more than one patient, and the door should be closed. In institutional settings, clinicians can confer with nursing staff or the patient to determine whether it is appropriate to have visitors leave or stay during the examination. If visitors remain, they should be away from the space needed to perform the examination unless the patient prefers their presence. It may be in the patient's best interest to excuse visitors so that they can focus on the examination and not perform for or entertain the visitors. On occasion the clinician may need to reschedule or ask if the visitors can be excused temporarily so the anthropometric and functional examination can be performed more safely and privately.

D CULTURAL CONSIDERATIONS

It is vital to recognize patient cultural practices, if possible, before performing an anthropometric or functional examination. Beliefs, practices, and related behaviors vary within and between patients and their cultures. No matter the patient's name, country or region of origin, religion, gender, or other personal beliefs, practices or behaviors, it is best not to assume cultural or family dynamics. These details may be noted in the medical record or known by caregivers or other clinicians, and therefore may be clarified before proceeding with the exam.

Beliefs and culture may influence anthropometric and functional examinations. Patients may require certain family members be present or absent. Family members related to the patient such as parents, grandparents or children may or may not insist upon remaining or departing during the examination. Patients may over or under perform during the examination depending on their relationship to family members, and their belief system regarding being ill or being well. While most often this does not impair the ability to complete examinations, clinicians are wise to be aware of and sensitive to cultural practices, and adjust the examination as needed to successfully obtain objective clinical results.

E CONSENT

Patients and family members are often unfamiliar with medical examinations and may have never experienced a nutrition-focused exam. Medications and stress related to hospitalization and illnesses may fog experiences and memories. Language and cultural misunderstandings may occur. Patients may not know the profession of the clinicians or the many other persons that care for them, and may mistake one profession for another. Past experience or unfamiliarity with medical systems may frighten patients that fear victimization. In consideration of all of these factors, it is the patient's right, and also clinically appropriate, to ensure they understand what the examination entails, the reason it is being performed, and how the clinician will use the information to treat them. Explanations need not be complex and should avoid medical jargon. The courtesy of verbal agreement by patients (and sometimes family members) to perform anthropometric and functional examinations is recommended. Documentation can include agreement (verbal consent) to the examination, any additional persons present, and that the purpose and method of the examination was explained to the patient. It is unnecessary to obtain formal or written consent for anthropometric and functional patient examinations unless a facility requires it.

F OTHER CONSIDERATIONS

The value of listening and asking questions cannot be overstated when obtaining the patient's anthropometric measurements and performing functional examinations. Information on changes in functional abilities, including time of onset and the severity of the change from baseline, adds significant depth to the nutritional assessment and provides useful information for accurate diagnosis and development of appropriate interventions. Patient appearance can be highly deceptive. For example, a young person of normal weight who presents as bright, cheerful and well-dressed may have a very weak hand grip strength (HGS) due to PEM, or an older adult who moves slowly with a cane may spend hours gardening and have an exceptionally strong HGS. Exploring this type of information with the patient can yield valuable facts and avoid erroneous assumptions based on appearance, age, medical diagnoses, or various social factors.

Finally, when performing anthropometric measurements and functional examinations it is important to be aware of other recent activities the patient has experienced. For example, if a rehabilitation patient recently completed an hour of intense physical therapy, and has not yet eaten lunch, their muscles will be fatigued, and they may be exhausted. Examination and measurement at this point in time would not provide meaningful results and may overwhelm the patient.

III EXAM METHODOLOGY

Exam methodology must be standardized and performed accurately, using validated methods and calibrated equipment by skilled clinicians. Various methods of examination, testing and equipment settings have been published. Some literature on specific diseases and conditions may describe different methodologies, such as in hand grip dynamometer settings. Methodology issues can be problematic for clinical practice and should be addressed by researching and selecting the most appropriate standardized methodology as applied to the target populations or professional practice standards.

National and profession-specific groups recognize standardized methods for many tests and examinations. For example, the American Society of Hand Therapists (ASHT)[2] and the American Society for Surgery of the Hand (ASSH)[3] recognize and adhere to the HGS examination method described in the *ASHT Clinical Assessment Recommendations*, 3rd edition, 2016.[4,5] The National Institutes of Health (NIH) also provides standardized methods for functional assessment and anthropometric measurements.[6] These organizations describe methodology in great detail, occasionally with video and diagrams to assist learners. Procedural methods may differ in subtle or distinct ways. Therefore, it is vital that clinicians learn the appropriate methodology and are able to reproduce results that align with that of their peers. This ensures that there is peer-to-peer consistency, as well as trust and reliability of the examination method, equipment, and reported results.

When equipment is used for functional examination, it must also be periodically checked for safety and recalibrated for accuracy as recommended by the manufacturer, and by qualified professionals such as biomedical engineers, who verify sensitivity and performance requirements.

IV   ANTHROPOMETRIC MEASUREMENTS

Anthropometric measurements are conducted using standardized methods to obtain objective and reliable clinical data. Results are interpreted and combined with other subjective and objective clinical information to help assess nutrition status and make a nutrition diagnosis. Measurements are then routinely monitored to gauge the patient's response to nutrition interventions. Commonly applied anthropometric measurements used in nutrition assessment, including height, weight, body mass index (BMI), calf circumference, and mid-upper arm circumference (MUAC), are described below. All have strengths and limitations to consider when assessing nutrition status.

A   HEIGHT

Height, recorded in inches or centimeters, is a standard measure to judge growth in children, adult height, changes in height related to aging or disease, and as a factor in numerous calculations such as BMI.[7] Adult height should be measured and re-measured periodically using a stadiometer (see Figure 5.1), as patient-reported height is often inaccurate and adults frequently lose height with age. Standing height should be measured with the head, shoulder, buttocks, and heels touching the wall or back of the stadiometer. Eyes are straight ahead, shoulders relaxed, arms at the side, legs straight with knees together, and feet flat on the ground and almost together.[8] If the patient has kyphosis or other body conformation that restricts the ability to touch the back of the stadiometer or wall, the clinician can measure the best they are able. Should the adult be unable to stand on a scale, other approaches to obtaining height are available and can be used as surrogates for standing height.[9,10] Should height

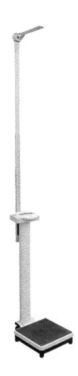

FIGURE 5.1   Stadiometer.

be stated and cannot be verified by measurement, documentation should include "reported" or "estimated".

1   Knee Height

Knee height is measured using a knee-height caliper, also called a rigid segmometer, or a flexible segmometer (see Figures 5.2–5.4), which tends to be less expensive and usable for more measurements than the rigid segmometer, such as demi-span, arm span and identifying the midpoint of the upper arm. This device is similar to a metal tape measure; however, a plastic or metal tip is attached to the end to place against the patient's joint or other body area, the floor, or the wall.[11] Once knee height is measured, population-specific equations are used to calculate height.[12,13]

2   Forearm Length

Forearm (ulna) length is the measured length between the point of the olecranon process (point of the elbow) and the midpoint of the styloid process 1 and 2 (prominent bone on the wrist), on the outside of the arm (see Figure 5.5).[11,14] This measurement is then compared to a height-estimate chart which differentiates between male and female and age ≥ 65 and < 65 years.

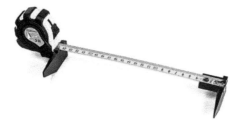

FIGURE 5.2 Rigid knee-height caliper.

(From Cescorf Equipamentos Para Esporte LTDA, Porto Alegre, Brazil, cescorf@cescorf.com.br. With permission.)

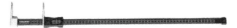

FIGURE 5.3 Flexible knee-height caliper (Holway rigid segmometer).

(From Structure & Function LLC, www.kinanthropometry.com. With permission.)

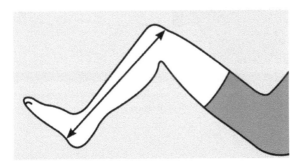

FIGURE 5.4 Knee-height measurement.

(From RxKinetics, www.rxkinetics.com. With permission.)

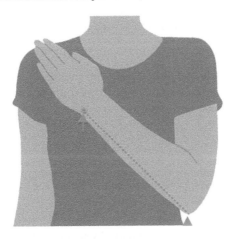

FIGURE 5.5 Forearm/ulna length measurement.

(The images are reproduced here with the kind permission of BAPEN [British Association for Parenteral and Enteral Nutrition]. For further information see www.bapen.org.uk. Copyright © BAPEN 2012.)

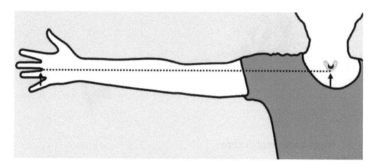

FIGURE 5.6   Demi-span measurement.

(The images are reproduced here with the kind permission of BAPEN [British Association for Parenteral and Enteral Nutrition]. For further information see www.bapen.org.uk. Copyright © BAPEN 2012.)

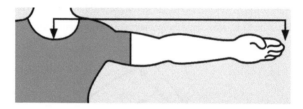

FIGURE 5.7   Half-arm span measurement.

(From RxKinetics, www.rxkinetics.com. With permission.)

3   Arm Span

Demi-span (mid-sternal notch to the web between the middle and ring finger; see Figure 5.6), arm span (tip of one middle finger to the tip of the other), and half-arm span (mid sternal notch at the top of the sternum to the tip of middle finger, multiplied by two; see Figure 5.7) can be used to determine height.[15] Use of arm spans can result in error, usually an over-estimation of the patient's actual height.[16]

4   Recumbent Length

Measurement is taken with the patient lying down without footwear, measuring from the top of the head to the base of the feet.[15] This position may be safest for patients who are wheelchair-bound or bedridden.[15,17]

B   WEIGHT

Weight, recorded in pounds or kilograms, is highly important for clinical care. Longitudinal tracking of weight is critical to understand fluid shifts and response to nutrition treatment, for various calculations, and changes may alert the clinician to a need for intervention. Scales must be calibrated periodically and patients should be weighed using a standardized procedure. In institutional settings, some beds allow the patient to be weighed while in the bed. Bed weights require that a tare weight first be set to "zero-out" the bed before the patient is placed. This method is relatively accurate when the same tare weight items are on the bed during subsequent measurements, but can be erroneous if items are removed or added. Weight should be measured when possible; if not, documentation should clarify the method used, i.e. "reported" or "estimated".

1 Weight History

Weight history is the longitudinal sequence of measured or stated body weights over time. These data can be correlated with medical and surgical events and provide supporting evidence to determine the etiology and severity of PEM, since starvation responses and stress response metabolism result in different patterns of loss.[18] Fluid shifts can confound the weight history pattern and need to be considered.

Often clinicians must depend on verbal reports from the patient or caregivers to assess weight history; however, this information is sometimes unreliable. For example, when asked for their usual weight, a patient may report one from decades ago, rather than a more recent usual weight. It may be necessary to probe for more information, such as asking the patient when they were last at their reported usual weight, or if they have noticed any changes in the fit of their clothing. Information from friends or family members about the patient's weight history may also offer insight. This baseline and subjective information can be documented and used to better assess the patient's weight history.

2 Weight Change

Percent of weight change is a critical measure of nutrition status as it is a characteristic included in many definitions of PEM. The time frame in which the change occurred is critical and should be documented, as it can help the clinician determine the etiology and severity of the change. For example, a weight change over a very short time frame such as one day can be interpreted as body fluid shifts. A longer time frame such as a week, or one, three, six or 12 months can indicate significant problems or changes in nutrition intake, activity levels, nutrient utilization, metabolism, or various medical conditions, especially those that are undiagnosed or poorly controlled. The time frame, amount, and percentage of weight lost or gained are highly important data points of the nutrition assessment, and must be documented and addressed, including the pattern of change and relationship to patient environmental and disease-related conditions. In situations where the clinician is not confident in measured weights, estimates and ranges may be utilized based on the information available, and documented as such.

$$\text{Percent weight change} = [(\text{Original weight} - \text{current weight}) / \text{original weight}] \times 100$$

The terms "significant" and "severe" have important clinical meaning and should be included when describing weight loss. The actual pounds or kilograms lost, percentage and timeframe of the loss, and loss severity should be documented.[19]

Significant weight loss: 5% loss in 1 month, 7.5% loss in 3 months, 10% loss in 6 months

Severe weight loss: > 5% loss in 1 month, > 7.5% loss in 3 months, > 10% loss in 6 months

3   Ideal Body Weight

Use of ideal body weight (IBW) is often necessary to identify patient-specific body weight targets to use in various nutrition calculations, such as energy and protein requirements. However, IBW has limitations, largely due to the wide variations in human body musculature and frame size. Further, the term "ideal" can imply weight bias and stigma.

a   Hamwi Formula

The Hamwi formula originated in 1964 in conjunction with other information used for diabetes management. The formula is quick and easy to calculate, and remains in common use in clinical nutrition practice.[20]

Males: 106 lbs + 6 lbs/inch over 5 feet for men

Females: 100 lbs + 5 lbs/inch over 5 feet for women

An adjustment of ±10% is made for small- and large-frame persons. Frame size is a relationship between a person's height and the wrist circumference of their dominant hand, or elbow breadth. Circumference of the wrist is measured with a thin measurement tape distal to the styloid process, before the hand itself. Frame size can then be determined by comparing the measure to male and female height-based tables.[21] (See Table 5.1.) Elbow breadth is an objective measurement that is not greatly affected by age or adiposity.[22] In addition to established tables, frame size using both wrist circumference and elbow breadth can be determined using online calculators. Weight adjusted for frame size, like any other estimated target weight, needs to be applied

TABLE 5.1

Frame Size as Determined by Wrist Circumference (Measurements in Inches)[21]

Sex	Height	Wrist circumference	Frame size
Women	< 62	< 5.5	Small
		5.5 to 5.75	Medium
		> 5.75	Large
	62 to 65	< 6	Small
		6 to 6.25	Medium
		> 6.25	Large
	> 65	< 6.25	Small
		6.25 to 6.5	Medium
		> 6.5	Large
Men	> 65	5.5 to 6.5	Small
		6.5 to 7.5	Medium
		> 7.5	Large

with clinical judgment, in consideration of each individual patient and realistic expectations.

b   Metropolitan Weight Tables

Metropolitan Weight Tables are infrequently used as target body weight goals in clinical practice. These weight ranges for males and females were based on actuarial insurance records that predicted mortality for insured persons from 1959 forward, with periodic adjustments.[23] In development of the tables, shoes and clothing were not considered in the measurement of height and weight. Additionally, a number of populations were underrepresented when the data were generated.[23] Therefore, this approach has generally fallen out of favor for clinical practice.

c   Challenges

As noted, use of IBW as an assessment of nutrition status is limited by its inability to account for differences in body composition and frame size in the general population. Several additional issues can pose challenges in the estimation of IBW, including changes in musculature associated with spinal cord injury, amputations, and measures used by other medical professions.

i   Spinal Cord Injury

Spinal cord injury (SCI) creates a challenging scenario for determination of target body weight. In 2009 the Academy of Nutrition and Dietetics' (Academy) Evidence Analysis Library (EAL) published recommendations for estimating IBW for those with SCI.[24]

Quadriplegia: 10–15% or 15–20 lbs lower than table weight
Paraplegia: 5–10% or 10–15 lbs lower than table weight

Additionally, BMI and skinfold measurements should not be used to assess weight status and body composition in those with SCI, as these methods were developed based on data from able-bodied persons only.[24]

ii   Amputations

The Amputee Coalition[25] and the Academy[26] recommend use of an adjusted BMI (i.e. what the BMI would have been had the patient not lost the limb) to more accurately assess weight classification for persons with limb loss. The person's weight is calculated by adding back the estimated weight of the absent limb, which is determined by an approximation of the limb's percent of the total body weight (see Table 5.2).[27] This estimated weight is used to calculate an adjusted BMI, which is then compared to the standard BMI cut points for underweight, normal, overweight, and obesity. All prosthetic devices should be removed prior to weight measurement.[25,26]

$$\text{Adjusted BMI} = [\text{current weight} + (\text{current weight} \times \text{percent of lost limb})] / \text{height}^2$$
(weight in kilograms, height in meters)

TABLE 5.2
Percent Body Weight for Amputations[27]

Amputation	Weight %
Foot	1.5
Below knee	5.9
Above knee	11
Entire leg	16
Hand	0.7
Below elbow	2.3
Above elbow	2.7
Entire arm	5

iii   Variations among Health Professions

Various health professions, such as anesthesia and pharmacy, may use different equations than registered dietitian nutritionists (RDNs) to determine IBW, and may not be familiar with commonly used nutrition-specific equations.[28,29] Dosing for some pharmaceuticals are based on IBW or other metrics obtained using historical equations of limited or unknown validity, including adjustments for patients with obesity.[30]

The RDN should be alert to these practice variations, as differing ideal weights between professions may potentially result in misaligned nutrition goals for parenteral and enteral nutrition dosing, nutrition modular product dosing, and nutrition care plan targets. Differing equations may be embedded in long-standing protocols, calculators or apps used by other professions and it may be difficult or inappropriate for the RDN to attempt to change these standard practices long-used by other professions.

For safe and consistent patient care, most notably between pharmacy and clinical nutrition, communication is critical to clarify and reconcile methods used for calculation of IBW. Clinicians should formally collaborate to define organizational policy within and between the various professions who deal with nutrition-related equations and calculation methods.

C   BODY MASS INDEX

BMI, also known as Quetelet's Index,[31] is a calculation that describes a mathematical relationship between weight and height and can be used for obesity-related screening purposes.[32] It is easy to obtain because height and weight are more easily measurable, as opposed to skinfold thickness or expensive technological tests which measure visceral and subcutaneous fat and require careful use of specific methodologies and equipment.

$$BMI = weight \ (kg)/ \ height \ (m^2)$$

$$BMI = weight \ (lbs)/height \ (in^2) \times 703$$

TABLE 5.3
NIH Classification of BMI[32]

BMI	Weight classification
< 18.5	Underweight
18.5–24.9	Normal
25–29.9	Overweight
30–34.9	Obesity grade I
35–39.9	Obesity grade II
≥ 40	Obesity grade III

Abbreviations: NIH = National Institutes of Health; BMI = body mass index.

The NIH weight categories are listed in Table 5.3. Additional categories for underweight have been published but are not currently espoused by the WHO or NIH.[33,34]

A significant drawback of BMI is that it does not account for body composition, therefore some experts suggest that it should not be used to assess nutrition status. This limitation is especially significant considering body composition differences between sexes and racial ethnicities.[35] BMI can be deceptive in patients whose weight is considered within a normal range, yet have a very low muscle mass and poor muscle quality (i.e. more intramuscular fat and visceral adipose tissue). While their BMI is normal, these patients may actually have, or be at significant risk of, PEM and/or sarcopenia.[36] This issue is especially problematic in patients with cancer. Research has shown poorer clinical outcomes, such as increased mortality, in cancer patients with low muscle mass and poor muscle quality as compared to those with the same BMI with normal muscle mass.[37]

In addition to body composition, BMI also does not account for age, as weight categories are the same for adults of all ages.[38] Research has shown seniors aged ≥ 65 years with a BMI of less than 23 have poorer clinical outcomes, including morbidity and mortality, suggesting an "ideal" BMI of 18.5 to 23 may not be an optimal range for this population.[39,40] These misperceptions related to BMI are one reason why the Academy of Nutrition and Dietetics/American Society for Parenteral and Enteral Nutrition (Academy/ASPEN) Consensus on Adult Protein-Calorie Malnutrition exclude BMI from the clinical characteristics.[41]

Another common diagnostic tool to identify disease-related PEM in adults, the Global Leadership Initiative on Malnutrition (GLIM) framework, is an international consensus intended to better align various local and traditional approaches, while not replacing long-standing local practices used to identify PEM.[18] Unlike the Academy/ASPEN clinical characteristics, the GLIM criteria include BMI as a phenotypic marker; however, the report recognizes regional variations. For example, BMI is not as widely used in North America due to high rates of obesity, which can mask muscle wasting.[18]

D   OTHER MEASURES

Other anthropometric measures may be utilized to assess nutritional status, although their use is uncommon in the inpatient clinical setting. These include circumference of the calf, mid upper arm, and waist.

1   Calf Circumference

The adult maximal calf circumference is an accessible, useful and likely under-utilized measurement that can be informative as to muscle mass.[42,43] The subject is seated and the widest circumference of the calf is measured with the measurement tape against the skin and at a right angle to the length of the calf (see Figure 5.8).[40] Measures greater than 31 cm are considered normal for both men and women.[44] However, Fernandes et al. found that that a calf circumference of less than 34.5 cm in seniors independently predicted increased mortality, suggesting that the 31 cm threshold is too low for this population. The authors concluded that calf circumfer-ence is an indirect measure of muscle mass and is therefore a more effective measure of nutrition status than BMI.[45] Other studies have found calf circumference to be associated with quality of life, disease severity, and mortality in patients with chronic obstructive pulmonary disease.[46,47]

2   Mid-Upper Arm Circumference

MUAC, also referred to as mid-arm circumference (MAC), is a proxy measure for body composition and infrequently utilized in adults;[43] however, it is accessible and easy to measure.[48] The measurement is the sum of the fat and muscle in the upper arm and is of interest because reductions in fat and muscle are frequently seen in patients with PEM. The right arm is usually measured; however, the left arm may need to be used in some circumstances, such as in patients with lymphedema of the

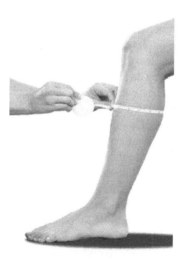

FIGURE 5.8   Calf circumference measurement.

(From RxKinetics, www.rxkinetics.com. With permission.)

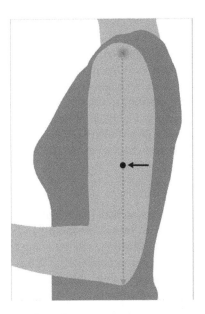

FIGURE 5.9 Mid-upper arm circumference measurement.

(The images are reproduced here with the kind permission of BAPEN [British Association for Parenteral and Enteral Nutrition]. For further information see www.bapen.org.uk. Copyright © BAPEN 2012.)

right arm. The length between the acromion process and the olecranon process is measured on the posterior (back) of the arm with the arm bent at 90 degrees. Midway (total length divided by 2) is marked. After determining the midpoint, the patient should be instructed to relax the arm at their side with muscles not flexed. The measuring tape is placed around the arm at the midway point, perpendicular to the arm, and not compressing the arm (see Figure 5.9).[48] Three measures should be taken and then averaged to obtain the result. Monthly measurements on the same arm are recommended because trends are meaningful when monitoring nutrition status.[49] Normal MUAC/MAC is > 23 cm in males and > 22 in females.[50] BMI may be estimated from the MUAC, according to the British Association of Parenteral and Enteral Nutrition (BAPEN), who describe:[50]

MUAC < 23.5 cm, BMI is likely to be < 20 kg/m^2
MUAC > 32 cm, BMI is likely to be > 30 kg/m^2

V FUNCTIONAL EXAMINATION

Declining muscle function and sarcopenia have emerged as significant problems due to the aging of the world's population.[51,52] Reduced physical function may limit a patient's ability to obtain, prepare, and consume food independently, which can impact their nutrition status and vice versa. Muscle mass, strength, and performance are altered in PEM, and often exacerbated by acute or chronic disease.[1] A vicious circle of declining nutrition status, disease burden, and associated declining functional ability contributes to physical dependency, more severe PEM, and further nutritional impairment.[36,53]

To identify performance in functional tasks such as walking, a number of standardized tests were initially developed for physical and occupational therapy. However, some of these tests are also associated with PEM, and can be clinically useful as part of a complete nutritional assessment. Some tests may be performed by the RDN or may be documented by other professionals.[54] Examples of functional examination tools include hand grip strength (HGS), gait speed (GS), the timed up and go (TUG), 4-m walk test, and chair stand test (CST).[55]

A HAND GRIP STRENGTH

HGS is the most commonly researched functional measure related to nutrition status, and is a proxy measure of muscle strength.[4] HGS, introduced in 1954, is useful for measuring upper body function, and assessing for PEM, age- or disease-related muscle function deficit, and sarcopenia.[56-59] It has also been identified as a meaningful data point (in conjunction with other data) by three international groups who have developed criteria for sarcopenia.[56,57,59,60] HGS is also used as an outcome measure in rehabilitation and clinical settings because it is responsive to changes over time.[4]

The Academy/ASPEN consensus characteristics for adult disease-related PEM recommend HGS as a preferred measure of functional ability because it is widely used, readily available, and represents the relationship between PEM and functional status in clinical practice settings.[41] The Academy/ASPEN consensus statement does not comment on specific HGS equipment or methodologies at this time. Low values are designated as minus 2 standard deviations below the mean for age, sex, and hand when compared to the normalization tables that come with the dynamometer. This level of weakness is noted as "measurably reduced".[41]

The GLIM work group noted that loss of muscle mass is generally accompanied by reduced muscle function, and that a decline in muscle strength exceeds changes in muscle size.[61] Therefore, GLIM concluded that when muscle mass cannot be readily assessed by phenotypic criteria (e.g. bioelectrical impedance analysis (BIA), ultrasound (US), computed tomography (CT), magnetic resonance imaging (MRI), dual-energy X-ray absorptiometry (DEXA or DXA)), HGS is an "appropriate supporting proxy".[61]

The ASHT published updated HGS methodology and equipment recommendations in 2016, which are also endorsed by the ASSH.[4] These recommendations include use of the Jamar® (manufactured by Sammons Preston) hand grip dynamometer (see Figure 5.10), which is reported to be the most commonly used brand in rehabilitation settings, and has strong test-retest reliability for grip strength measurement.[4] Other devices are compared against it as the "gold standard".[4]

As with any measured clinical test or physical examination, methodology is critical to accuracy and to obtain meaningful results that can be repeated by future clinicians. Hand grip strength examination requires systematic, reproducible, and standardized examination methods to ensure reliable results and inter-rater consistency.[5]

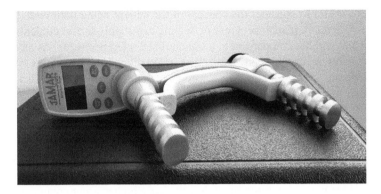

FIGURE 5.10 Hand grip dynamometer.

B OTHER FUNCTIONAL MEASURES

In addition to HGS, other commonly used measures of functional ability are part of the Short Physical Performance Battery (SPPB), which measures physical performance.[55] The SPPB tests include the Balance Test, Gait Speed (4-meter test), and Chair Stand (Sit-to-Stand). The Balance Test includes the Tandem Stand, Semi-tandem Stand, Side-by-Side Stand, and Stand on One Foot tests. These test results are associated with many health conditions including PEM and skeletal muscle deficit, e.g. sarcopenia.[60,62] At present HGS and gait speed are the preferred measures of sarcopenia according to criteria published by the European Working Group, the Sarcopenia Definition and Outcomes Consortium, and the Asian Working Group.[56,57,59]

VI DATA INTERPRETATION

After obtaining anthropometric and functional data, they must then be compared to appropriate reference data. However, comparing the patient to what is considered "normal" is an ongoing challenge of using anthropometric measurements or tests of functional ability. Humans do not all always fall into specific categories and present innumerable variations within normal ranges. Therefore, all measurements must be thoughtfully interpreted for clinical application. One-time measures are rarely definitive. Typically, nutrition-related trends and patterns over the course of time are more meaningful. Anthropometric and functional measures are therefore especially useful longitudinally.

Standardized/normalized references for examination measures usually compare the results to standardized age, sex-matched or other parameters of peer testing groups, and ranges are typically based on normal distributions in a bell curve. Hand grip dynamometers usually include reference tables specific for the device. However, reference tables for any test or device may include or exclude various ethnic groups, particular diseases or conditions, ages, or other patient characteristics; therefore, before choosing a reference table, it is important to determine how it was developed and validated. Regardless of the tables used, the clinician should always use clinical judgment in the interpretation of results.

It is also useful to consider the concept of the patient being their own "normal". Trends or patterns in patient progress or decline can supply useful clinical information, with and without comparison to a standardized reference value. As an example, grip strength reference tables provide a comparison of the patient's results to age, sex, and handedness, whereas monitoring a specific patient's trend in results also provides data on their performance over time in comparison to their own "normal".[63–66]

VII TECHNOLOGICAL TOOLS

BIA is the most commonly used technology to assess body composition. BIA uses electrical resistance to estimate body muscle and fat mass, and is the most practical tool for body composition assessment. Muscle has a higher water content, so when a weak electric current passes through various parts of the body, the resistance (impedance) will differentiate muscle and other fat-free mass from fat mass. Muscle has a low resistance because of its water content, and fat does not hold water so has a higher resistance.[67] Limitations to BIA include variability in test methods, hydration status, and physical activity, among other factors. Standardized methodology and procedures must be followed and the test performed by trained personnel.[51,68,69]

BIA testing equipment is available in some healthcare institutions. Reliability of BIA results has generally improved in recent years as manufacturing and technology have advanced; however, ASPEN guidelines do not recommend a specific device because there is too much variability in measures used to compare equipment.[70,71] When considering purchase of various BIA devices such as foot scales, handheld devices (see Figure 5.1), whole body devices (see Figures 5.12 and 5.13) and the more sophisticated and expensive direct segmental multi-frequency bioelectrical impedance devices,[72] the validity and accuracy of results, equations used, equipment calibration and maintenance, patient comfort, and cost should be considered.

BIA equipment reliability and accuracy, as well as various equations and their application to specific populations, have been debated.[67] The current state of research is not adequate to support the use of imaging results in routine clinical nutrition practice in most settings. However, there is movement in this general direction as clinicians are eager to use imaging results to better assess skeletal mass, visceral

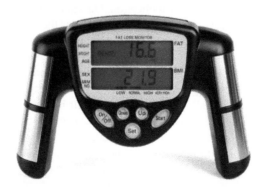

FIGURE 5.11   Bioelectrical impedance analysis – handheld device.

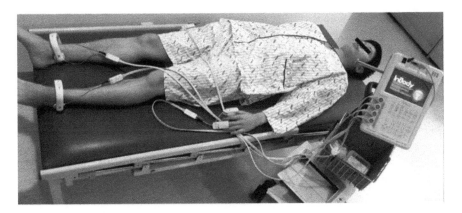

FIGURE 5.12   Bioelectrical impedance analysis – whole body reclining.

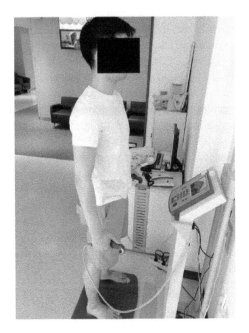

FIGURE 5.13   Bioelectrical impedance analysis – whole body standing.

fat, and muscle mass and quality to understand PEM, treatment risks, medication dosing, and clinical outcomes. The potential application of these tests in the nutrition arena is progressing rapidly, with significant ongoing research, especially in the areas of cancer outcomes, muscle wasting, and sarcopenia.[36,73–75] Of note, the relationship between the hands-on nutrition-focused physical examination (NFPE) and results of these imaging tools has not yet been validated. Nevertheless, the NFPE at this time remains the most available and practical method of examination for routine use in clinical nutrition practice.

Researchers have studied the validity and efficacy of other advanced body composition imaging and measurement tools, including CT, MRI, DXA/DEXA, and US. Rarely will the RDN be able to independently order and obtain a body composition test using these imaging tools, and they are not often utilized for this purpose outside the research setting. In most settings in the United States, these tests are only orderable by physicians and are typically not intended for nutrition-specific assessment of body composition, but rather for diagnostic or other medical reasons. Progress is being made to advance these technological approaches and statistical analyses are ongoing to determine the usability of these images for assessment of PEM and clinical outcomes.[76–78] ASPEN has published a clinical guideline on the validity of body composition assessment in clinical populations.[70]

VIII   CONCLUSION

Anthropometric measurements and functional exams are useful to assess and reassess nutrition status, sarcopenia, and frailty, to provide evidence of a PEM diagnosis, direct appropriate interventions, and monitor patient progress and outcomes. Muscle quality, which changes with age due to myosteatosis and connective tissue changes, as well as other factors in aging and disease, underlies impaired muscle performance that affects the individual's ability to be independent, recover from illness, and their quality of life. Discovery of functional deficits related to PEM can prompt the clinician to promote activities to improve nutrition intake and physical activity, to slow the rate of deficit, maintain, or ideally improve, skeletal muscle mass, muscle quality, strength, and performance.[79] Conversely, early discovery of nutrition deficits can trigger awareness of potential functional deficits, especially in less active patients, older adults, and those with complex diagnoses. Nutrition therapy and physical activity can often help improve functional ability, patient independence, and quality of life. Inclusion and analysis of these measures adds to the importance, depth, and strength of a thorough nutrition assessment of the malnourished patient as well as early identification of functional conditions of those at risk of PEM, sarcopenia, and frailty so that early and prompt intervention can be implemented to maintain or improve declines in health and clinical outcomes.

REFERENCES

1. Heymsfield S, Gonzalez M, Lu J, Jia G, Zheng J. Skeletal muscle mass and quality: Evolution of modern measurement concepts in the context of sarcopenia. *Proc Nutr Soc.* 2015;74(4):355–366.
2. American Society of Hand Therapists. Accessed November 23, 2021. www.asht.org.
3. American Society for Surgery of the Hand. Accessed November 23, 2021. www. assh.org.
4. Schectman O, Sindhu BS. Grip Assessment. In: MacDermid J, ed. *Clinical Assessment Recommendations and Online Companion.* 3rd ed. American Society of Hand Therapists. 2015.

5. Scollard T. Handgrip strength assessment: a skill to enhance diagnosis of disease-related malnutrition. *Support Line*. 2011;39(2):7–13.

6. National Institutes of Health toolbox. Accessed November 23, 2021. www.healthmeasures.net/explore-measurement-systems/nih-toolbox.

7. Casadei K, Kiel J. Anthropometric Measurement. In: StatPearls [Internet]. Updated October 1, 2021. Accessed January 20, 2022. www.ncbi.nlm.nih.gov/books/NBK537315/.

8. Centers for Disease Control and Prevention. Published January 2017. Accessed January 20, 2022. wwwn.cdc.gov/nchs/data/nhanes/2017-2018/manuals/2017_Anthropometry_Procedures_Manual.pdf.

9. RxKinetics. Estimating height in bedridden patients. Accessed January 20, 2022. https://rxkinetics.com/height_estimate.html.

10. Gordon SA, Fredman L, Orwig DL, Alley DE. Comparison of methods to measure height in older adults. *J Am Geriatr Soc*. 2013;61(12):2244–2246.

11. Nutriactiva. Segmometer for knee height measurement, ulna/forearm length, demi span. Published January 29, 2021. Accessed January 20, 2022. https://nutriactiva.com/blogs/anthropometry/segmometer-for-knee-height-measurement-forearm-length.

12. Chumlea WC, Guo SS, Wholihan K, Cockram D, Kuczmarski RJ, Johnson CL. Stature prediction equations for elderly non-Hispanic white, non-Hispanic black, and Mexican-American persons developed from NHANES III data. *J Am Diet Assoc*. 1998;98(2):137–142.

13. Chumlea WC, Guo SS, Steinbaugh ML. Prediction of stature from knee height for black and white adults and children with application to mobility-impaired or handicapped persons. *J Am Diet Assoc*. 1994;94(12):1385–1391.

14. British Association for Parenteral and Enteral Nutrition. Alternative measurements: instructions and tables. Accessed January 20, 2022. https://www.bapen.org.uk/pdfs/must/must_page6.pdf.

15. Cirillo D, Hart S, Reich R, Mason T. Height measures: evaluating alternatives to standing height in the ambulatory setting. *Clin J Oncol Nurs*. 2018;22(5):529–533.

16. Weinbrenner T, Vioque J, Barber X, Asensio L. Estimation of height and body mass index from demi-span in elderly individuals. *Gerontology*. 2006;52(5):275–281.

17. Froehlich-Grobe K, Nary DE, Van Sciver A, Lee J, Little TD. Measuring height without a stadiometer: empirical investigation of four height estimates among wheelchair users. *Am J Phys Med Rehabil*. 2011;90(8):658–666.

18. Jensen GL, Cederholm T, Correia MIT, et al. GLIM criteria for the diagnosis of malnutrition: a consensus report from the global clinical nutrition community. *JPEN J Parenter Enteral Nutr*. 2019;43(1):32–40.

19. Blackburn GL, Bistrian BR, Maini BS, Schlamm HT, Smith MF. Nutritional and metabolic assessment of the hospitalized patient. *JPEN J Parenter Enteral Nutr*. 1977;1(1):11–22.

20. Hamwi GJ. Therapy: changing dietary concepts. In: Danowski TS, ed. *Diabetes Mellitus: Diagnosis and Treatment*. Vol 1. American Diabetes Association; 1964:73–78.

21. Academy of Nutrition and Dietetics. Nutrition Care Manual. Anthropometric measurements: frame size. Accessed January 20, 2022. www.nutritioncaremanual.org/topic.cfm?ncm_toc_id=267413.

22. Frisancho AR, Flegel PN. Elbow breadth as a measure of frame size for US males and females. *Am J Clin Nutr*. 1983;37(2):311–314.

23. Assessment Psychology Online. Accessed November 23, 2021. www.assessmentpsychology.com/metlife.htm.

24. Academy of Nutrition and Dietetics Evidence Analysis Library. Accessed November 23, 2021. www.andeal.org/.

25. Amputee Coalition. Accessed November 5, 2021. www.amputee-coalition.org.

26. Academy of Nutrition and Dietetics. Estimating BMI for patients with amputations. Published online June 2, 2021. Accessed November 5, 2021. www.eatrightpro.org/news-center/nutrition-trends/nutrition-assessment/estimating-bmi-for-patients-with-amputations.

27. Osterkamp LK. Current perspective on assessment of human body proportions of relevance to amputees. *J Am Diet Assoc.* 1995;95(2):215–218.

28. Moreault O, Lacasse Y, Bussières JS. Calculating ideal body weight: keep it simple. *Anesthesiology.* 2017;127(1):203–204.

29. Robinson JD, Lupkiewicz SM, Palenik L, Lopez LM, Ariet M. Determination of ideal body weight for drug dosage calculations. *Am J Hosp Pharm.* 1983;40(6):1016–1019.

30. Boullata J, Armenti VT, eds. *Handbook of Drug-Nutrient Interactions (Nutrition and Health).* 2nd ed. Humana Press; 2010.

31. Quetelet A. *Physique sociale ou essai sur le developpement des facultes de l'homme.* C. Muquardt; 1869.

32. Khosla T, Lowe CR. Indices of obesity derived from body weight and height. *Br J Prev Soc Med.* 1967;21(3):122–128.

33. World Health Organization. Body mass index – BMI. Accessed February 17, 2022. www.euro.who.int/en/health-topics/disease-prevention/nutrition/a-healthy-lifestyle/body-mass-index-bmi..

34. National Institutes of Health. Calculate your body mass index. Accessed February 17, 2022. www.nhlbi.nih.gov/health/educational/lose_wt/BMI/bmi-m.htm.

35. Heymsfield SB, Peterson CM, Thomas DM, Heo M, Schuna JM Jr. Why are there race/ethnic differences in adult body mass index-adiposity relationships? A quantitative critical review. *Obes Rev.* 2016;17(3):262–275.

36. Prado CM, Purcell SA, Alish C, et al. Implications of low muscle mass across the continuum of care: a narrative review. *Ann Med.* 2018;50(8):675–693.

37. Brown JC, Caan BJ, Prado CM, et al. The association of abdominal adiposity with mortality in patients with stage I-III colorectal cancer. *J Natl Cancer Inst.* 2020;112(4):377–383.

38. Centers for Disease Control and Prevention. Accessed November 23, 2021. www.cdc.gov/healthyweight/assessing/bmi/adult_bmi/index.html.

39. Winter JE, MacInnis RJ, Wattanapenpaiboon N, Nowson CA. BMI and all-cause mortality in older adults: a meta-analysis. *Am J Clin Nutr.* 2014;99(4):875–890.

40. Nestle Nutrition Institute. Mini Nutritional Assessment. Accessed November 23, 2021. https://mna-elderly.com/sites/default/files/2021-10/mna-guide-english.pdf.

41. White JV, Guenter P, Jensen G, et al. Consensus statement: Academy of Nutrition and Dietetics and American Society for Parenteral and Enteral Nutrition: characteristics recommended for the identification and documentation of adult malnutrition (undernutrition). *JPEN J Parenter Enteral Nutr.* 2012;36(3):275–283.

42. Bahat G. Measuring calf circumference: a practical tool to predict skeletal muscle mass via adjustment with BMI. *Am J Clin Nutr.* 2021;113(6):1398–1399.

43. Gonzalez MC, Mehrnezhad A, Razaviarab N, Barbosa-Silva TG, Heymsfield SB. Calf circumference: cutoff values from the NHANES 1999–2006. *Am J Clin Nutr.* 2021;113(6): 1679–1687.

44. Tsai AC, Ku PY. Population-specific Mini Nutritional Assessment effectively predicts the nutritional state and follow-up mortality of institutionalized elderly Taiwanese regardless of cognitive status. *Br J Nutr.* 2008;100(1):152–158.

45. Fernandes DPdS, Juvanhol LL, Lozano M, Ribeiro AQ. Calf circumference is an independent predictor of mortality in older adults: An approach with generalized additive models. *Nutr Clin Pract*. October 14, 2021. Published online ahead of print. doi: 10.1002/ncp.10780.

46. Bernardes S, Silva FM, da Costa CC, de Souza RM, Teixeira PJZ. Reduced calf circumference is an independent predictor of worse quality of life, severity of disease, frequent exacerbation, and death in patients with chronic obstructive pulmonary disease admitted to a pulmonary rehabilitation program: A historic cohort study. *JPEN J Parenter Enteral Nutr*. June 26, 2021. Published online ahead of print. doi.org/10.1002/jpen.2214.

47. Ho SC, Wang JY, Kuo HP, et al. Mid-arm and calf circumferences are stronger mortality predictors than body mass index for patients with chronic obstructive pulmonary disease. *Int J Chron Obstruct Pulmon Dis*. 2016;11:2075–2080.

48. Centers for Disease Control and Prevention. National Health and Nutrition Examination Survey (NHANES) Anthropometry Procedures Manual. Published January 2013. Accessed February 2022. https://cdc.gov/nchs/data/nhanes/2017-2018/manuals/2017_Anthropometry_Procedures_Manual.pdf.

49. National Institute for Health Research, Cambridge Biomedical Research Centre. DAPA measurement toolkit: simple measures – arm anthropometry. Accessed November 23, 2021. https://dapa-toolkit.mrc.ac.uk/anthropometry/objective-methods/simple-measures-muac.

50. Benítez Brito N, Suárez Llanos JP, Fuentes Ferrer M, et al. Relationship between mid-upper arm circumference and body mass index in inpatients. *PLoS One*. 2016;11(8):e0160480.

51. Peterson SJ, Braunschweig CA. Prevalence of sarcopenia and associated outcomes in the clinical setting. *Nutr Clin Pract*. 2016;31(1):40–48.

52. Landi F, Camprubi- Robles M, Bear DE, et al. Muscle loss: The new malnutrition challenge in clinical practice. *Clin Nutr*. 2019;38(5):2113–2121.

53. Goodpaster BH, Park SW, Harris TB, et al. The loss of skeletal muscle strength, mass, and quality in older adults: the health, aging and body composition study. *J Gerontol A Biol Sci Med Sci*. 2006;61(10):1059–1064.

54. Russell MK. Functional assessment of nutrition status. *Nutr Clin Pract*. 2015;30(2):211–218.

55. National Institute on Aging. Short Physical Performance Battery (SPPB). Accessed November 23, 2021. www.nia.nih.gov/research/labs/leps/short-physical-performance-battery-sppb.

56. Cruz-Jentoft AJ, Bahat G, Bauer J, et al. Sarcopenia: revised European consensus on definition and diagnosis [published correction appears in *Age Ageing*. 2019;48(4):601]. *Age Ageing*. 2019;48(1):16–31.

57. Chen LK, Woo J, Assantachai P, et al. Asian Working Group for Sarcopenia: 2019 consensus update on sarcopenia diagnosis and treatment. *J Am Med Dir Assoc*. 2020;21(3):300–307.

58. Sipers WMWH, de Blois W, Schols JMGA, van Loon LJC, Verdijk LB. Sarcopenia Is related to mortality in the acutely hospitalized geriatric patient. *J Nutr Health Aging*. 2019;23(2):128–137.

59. Bhasin S, Travison TG, Manini TM, et al. Sarcopenia definition: the position statements of the Sarcopenia Definition and Outcomes Consortium. *J Am Geriatr Soc*. 2020;68(7):1410–1418.

60. Meza-Valderrama D, Marco E, Davalos-Yerovi V, et al. Sarcopenia, malnutrition, and cachexia: adapting definitions and terminology of nutritional disorders in older people with cancer. *Nutrients*. 2021;13(3):761.

61. Cederholm T, Jensen GL, Correia MITD, et al. GLIM criteria for the diagnosis of malnutrition – A consensus report from the global clinical nutrition community. *J Cachexia Sarcopenia Muscle.* 2019;10(1):207–217.

62. Phu S, Kirk B, Bani Hassan E, et al. The diagnostic value of the Short Physical Performance Battery for sarcopenia. *BMC Geriatr.* 2020;20(1):242.

63. Mathiowetz V, Kashman N, Voland G, Weber K. Grip and pinch strength: normative data for adults. *Arch Phys Med Rehabil.* 1985;66(2):69–74.

64. Mathiowetz V, Wiemer DM, Federman SM. Grip and pinch strength: norms for 6–19-year-olds. *Arch Phys Med Rehabil.* 1986;40(10):705–711.

65. Bohannon RW, Bear-Lehman J, Desrosiers J, Massy-Westropp N, Mathiowetz V. Average grip strength: a meta-analysis of data obtained with a Jamar dynamometer from individuals 75 years or more of age. *J Geriatr Phys Ther.* 2007;30(1):28–30.

66. Dodds RM, Syddall HE, Cooper R, et al. Grip strength across the life course: normative data from twelve British studies. *PLoS One.* 2014;9(12):e113637. Published 2014 December 4. doi:10.1371/journal.pone.0113637.

67. Lustgarten MS, Fielding RA. Assessment of analytical methods used to measure changes in body composition in the elderly and recommendations for their use in phase II clinical trials. *J Nutr Health Aging.* 2011;15(5):368–375.

68. Marra M, Sammarco R, De Lorenzo A, et al. Assessment of body composition in health and disease using bioelectrical impedance analysis (BIA) and dual energy x-ray absorptiometry (DXA): A critical overview. *Contrast Media Mol Imaging.* May 29;2019:3548284. doi: 10.1155/2019/3548284.

69. Ward LC. Bioelectrical impedance analysis for body composition assessment: reflections on accuracy, clinical utility, and standardisation. *Eur J Clin Nutr.* 2019;73(2):194–199.

70. Sheean P, Gonzalez MC, Prado CM, McKeever L, Hall AM, Braunschweig CA. American Society for Parenteral and Enteral Nutrition clinical guidelines: the validity of body composition assessment in clinical populations. *JPEN J Parenter Enteral Nutr.* 2020;44(1):12–43.

71. Khalil SF, Mohktar MS, Ibrahim F. The theory and fundamentals of bioimpedance analysis in clinical status monitoring and diagnosis of diseases. *Sensors (Basel).* 2014;14(6):10895–10928.

72. Ling CHY, de Craen AJM, Slagboom PE, et al. Accuracy of direct segmental multi-frequency bioimpedance analysis in the assessment of total body and segmental body composition in middle-aged adult population. *Clin Nutr.* 2011;30(5):610–615.

73. Earthman CP. Body composition tools for assessment of adult malnutrition at the bedside. *JPEN J Parenter Enteral Nutr.* 2015:39(7):787–822.

74. Wilkinson DJ, Piasecki M, Atherton PJ. The age-related loss of skeletal muscle mass and function: Measurement and physiology of muscle fibre atrophy and muscle fibre loss in humans. *Ageing Res Rev.* 2018;47:123–132.

75. Sheean PM, Peterson SJ, Gomez Perez S, et al. The prevalence of sarcopenia in patients with respiratory failure classified as normally nourished using computed tomography and Subjective Global Assessment. *J Parenter Enteral Nutr.* 2014;38(7):873–879.

76. Teigen LM, Kuchnia AJ, Mourtzakis M, Earthman CP. The use of technology for estimating body composition. *Nutr Clin Pract.* 2017;32(1):20–29.

77. Perkisas S, Bastijns S, Sanchez-Rodriguez D, et al. Application of ultrasound for muscle assessment in sarcopenia: 2020 SARCUS update: reply to the letter to the editor: SARCUS working group on behalf of the Sarcopenia Special Interest Group of the European Geriatric Medicine Society. *Eur Geriatr Med.* 2021;12(2):427–428.

78. Mulasi U, Kuchnia AJ, Cole AJ, Earthman CP. Bioimpedance at the bedside. [Correction in: *Nutr Clin Pract.* 2015;30(4):589.] *Nutr Clin Pract.* 2015;30(2):180–193.

79. McGregor RA, Cameron-Smith D, Poppitt SD. It is not just muscle mass: a review of muscle quality, composition and metabolism during ageing as determinants of muscle function and mobility in later life. *Longev Healthspan.* 2014;3(1):9.

6 Assessment – Nutrition-Focused Physical Exam to Detect Macronutrient Deficiencies

Sunitha Zechariah

CONTENTS

I INTRODUCTION

Nutrition-focused physical exam (NFPE) is a systematic, head-to-toe examination of the body to determine whether a patient's muscle, subcutaneous fat, fluid, and micronutrient status has diminished due to poor nutritional intake, inflammation,

DOI: 10.1201/9781003177586-6

and/or other causes.[1] With a 30–50% malnutrition prevalence among hospitalized patients in the United States,[2–4] Registered Dietitian Nutritionists (RDNs) play a critical role in recognizing and diagnosing malnutrition in this population. Early identification of malnutrition and timely nutritional intervention are crucial as they aid in reducing medical complications, allow for faster recovery, improve wound healing, reduce the hospital length of stay and readmission rates, and decrease the overall cost of care.[5–8]

The malnutrition diagnostic criteria recommended by the Academy of Nutrition and Dietetics (the Academy) and the American Society of Parenteral and Enteral Nutrition (ASPEN) requires RDNs to utilize NFPE as a vital tool to detect muscle wasting, subcutaneous fat loss, accumulation of fluid, and reduced strength.[9,10] Traditionally, physicians, physician assistants, and nurse practitioners perform physical exams to establish a medical diagnosis; however, these healthcare professionals focus on identifying the present medical concerns and may fail to recognize signs of malnutrition.[11,12] On the other hand, the NFPE performed by RDNs focuses on macro- and micronutrient-related clinical changes and characteristics, enabling RDNs to determine the presence and severity of malnutrition and micronutrient deficiencies.[13]

RDNs who work in inpatient acute care, outpatient clinics, and long-term care settings can utilize the NFPE as part of their routine nutrition assessment and re-assessment to elicit supportive information to gather baseline data, compare data with historical information obtained from medical records, uncover clues for the presence of nutritional deficiencies, evaluate the patient's changing nutritional status, and assess clinical outcomes of care.

II   BASIC EXAM TECHNIQUES

The four basic techniques used in a physical examination are inspection (observing), palpation (touching), percussion (tapping to evoke sound waves), and auscultation (listening to internal sounds using a stethoscope). Occasionally, two additional techniques are used: mensuration (measuring) and manipulation (moving of body parts). Of these techniques, RDNs most often use inspection and palpation in the inpatient settings, as well as auscultation if assessing bowel sounds. Mensuration is commonly used in the outpatient areas to measure adult patients' height, weight, and waist circumference. In the inpatient setting, anthropometric data are generally obtained from the patient's verbal report during admission, and subsequently weight is measured using bed scales.

Sequencing of the physical exam techniques in clinical practice is critical. Following a sequence allows the clinician to better remember all necessary components of the exam and ensures the patient's comfort. The best sequence of the physical exam is inspection, palpation, percussion, and auscultation.[14] However, in an abdominal examination, this sequence should be changed to inspection, auscultation, percussion, and finally palpation as palpation and percussion can alter bowel sounds, resulting in inaccurate assessment. The details of each basic exam technique are outlined in Table 6.1.

TABLE 6.1

Basic Physical Exam Techniques

Technique	Action	Exam details
Inspection	Observe	Visually examine the patient's appearance, general state of health, height, build, grooming, hygiene, posture, facial expressions, body language, motor activity, visible signs such as jaundice or poor dentition, alertness and orientation to place, person, time and situation, signs of pain such as grimacing, rapid blinking or tightly closed eyes and signs of distress such as dyspnea or cyanosis etc.
Palpation	Touch	Touch and feel the patient using hands or fingerpads to examine the body to identify muscle and fat loss, fluid accumulation, temperature, skin elevation as seen with follicular hyperkeratosis or acanthosis nigricans, pulse, contours, size of organs, and presence of any masses.
		Palpation can be light or deep. Light palpation is gentle depression of skin by 1–2 cm while deep palpation is firm, deep depression of skin by 4–5 cm.
Percussion	Tap body surfaces to evoke sounds	Tap the patient's body surfaces to evoke and hear the sounds from underlying tissues and organs. Use the middle finger of the dominant hand as the striking finger to tap against the non-striking finger, usually the middle finger of the non-dominant hand. Alternatively, use a plexor (small hammer with a rubber head) to tap against a distal pleximeter (small hard flat plate placed in contact with the body).
		The sound waves help to establish whether the underlying area is air-filled, fluid-filled, or solid. The sounds heard with percussion are:
		• Resonance – low-pitched, hollow sound heard over normal lung tissue
		• Hyper resonance – loud, booming sound heard in over-inflated lungs as seen in emphysema
		• Dullness – thud-like sound heard over organs and solid masses
		• Flatness – extremely dull sound heard over bones and muscles
		• Tympany – loud, high-pitched, drum-like sound heard over air-filled spaces such as the small and large intestines.
Auscultation	Listen with a stethoscope	Listen to the patient's body sounds using a stethoscope to determine the characteristics of bowel, heart, or lung sounds. Listen to bowel sounds in each abdominal quadrant. If bowel sounds are not immediately audible, listen for at least five minutes. Normal bowel sounds will have a low to moderate gurgling or rumbling pitch. Hypoactive bowel sounds are soft, barely audible sounds while hyperactive bowel sounds are loud, frequent gurgling sounds.

(Continued)

TABLE 6.1 (Continued)
Basic Physical Exam Techniques

Technique	Action	Exam details
Mensuration	Measure	Measure and record the patient's height, weight, waist circumference, mid-arm circumference, grip strength using a dynamometer, and size and depth of a wound.
Manipulation	Move body parts	Move patient's extremities to assess range of motion to check for abnormalities that affect movement.

Source: Adapted from Bickley et al.[14]

III   PREPARING FOR NFPE

Prior to examining the patient, take time to prepare for the NFPE, which will ease the process for both the clinician and the patient. Discuss with the patient, caregiver, or a nurse to assess the patient's ability to participate in the physical exam. In addition, determine the patient's level of orientation, alertness, and physical distress such as pain prior to initiating the exam. Here are some simple steps to follow:

- Wash or sanitize hands before beginning the NFPE
- Wear personal protective equipment (PPE) if the patient is in isolation or if standard precautions are required
- Ensure all instruments are available within reach (see Table 6.2)
- Check for adequate lighting in the room
- Ensure that the curtains are drawn, and doors are properly closed to protect patients' privacy and dignity
- Greet the patient to make them feel comfortable
- Introduce self to the patient and/or family members and explain the need for the visit
- Inform the patient about NFPE as some patients may feel anxious about being touched during an examination, and ask the patient if they would prefer visitors to step out during the exam
- Obtain verbal consent from the patient and/or family members when applicable

IV   ETIQUETTE

Practicing proper etiquette through patient engagement, comfort, and clear communication is crucial while performing a physical exam. A pleasant encounter will allow the clinician to build rapport with the patient, positively impact patient satisfaction, and gain more accurate information. Prior to beginning the exam, introduce yourself and warmly greet the patient with a smile and shake the patient's hand, if feasible. Address the patient by name and make eye contact throughout the encounter. Explain the purpose of the exam and ask the patient for permission to proceed. Listen

TABLE 6.2
Instruments for Nutrition-Focused Physical Exam

Instrument	Purpose
Gloves	Standard precaution infection prevention
Penlight	Examination of eyes and oral cavity
Tongue blade	Examination of oral cavity
Cotton swabs	Assessment of sharp and dull sensation
Sphygmomanometer	Measurement of blood pressure
Pulse oximeter	Measurement of pulse and oxygen saturation
Glucometer	Measurement of blood glucose
Stethoscope	Auscultation of bowel sounds
Hand held dynamometer	Measurement of hand grip strength

with empathy while taking note of the patient's non-verbal expressions. If the patient shows signs of pain or discomfort during the exam, stop and address the immediate concern and delay the exam until the patient is ready to continue.

While performing the NFPE, maintain patient dignity by uncovering the patient only as needed and examining all the necessary surrounding areas to minimize uncovering the patient repeatedly. Ensure patient comfort and be gentle when moving the patient's arms and legs during the examination or when rolling the patient over for the back exam. Always return the patient's arms and legs to the original position after completing the exam.

It is important to be sensitive while discussing any distressing findings with the patient.[13] It is best to evaluate the patient's capability to accept their present status before informing them of such sensitive information.[13] In the circumstance that the patient is ready to receive the information, communicate clearly and compassionately. If time permits, discuss the findings with the physician and/or during interdisciplinary team meetings prior to bringing them to the attention of the patient and their caregivers. If malnutrition is evident, provide a comprehensive treatment plan and offer reassurance to stave off any apprehension. In the outpatient setting, where immediate access to the referring physician is not possible, inform the patient about the muscle and fat loss findings in a truthful, yet empathetic manner. Avoid words that might hurt or alarm the patient like "severe wasting" or "severe malnutrition" and instead replace with less intimidating phrases such as "less muscle" or "unintentional weight loss".[13] Reassure the patient and offer appropriate nutritional recommendations and treatment to alleviate their condition.

V INTERVIEW TECHNIQUES

Patient health history provides important supportive information for nutrition assessment and malnutrition diagnosis. Skilled interviewing during a physical exam is an art that is developed through practice and experience. RDNs who are unable to simultaneously interview while performing the physical exam may need to focus on completing the patient interview prior to beginning the NFPE. RDNs may ask follow-up questions at the conclusion of the exam if needed.

Patient interviewing is an effective method of gathering essential information primarily through active listening. Listening is paying attention not only to the patient's verbal communication but also to non-verbal indications such as facial expressions, posture, gestures, behaviors, and emotions. Recognizing and understanding these non-verbal cues will allow RDNs to appreciate patients more fully and to provide a holistic approach to the treatment plan.

Interviews may include a mixture of open-ended and closed-ended questions. Open-ended questions will aid in eliciting the patient's thoughts and feelings and are useful in building rapport. On the other hand, closed-ended questions allow the examiner to determine focused, specific details in a time-efficient manner. Questions should be customized to each patient's situation and health condition. In general, questions should be sequenced to flow from the general (open-ended) to focused (closed-ended) questions. For example, ask open-ended questions such as "Can you tell me more about your poor appetite?" or "How would you describe your daily eating pattern?" to more specific questions such as "Have you lost weight without trying?" or "Have you seen any recent hair changes?" Avoid leading questions such as "Has your appetite been improving?" or "You do not have any nausea, do you?" Be sensitive to the patient's culture and gender identity and incorporate pertinent questions as necessary to confirm the findings from the physical exam.

VI HEAD-TO-TOE APPROACH

In general, a good approach to conduct a physical examination is to start from the patient's head, and move down the body to the toes, using a systematic head to toe approach.[13-15] This helps to maintain better hygiene by avoiding examination of the patient's feet before examining the patient's face and mouth.[14] Also, this sequence allows for a continuous movement from top down, maximizing the patient's comfort, and avoiding unnecessary positioning and repositioning of the patient. Tables 6.3 through 6.7 describe the examination techniques and physical signs of macronutrient deficiency by body area.

Approach the patient from the right side particularly in an inpatient setting as the inpatient beds are frequently positioned to accommodate a right-sided approach.[14] Examine the patient's right side first and then move to the opposite side. Assess patients bilaterally to evaluate whether a weakness may be present on one side of the body compared to the other side.[13] For instance, patients following a cerebrovascular accident may have hemiparesis resulting in one-sided weakness or hemiplegia with complete loss of strength or paralysis on one side of the body.

The clinician may have to modify their examination technique to accommodate the patient's condition, as hospitalized patients may be restricted to bed rest or sedated, which affects their mobility. Such patients frequently cannot sit up in bed for their exams. The examiner may have to inspect and palpate while the patient is lying supine and can gently roll the patient over to examine the back if necessary.

VII EXAMINATION FOR MUSCLE ATROPHY

Muscle atrophy is defined as a reduction in muscle mass, which can be a partial or significant loss.[16] Muscle atrophy occurs when the body loses protein at an excessive rate while protein synthesis is diminished and where catabolism exceeds synthesis. Muscle loss is commonly observed in disease-related malnutrition, particularly in diseases such as cancer, chronic obstructive pulmonary disease, heart failure, chronic renal failure, gastrointestinal disorders, and severe burns. Muscle atrophy can also occur due to reduced physical activity, immobility, poor nutritional intake, increased energy and protein needs, and decreased nutrient utilization or absorption. Muscle weakness and atrophy may also develop during the course of hospitalization in the intensive care unit (ICU) and is termed "intensive care unit acquired weakness".[17,18] One study has shown that when patients are admitted and treated in the ICU for 7–10 days, the incidence of ICU-induced muscle weakness increases by 24–55%.[18]

Muscle wasting is identified through inspection and palpation for muscle volume and strength. Inspection of muscles involves visualizing various parts of the body for signs of muscle loss such as hollowing, scooping, and/or concave depression, which may suggest muscle atrophy. Palpation requires touching and feeling the muscles for flaccidity and strength. Muscle strength is the muscle's ability to contract and generate force in response to resistance. The amount of force generated is dependent on the amount of muscle mass. A strong forceful response indicates sufficient muscle mass while a weak response may signify muscle weakness and wasting. On palpation, strong, well-developed muscles will feel firm and rigid, while weak, wasted muscles will feel flaccid and soft.

For some of the muscle-wasting examination techniques, the patient may need to be placed in a sitting position. However, if the patient is unable to sit up, patients can still be examined with the patient in the lying down position. Safely move the patient as required to access the areas needed for inspection and palpation. Inform the patient prior to moving them and return them to the original position as soon as the exam is completed.

Twelve superficial muscle groups can be inspected and palpated for muscle atrophy during the NFPE. Beginning with the temporalis muscle in the temple region, the examiner can work their way down to the trunk area to examine the trapezius, deltoid, pectoralis, intercostal muscles, muscles along the midaxillary line, continue to the back to assess scapular muscles (supraspinatus and infraspinatus), then move to upper extremities to examine interosseous, thenar eminence and finally continue down to the lower extremities to assess quadriceps and gastrocnemius muscle groups.[13] See Figure 6.1 for an overview of the major muscle groups. See Tables 6.3 to 6.7 for exam techniques and descriptions of findings for the head/face, anterior upper body, posterior upper body, upper extremities, and lower extremities.

A TEMPORALIS MUSCLE EXAM

The temporalis muscle is one of the muscles of mastication and is located along the side of the head occupying the temporal fossa. Clenching and unclenching the jaws

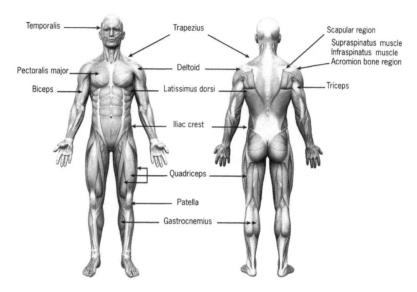

FIGURE 6.1 Major muscle groups.

(Reproduced with permission from the Cleveland Clinic and the American Society of Parenteral and Enteral Nutrition from Hamilton, C. *Nutrition-Focused Physical Exam for Adults: An Illustrated Handbook.* 2nd ed. 2022. Images created and owned exclusively by Cleveland Clinic's Center for Medical Art and Photography. Copyright 2022 Cleveland Clinic.)

or teeth contracts this muscle. Standing directly in front of the patient, the examiner should inspect the temporalis muscle for signs of hollowing, scooping, or concave depression. To palpate the temporalis, ask the patient to clench the teeth for muscle engagement. Using the index and middle fingers, palpate the muscle over the temporal bone in a scooping motion forward, backward, and diagonally. In well-nourished patients, there will be ample temporalis muscle and no apparent hollowing or scooping. In severely malnourished patients, inspection will reveal hollowing temples with concave depression. Palpation of the engaged temporalis muscle will feel firm and rigid on well-nourished patients and will feel flaccid and limp in malnourished patients. See Figures 6.2–6.4.

B UPPER BODY MUSCLE EXAM

The muscles in the upper body are more vulnerable to atrophy during nutritional deprivation as they are more sensitive to wasting compared to the lower parts of the body.[13] Inspect the clavicular region bilaterally by standing directly in front of the patient with arms at their sides. If able, the patient should be placed in a sitting position for inspection. Inspect for bone protrusion and muscle wasting in the anterior neck triangle and area behind the clavicle. Deep hollowing in the anterior neck triangle may indicate muscle wasting. Protrusion of the clavicular bone may indicate muscle wasting; however, it is important to note that some women may have prominent clavicular bone structure naturally. In severe malnutrition, the clavicular

TABLE 6.3

Head and Face: Exam Techniques and Physical Signs of Macronutrient Deficiencies

Exam areas	Technique Inspection	Technique Palpation	Normal appearance	Mild-moderate loss	Severe loss
Temporalis muscle	Inspect temporalis muscle bilaterally directly from front (as feasible) for hollowing/scooping	Palpate the temple region using index/middle fingers while patient clenches teeth	Well-defined muscle, firm muscle felt on palpation	Slight hollowing and depression	Deep hollowing and scooping; depressed temples
Orbital fat pads	Inspect eye sockets bilaterally from front (as feasible) for hollowing and bony prominence	Using index and middle fingers, gently palpate around the eye sockets	Bulged fat pads, well-defined muscle	Slight hollow look and slight scooping, slight depression, and some loose skin	Deep hollow look, scooped shape, depressed, loose skin
Buccal fat pads	Inspect cheeks bilaterally from front (as feasible)	Palpate fat pads under the cheekbone	Full cheeks, bulged fat pads, good bounce	Slight hollow appearance with minimal bounce	Hollow and sunken appearance, depressed on touch, no bounce

bone protrusion will be prominent with the area behind the clavicle significantly depressed.

Using the fingerpads, palpate the pectoralis major muscles right below the clavicles. Using the index and middle fingers, palpate the upper trapezius along the shoulders, from the acromion process to the border of the neck. The pectoralis major and upper trapezius muscles will feel firm in well-nourished patients, and weak and flaccid in malnourished patients.

With the patient in the sitting position, if able, inspect the deltoid muscles around the shoulder region for muscle volume and roundness. Well-nourished patients will have rounded shoulders without a prominent acromion process. Conversely, squared shoulders with a protruding acromion process may indicate muscle wasting. Cup hands to palpate the area around the shoulders to assess for deltoid muscle loss. In well-nourished patients, the muscles will feel firm without sharp bony prominences. In severely malnourished patients, the deltoids will feel less firm, and sharp and angular bony edges may be felt on palpation. See Figures 6.5–6.7.

While the patient remains in the sitting position, inspect the serratus anterior along the midaxillary line, which is a fan-shaped muscle that originates on the superolateral

TABLE 6.4

Anterior Upper Body: Exam Techniques and Physical Signs of Macronutrient Deficiencies

Exam areas	Technique		Normal appearance	Mild-moderate loss	Severe loss
	Inspection	Palpation			
Trapezius	Ask patient to sit up if able, with arms at sides; inspect directly from the front as feasible	Palpate trapezius along the shoulders from the acromion process to the border of the neck	Well-defined muscles, firm rounded appearance along shoulder line	Slightly flat shoulder line with slightly low muscle mass	Very flat shoulder line with very low muscle mass
Pectoralis major	Ask patient to sit up if able, with arms at sides; inspect directly from the front as feasible	Palpate muscles above and right below clavicles	Minimal protrusion, well-defined muscles	Some clavicular protrusion, low muscle mass above and below clavicle, slight depression behind clavicle	Prominent bone, low muscle mass above and below clavicle, area behind clavicle significantly depressed
Deltoids	Inspect for rounded versus squared shoulders	Cup hands to palpate around deltoids	Rounded curves at arm, shoulder, and neck	Shoulders slightly squared off	Shoulder joints look square, bones prominent
Acromion process	Inspect for prominent protrusion of acromion process	—	No protrusion of acromion process	Acromion process slightly protruding	Acromion process prominent and clearly visible
Intercostal muscles	Inspect for concave shape and depression between ribs	Palpate between the ribs for depression	Chest is full, ribs do not show	Slight depression between ribs	Depression between ribs is very apparent
Serratus anterior	Inspect for bony prominence and concave depressions between 1st and 8th ribs directly under the axilla (armpit)	Palpate muscles between 1st and 8th ribs around midaxillary line	Ribs do not show, rounded appearance	Slight depression between ribs	Depression between ribs is very apparent
Iliac crest skinfolds	Ask patient to sit up if able. Inspect top of hip bone for prominent iliac crest	Pinch and roll iliac crest skinfolds between index finger and thumb to determine the amount of fat	Ample fat tissue between folds of skin, ample spacing between fingers, iliac crest not prominent	Some loose skin, some space between fingers, iliac crest slightly prominent	Loose skin, very little space between fingers, very prominent iliac crest

TABLE 6.5
Posterior Upper Body: Exam Techniques and Physical Signs of Macronutrient Deficiencies

Exam areas	Technique		Normal appearance	Mild-moderate loss	Severe loss
	Inspection	Palpation			
Posterior trapezius muscles	Inspect posterior trapezius around upper back bilaterally	Palpate posterior trapezius around upper back	Adequate muscle mass, rounded back	Slightly low muscle mass, somewhat flat back	Very low muscle mass, very flat back with poorly defined muscles
Scapulary muscles (supraspinatus and infraspinatus)	Inspect scapula for bony prominence while asking patient to extend arms out and push against examiner's hand	Palpate around scapula bilaterally as patient's arm pushes against examiner's hand	Bones not prominent, no significant depression	Mild depression, bones slightly visible	Prominent, visible bones, apparent depressions between the scapula and spine

TABLE 6.6
Upper Extremities: Exam Techniques and Physical Signs of Macronutrient Deficiencies

Exam areas	Technique		Normal appearance	Mild-moderate loss	Severe loss
	Inspection	Palpation			
Biceps/triceps	Inspect biceps/triceps area for loose skin	Ask patient to bend arm at 90-degree angle, gently grab biceps/triceps between thumb and index finger and roll and pinch to determine amount of fat. Support patient's elbow if needed	Ample fat tissue between folds of skin	Slightly loose skin, some space between fingers around skinfolds	Loose skin, very little space between fingers around skinfolds
Interosseous muscles	Inspect the area between the index finger and thumb on the dorsal side of hand while patient presses the pads of thumb against the other four fingers or pretends to hold a pencil/pen	Palpate the area between the index finger and thumb, near metacarpal bone on the dorsal side of hand while patient engages muscle	Adequate, firm musculature, no depression	Slightly depressed between index finger and thumb	Deep depression between index finger and thumb
Thenar muscles	Inspect the base of the thumb on the palmer side while patient presses the pads of thumb against the other four fingers	Palpate the base of the thumb on the palmer side while patient presses the pads of thumb against the other four fingers	Rounded thumb base, no depression	Slightly depressed thumb base	Deep depression on thumb base

TABLE 6.7

Lower Extremities: Exam Techniques and Physical Signs of Macronutrient Deficiencies

| Exam areas | Technique | | Normal appearance | Mild-moderate loss | Severe loss |
	Inspection	Palpation			
Quadriceps	With patient's leg propped up and slightly bent at knee, inspect for concave depression	Palpate quadriceps bilaterally, may ask patient to lift leg for muscle engagement	Rounded, well-developed muscles, bones not prominent	Slightly prominent patella, slight depressions	Prominent patella, apparent concave depressions
Gastrocnemius	Inspect the calf area for thinning and loose skin	Gently grasp calf muscle and assess for bulk or thinning, ask patient to point toes to engage muscle	Rounded, well developed, firm calf	Not well developed, slightly thin calf, not firm on touch	Poorly developed calf, thin to minimal bulk

FIGURE 6.2 Head and face – normal.

(Reproduced with permission from the Cleveland Clinic and the American Society of Parenteral and Enteral Nutrition from Hamilton, C. *Nutrition-Focused Physical Exam for Adults: An Illustrated Handbook.* 2nd ed. 2022. Images created and owned exclusively by Cleveland Clinic's Center for Medical Art and Photography. Copyright 2022 Cleveland Clinic.)

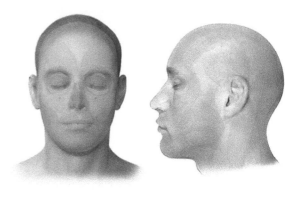

FIGURE 6.3 Head and face – mild/moderate wasting.

(Reproduced with permission from the Cleveland Clinic and the American Society of Parenteral and Enteral Nutrition from Hamilton, C. *Nutrition-Focused Physical Exam for Adults: An Illustrated Handbook.* 2nd ed. 2022. Images created and owned exclusively by Cleveland Clinic's Center for Medical Art and Photography. Copyright 2022 Cleveland Clinic.)

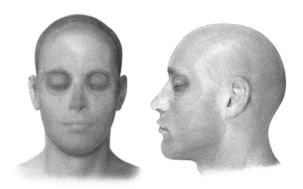

FIGURE 6.4 Head and face – severe wasting.

(Reproduced with permission from the Cleveland Clinic and the American Society of Parenteral and Enteral Nutrition from Hamilton, C. *Nutrition-Focused Physical Exam for Adults: An Illustrated Handbook.* 2nd ed. 2022. Images created and owned exclusively by Cleveland Clinic's Center for Medical Art and Photography. Copyright 2022 Cleveland Clinic.)

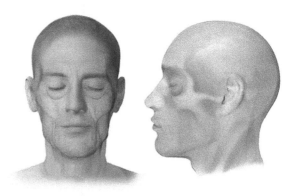

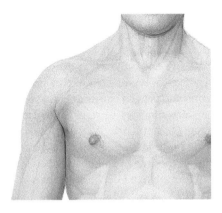

FIGURE 6.5 Clavicle and shoulder – normal.

(Reproduced with permission from the Cleveland Clinic and the American Society of Parenteral and Enteral Nutrition from Hamilton, C. *Nutrition-Focused Physical Exam for Adults: An Illustrated Handbook*. 2nd ed. 2022. Images created and owned exclusively by Cleveland Clinic's Center for Medical Art and Photography. Copyright 2022 Cleveland Clinic.)

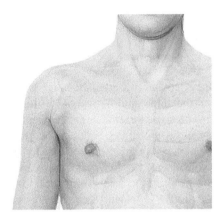

FIGURE 6.6 Clavicle and shoulder – mild/moderate wasting.

(Reproduced with permission from the Cleveland Clinic and the American Society of Parenteral and Enteral Nutrition from Hamilton, C. *Nutrition-Focused Physical Exam for Adults: An Illustrated Handbook*. 2nd ed. 2022. Images created and owned exclusively by Cleveland Clinic's Center for Medical Art and Photography. Copyright 2022 Cleveland Clinic.)

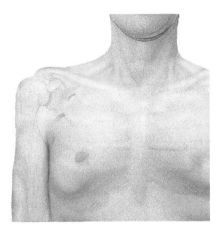

FIGURE 6.7 Clavicle and shoulder – severe wasting.

(Reproduced with permission from the Cleveland Clinic and the American Society of Parenteral and Enteral Nutrition from Hamilton, C. *Nutrition-Focused Physical Exam for Adults: An Illustrated Handbook*. 2nd ed. 2022. Images created and owned exclusively by Cleveland Clinic's Center for Medical Art and Photography. Copyright 2022 Cleveland Clinic.)

surfaces of the first to eighth ribs at the lateral wall of the thorax. This muscle can also be inspected while the patient is in the standing position, as shown in Figures 6.8–6.10. Inspect for bony prominence and concave depressions between the first and eighth ribs. Palpate the serratus anterior, directly under the axilla, between the pectoralis major and latissimus dorsi to identify muscle wasting. In well-nourished patients, the muscles will appear full on inspection and firm on palpation. In severely malnourished patients, concave depressions between ribs may be seen and muscles will feel flaccid on palpation.

Similarly, the external intercostal muscles can be inspected with the patient in the sitting position. Intercostal muscles lie in the intercostal spaces between the ribs. Inspect the thoracic region for protruding ribs and depressions between the ribs. A severe depression between the ribs may indicate muscle loss. Palpate the muscles between the ribs with the index finger to identify whether loss of chest wall muscle mass is apparent. In well-nourished patients, the chest muscles will be well-defined with no apparent depressions. In severely malnourished patients, the apparent depression between ribs will be visible and can be felt on palpation.

C   BACK MUSCLE EXAM

With the patient sitting up, if able, inspect the scapular area (the shoulder blade) for prominent bones and a depression between the spine and the scapula. Patients who are unable to sit up can be gently rolled over for back examination. Inspect the trapezius, supraspinatus, and infraspinatus muscles for protruding bones and depression between the spine and scapula. Prior to palpation, ask the patient to extend the arm forward and press against the examiner's hand in order to engage the scapulary muscles. Palpate around the engaged scapular muscles to assess for muscle loss. Engage the trapezius by asking the patient to shrug the shoulders against the resistance of the examiner's hand. In well-nourished patients, the trapezius and the scapulary muscles will be well-defined with no apparent depressions or bony protrusions. In severely malnourished patients, the spine and the bone around the scapula will be prominently visible and significant depressions between the spine and scapula will be noted on palpation. See Figures 6.8–6.10.

D   HAND MUSCLE EXAM

Examination of the hand is performed on the dorsal interosseous muscles and the palmar thenar eminence. The dorsal interosseous muscles are a group of muscles between the metacarpal bones of the hand. Muscle wasting in the hand can be generalized or localized. Generalized wasting is often seen with malnutrition while localized wasting may be due to nerve lesions, inadequate blood perfusion, or myopathy. Inspect the interosseous muscles between the thumb and the index finger. Palpate the area between the thumb and index finger by asking the patient to engage the muscle by pressing the thumb against the other four fingerpads. Alternatively, you can also ask the patient to hold a small object like a pencil or pen to engage the

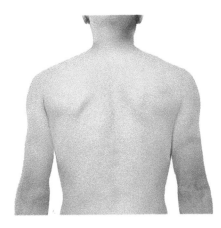

FIGURE 6.8 Back – normal.

(Reproduced with permission from the Cleveland Clinic and the American Society of Parenteral and Enteral Nutrition from Hamilton, C. *Nutrition-Focused Physical Exam for Adults: An Illustrated Handbook.* 2nd ed. 2022. Images created and owned exclusively by Cleveland Clinic's Center for Medical Art and Photography. Copyright 2022 Cleveland Clinic.)

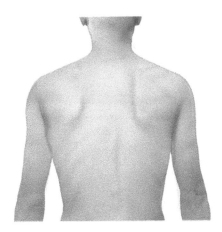

FIGURE 6.9 Back – mild/moderate wasting.

(Reproduced with permission from the Cleveland Clinic and the American Society of Parenteral and Enteral Nutrition from Hamilton, C. *Nutrition-Focused Physical Exam for Adults: An Illustrated Handbook.* 2nd ed. 2022. Images created and owned exclusively by Cleveland Clinic's Center for Medical Art and Photography. Copyright 2022 Cleveland Clinic.)

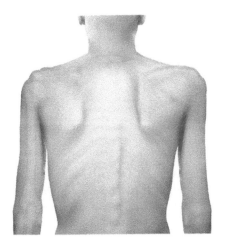

FIGURE 6.10 Back – severe wasting.

(Reproduced with permission from the Cleveland Clinic and the American Society of Parenteral and Enteral Nutrition from Hamilton, C. *Nutrition-Focused Physical Exam for Adults: An Illustrated Handbook.* 2nd ed. 2022. Images created and owned exclusively by Cleveland Clinic's Center for Medical Art and Photography. Copyright 2022 Cleveland Clinic.)

FIGURE 6.11   Dorsal hand – normal.

(Reproduced with permission from the Cleveland
Clinic and the American Society of Parenteral and
Enteral Nutrition from Hamilton, C. *Nutrition-
Focused Physical Exam for Adults: An Illustrated
Handbook.* 2nd ed. 2022. Images created and
owned exclusively by Cleveland Clinic's Center
for Medical Art and Photography. Copyright 2022
Cleveland Clinic.)

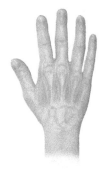
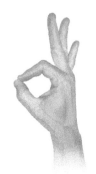

FIGURE 6.12   Dorsal hand – mild/moderate
wasting.

(Reproduced with permission from the Cleveland
Clinic and the American Society of Parenteral and
Enteral Nutrition from Hamilton, C. *Nutrition-
Focused Physical Exam for Adults: An Illustrated
Handbook.* 2nd ed. 2022. Images created and
owned exclusively by Cleveland Clinic's Center
for Medical Art and Photography. Copyright 2022
Cleveland Clinic.)

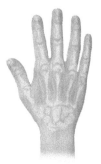
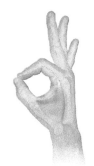

FIGURE 6.13   Dorsal hand – severe wasting.

(Reproduced with permission from the Cleveland
Clinic and the American Society of Parenteral and
Enteral Nutrition from Hamilton, C. *Nutrition-
Focused Physical Exam for Adults: An Illustrated
Handbook.* 2nd ed. 2022. Images created and owned
exclusively by Cleveland Clinic's Center for Medical
Art and Photography. Copyright 2022 Cleveland
Clinic.)

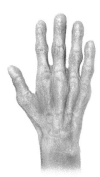
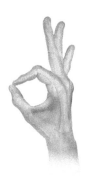

interosseous muscles. The strength of the muscles can also be assessed by asking the
patient to keep the fingers pressed as tight as possible and the examiner can attempt
to pull the patient's fingers apart. See Figures 6.11–6.13.

The palmar thenar muscles are a group of muscles at the base of the thumb
and are used for thumb movement. Inspect the base of the thumb for muscle bulk.
A well-defined thenar eminence will appear as a mound at the base of the thumb. The
thenar muscles can be palpated using the same technique described above for muscle

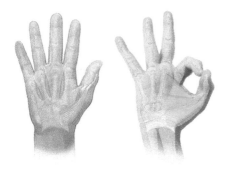

FIGURE 6.14 Palmar hand – normal.

(Reproduced with permission from the Cleveland Clinic and the American Society of Parenteral and Enteral Nutrition from Hamilton, C. *Nutrition-Focused Physical Exam for Adults: An Illustrated Handbook.* 2nd ed. 2022. Images created and owned exclusively by Cleveland Clinic's Center for Medical Art and Photography. Copyright 2022 Cleveland Clinic.)

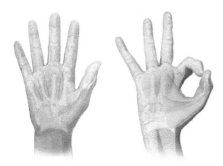

FIGURE 6.15 Palmar hand – mild/ moderate wasting.

(Reproduced with permission from the Cleveland Clinic and the American Society of Parenteral and Enteral Nutrition from Hamilton, C. *Nutrition-Focused Physical Exam for Adults: An Illustrated Handbook.* 2nd ed. 2022. Images created and owned exclusively by Cleveland Clinic's Center for Medical Art and Photography. Copyright 2022 Cleveland Clinic.)

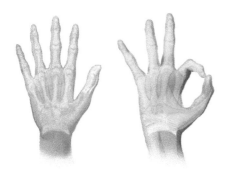

FIGURE 6.16 Palmar hand – severe wasting.

(Reproduced with permission from the Cleveland Clinic and the American Society of Parenteral and Enteral Nutrition from Hamilton, C. *Nutrition-Focused Physical Exam for Adults: An Illustrated Handbook.* 2nd ed. 2022. Images created and owned exclusively by Cleveland Clinic's Center for Medical Art and Photography. Copyright 2022 Cleveland Clinic.)

engagement. While the patient is holding their thumb pressed against the other four fingerpads, palpate the base of the thumb on the palmar side to assess the musculature. Well-nourished patients will have adequate muscle bulk between the metacarpal bones and thumb base with no apparent depressions. In severely malnourished patients, an apparent depression will be seen between the metacarpal bones and the base of the thumb. Lack of muscle bulk can also be felt on palpation. See Figures 6.14–6.16.

FIGURE 6.17   Lateral lower
extremity – normal.

(Reproduced with permission
from the Cleveland Clinic and the
American Society of Parenteral
and Enteral Nutrition from
Hamilton, C. *Nutrition-Focused
Physical Exam for Adults: An
Illustrated Handbook.* 2nd ed.
2022. Images created and owned
exclusively by Cleveland Clinic's
Center for Medical Art and
Photography. Copyright 2022
Cleveland Clinic.)

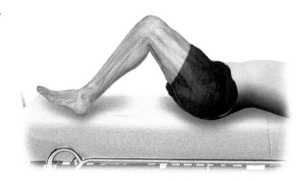

FIGURE 6.18   Lateral lower
extremity – mild/moderate
wasting.

(Reproduced with permission
from the Cleveland Clinic and the
American Society of Parenteral
and Enteral Nutrition from
Hamilton, C. *Nutrition-Focused
Physical Exam for Adults: An
Illustrated Handbook.* 2nd ed.
2022. Images created and owned
exclusively by Cleveland Clinic's
Center for Medical Art and
Photography. Copyright 2022
Cleveland Clinic.)

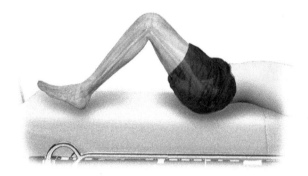

FIGURE 6.19   Lateral lower
extremity – severe wasting.

(Reproduced with permission
from the Cleveland Clinic and the
American Society of Parenteral
and Enteral Nutrition from
Hamilton, C. *Nutrition-Focused
Physical Exam for Adults: An
Illustrated Handbook.* 2nd ed.
2022. Images created and owned
exclusively by Cleveland Clinic's
Center for Medical Art and
Photography. Copyright 2022
Cleveland Clinic.)

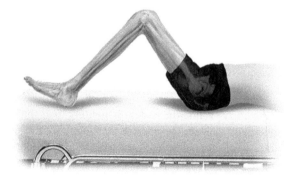

E LOWER BODY MUSCLE EXAM

Examining the muscles in the lower body includes evaluating the quadriceps around the patellar region and the gastrocnemius muscles on the posterior calf region. The quadriceps are a group of four muscles, which are the largest and strongest muscles in the body. These muscles help with standing, walking, running, and other movements. Inspect the quadriceps with the patient's legs bent and propped up if able. Visually inspect for rounded musculature and shape of the quadriceps. Poorly defined muscles and a concave depression may indicate muscle loss. Palpate by cupping the hand above, below, and around the thighs to assess the quadriceps. Exercise caution while uncovering the patient to palpate for the quadriceps. Uncover only the necessary area to maintain patient privacy and dignity and cover exposed areas immediately upon completion of the exam.

The gastrocnemius is the major muscle at the back of the lower legs and is responsible for plantar flexion of the foot and the ankle. Again, with the patient's leg propped up, inspect the muscles in the calf area for thinning or bulking of the gastrocnemius muscles. Ask the patient to flex their toes to engage the muscles and palpate by grasping the calf region. Thin to minimally defined muscles may indicate muscle loss. See Figures 6.17–6.22.

VIII EXAMINATION FOR SUBCUTANEOUS FAT LOSS

Subcutaneous fat is the layer of adipose tissue widely distributed directly under the skin. This layer of padding acts as a shock absorber and an energy reserve. The amount of adipose tissue in different areas of the body varies depending on an individual's nutritional state. There are four areas where subcutaneous fat deposition can be examined to identify malnutrition. These regions include the orbital and buccal fat pads, the biceps and triceps region in the upper arm, and the suprailiac skinfold above the iliac crest.

A ORBITAL FAT PAD EXAM

Standing directly in front of the patient, inspect the orbital fad pads around the eye sockets to observe for depressions, hollowing, and loose skin. Using the index and middle fingers, palpate above the cheekbone, around the eyes and along the supraorbital foramen for fat loss. Examine for any bony prominence. Well-nourished patients will have bulgy orbital fat pads with no apparent bony prominence. Severely malnourished patients will have a pronounced hollow appearance with a sunken look, loose skin, and prominent eye sockets indicating fat loss. Caution should be applied when examining elderly patients as some elderly patients may have a sunken look due to the loss of collagen as a result of the natural aging process. See Figures 6.2–6.4.

FIGURE 6.20   Anterior lower extremity – normal.

(Reproduced with permission from the Cleveland Clinic
and the American Society of Parenteral and Enteral
Nutrition from Hamilton, C. *Nutrition-Focused Physical
Exam for Adults: An Illustrated Handbook.* 2nd ed. 2022.
Images created and owned exclusively by Cleveland
Clinic's Center for Medical Art and Photography.
Copyright 2022 Cleveland Clinic.)

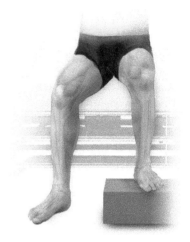

FIGURE 6.21   Anterior lower extremity – mild/
moderate wasting.

(Reproduced with permission from the Cleveland Clinic
and the American Society of Parenteral and Enteral
Nutrition from Hamilton, C. *Nutrition-Focused Physical
Exam for Adults: An Illustrated Handbook.* 2nd ed. 2022.
Images created and owned exclusively by Cleveland
Clinic's Center for Medical Art and Photography.
Copyright 2022 Cleveland Clinic.)

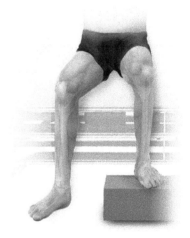

FIGURE 6.22   Anterior lower extremity – severe
wasting.

(Reproduced with permission from the Cleveland Clinic
and the American Society of Parenteral and Enteral
Nutrition from Hamilton, C. *Nutrition-Focused Physical
Exam for Adults: An Illustrated Handbook.* 2nd ed. 2022.
Images created and owned exclusively by Cleveland
Clinic's Center for Medical Art and Photography.
Copyright 2022 Cleveland Clinic.)

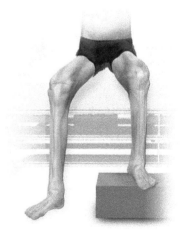

B BUCCAL FAT PAD EXAM

Again, standing directly in front of the patient, inspect the buccal fat pad region for hollowing and depressed/sunken appearance along the cheek lines. Using the index and middle fingers, palpate the buccal fat pads under the cheekbones to assess fullness and bounce. Well-nourished patients will have full, round, and filled-out cheeks and will have a good bounce on palpation. Severely malnourished patients will have hollow, sunken depression with minimal bounce on palpation, indicating fat loss. See Figures 6.2–6.4.

C BICEPS AND TRICEPS SKINFOLD EXAM

With the patient's arm at a 90-degree angle, inspect the biceps and triceps in the upper arm region. Support the arm under the patient's elbow if needed. Inspect for loose skin. Using the index finger and the thumb, gently roll down the triceps to separate the muscle from the fat. Pinch the fat between fingers to assess the amount of fat and space between skinfolds. Similarly, gently roll up around the bicep area to separate fat from muscle and assess the space between fingers. Well-nourished patients will have ample fat around the biceps and triceps areas with good space between fingers around skinfolds. In severely malnourished patients, loose skin will be apparent with very little space between fingers around skinfolds, and the examiner's fingers may almost touch, indicating subcutaneous fat loss. See Figures 6.23–6.25.

D ILIAC CREST SKINFOLD EXAM

Inspect the iliac crest (top of the hip bone) for bony prominence. To palpate the iliac crest skinfold, locate the diagonal skinfold raised immediately above the crest of the ilium along the mid-axillary line. Using the thumb and index finger, pinch and roll to determine the amount of fat at the iliac crest. Very little fat on pinch and very little space between fingers may indicate subcutaneous fat loss. Well-nourished patients will have ample fat with no bony prominence. Severely malnourished patients will have a prominent iliac crest and very little fat on the pinch.

IX EXAMINATION FOR FLUID ACCUMULATION

Edema is an accumulation of fluid in the intercellular tissue that results from an abnormal expansion of interstitial fluid volume and can be categorized as pitting or non-pitting edema. Pitting edema is palpable swelling that leaves a pit in the edematous area when pressure is applied. Pitting edema is seen in malnutrition, heart failure, renal failure, and severe lung diseases. Low serum protein levels can cause edema in malnourished patients. Proteins help retain sodium and water within the blood vessels. When blood proteins are too low, fluid can leak into the interstitial tissue spaces, leading to edema, especially in the lower legs, ankles, and feet. Although low serum proteins may trigger edema, these protein levels should not be considered as a nutritional biomarker to assess change in nutritional status. Serum hepatic protein levels of albumin, prealbumin, and transferrin decrease in response to an acute

FIGURE 6.23   Upper extremity – normal.

(Reproduced with permission from the Cleveland Clinic and
the American Society of Parenteral and Enteral Nutrition
from Hamilton, C. *Nutrition-Focused Physical Exam for
Adults: An Illustrated Handbook*. 2nd ed. 2022. Images
created and owned exclusively by Cleveland Clinic's Center
for Medical Art and Photography. Copyright 2022 Cleveland
Clinic.)

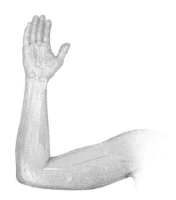

FIGURE 6.24   Upper extremity – mild/moderate
wasting.

(Reproduced with permission from the Cleveland Clinic and
the American Society of Parenteral and Enteral Nutrition
from Hamilton, C. *Nutrition-Focused Physical Exam for
Adults: An Illustrated Handbook*. 2nd ed. 2022. Images
created and owned exclusively by Cleveland Clinic's Center
for Medical Art and Photography. Copyright 2022 Cleveland
Clinic.)

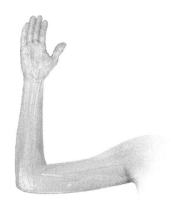

FIGURE 6.25   Upper extremity – severe wasting.

(Reproduced with permission from the Cleveland Clinic and
the American Society of Parenteral and Enteral Nutrition
from Hamilton, C. *Nutrition-Focused Physical Exam for
Adults: An Illustrated Handbook*. 2nd ed. 2022. Images
created and owned exclusively by Cleveland Clinic's Center
for Medical Art and Photography. Copyright 2022 Cleveland
Clinic.)

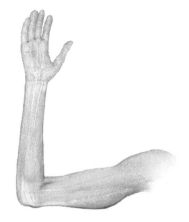

infection, injury, or trauma; however, they are not useful nutritional markers.[19] The significant drop in albumin and prealbumin levels during an acute inflammatory phase can be used by clinicians to monitor a patient's response to medical treatment, but not for nutritional treatment as the serum levels do not increase in response to the provision of protein and energy.[19]

Non-pitting edema is commonly seen in patients with lymphedema and myxedema. Edema also occurs in chronic disease states such as chronic lung diseases, heart failure and renal diseases where high blood pressure causes vascular damage in which the heart can no longer pump efficiently, resulting in peripheral edema.

Edema resulting from malnutrition should not be confused with that caused by chronic diseases. Hence, caution should be exercised when utilizing edema as a criterion for diagnosing malnutrition using the Academy/ASPEN characteristics. Clinicians should investigate the causes of peripheral edema thoroughly. In the absence of any diseases that can cause edema and in the presence of severe protein-calorie malnutrition, peripheral edema can be attributed to malnutrition.

TABLE 6.8
Measurement of Pitting Edema

Pitting edema scale		
Edema grade	Pitting depth	Rebound time
1+	Less than 2 mm, slight pitting, barely visible	Pit rebounds rapidly
2+	2 mm, somewhat deeper pit	Pit rebounds in 10–15 seconds
3+	4 mm, noticeably deep pit	Pit rebounds in 30 seconds
4+	6 mm or more, deep pit	Pit takes >30 seconds to rebound

Abbreviation: mm = millimeters.

Source: Adapted from O'Sullivan, S.B. and Schmitz T.J. (Eds.). (2007). Physical rehabilitation: assessment and treatment (5th ed.). Philadelphia: F. A. Davis Company. p. 659.

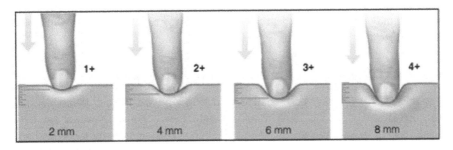

FIGURE 6.26 Pitting edema.

(From www.med-health.net/Edema-Grading.html.)

Inspect the lower extremities for pitting edema. Using the thumb, press down on the pretibial area, around the ankles and feet. If the skin is indented, assess the depth of the pit and the time it takes for the skin to bounce back to its original position. Grade the depth of the pit and the rebound time using the edema scale to determine the severity of pitting edema. See Table 6.8 and Figure 6.26.

X   HAND GRIP STRENGTH

Functional assessment and grip strength using objective hand grip measurements are discussed in detail in Chapter 5. In settings where a handgrip dynamometer or other objective grip strength measures are unavailable, clinicians can utilize a subjective grip strength measure by asking the patient to grasp the examiner's middle and index finger. This tests for strength of the four intrinsic hand muscle groups, which are the thenar, hypothenar, interossei, and the lumbrical muscles.[14] Clinicians must note that this is a highly subjective measure and is gauged solely on the clinician's judgment. Clinicians can confirm their clinical judgment by asking appropriate questions about the patient's functional state. For example, questions about the patient's ability to climb stairs, cook, shower, and walk short distances can give additional clues to the patient's functional state. However, using standardized tools to measure handgrip strength is highly recommended in order to obtain an accurate measurement and to avoid subjective interpretation by the clinician.

XI   CHALLENGES – OBESITY

Obesity may pose challenges for an examiner while performing the NFPE. Patients with excessive overlaying adipose tissues may not readily show signs of muscle loss and, in fact, may look normal on inspection.[13] Palpation on morbidly obese patients may be challenging particularly with proper positioning of the patient for the exam. In addition, it may be difficult to turn obese patients who are unable to stand or sit up, limiting the ability to examine the scapulary region and to grasp areas around intertriginous folds.

NFPE in obese adults should be adapted to accommodate the patient's body habitus. Inspection of obese patients should be similar to a normal physical examination; however, palpation may be modified depending on the patient's mobility. Although obese patients may not have a visibly sunken appearance on inspection, palpation may quickly reveal depressions in muscle areas, and muscles with a soft, flaccid texture.

XII   CHALLENGES – AGE-RELATED SARCOPENIA

Age-related changes may pose challenges during a physical exam. Sarcopenia, the age-related loss of skeletal muscles and strength, may begin at a younger age but is accelerated between the ages of 60 and 70 years.[20] Muscle atrophy associated with aging leads to reduction in functional capacity, which in turn results in physical impairment and subsequently other adverse health problems.[21] As sarcopenia progresses, it leads to rapid replacement of lost muscle mass with fatty adipose tissue especially around the abdominal area, resulting in sarcopenic obesity. Aging and sarcopenic obesity act synergistically, leading to an overall decrease in physical mobility, functional impairment, and poor quality of life.[22] In the elderly, distinguishing malnutrition from age-related sarcopenia may pose a challenge. It is important to note that malnutrition involves both muscle and subcutaneous fat loss, while sarcopenia is associated mainly with muscle loss and often an increase in adipose tissue. In addition, anorexia is common in malnourished elderly patients, while age-related sarcopenia may occur despite adequate nutritional intake.[23]

Inspection of elderly patients may show loose skin with decreased skin turgor. Palpation may show muscle rigidity with sufficient lean tissue in well-nourished elderly and areas of depression with muscle wasting in undernourished elderly patients. Use gentle palpation for elderly patients due to their frail and delicate skin; however, palpate hard enough to distinguish between skin and muscle.

Examiners should not automatically assume and equate advanced age to malnutrition and vice versa. Although loss of muscle mass is an inevitable part of aging, adequate nutrition and activity can allow healthy elderly individuals to age without losing significant amounts of muscle and fat. Clinicians should examine elderly patients thoroughly and ask pertinent questions to distinguish between malnutrition and sarcopenia. Appropriate nutrition intervention and treatment should be provided based on the findings.

XIII NFPE COMPETENCE

Initial and ongoing competency evaluation of RDNs is essential to ensure that safe and effective patient care is provided, and to satisfy the verification of skills required by healthcare accreditation and regulatory agencies. Competency is defined as "the knowledge, skills, ability and behaviors that a person possesses in order to perform skills correctly and skillfully".[24] Evaluating the RDN's initial hands-on NFPE skills should be part of a comprehensive competency assessment, and it is critical to re-assess competence at regular intervals to maintain and improve their skills. A focus-group study among NFPE experts in 2021 suggested that the NFPE competency evaluation should be conducted annually and is best administered by the RDN's direct supervisor, provided that the supervisor is also competent to perform an NFPE. If time is an issue, the NFPE experts agreed that at a minimum alternate-year evaluation should be considered.[25]

Competency assessment goes beyond checking boxes on a checklist or administering a graded test. It is an ongoing process of initial education, evaluation at regular intervals, remediation, and retraining as needed.[26] Despite the need for ongoing NFPE competency evaluation, the availability of a standardized and validated NFPE competency tools is severely limited. At this time, there has been only one recently published study investigating a tool developed based on literature review and validated with a small number of experts.[27] However, there is promising, ongoing research in the development and validation of additional NFPE competency tools.[25] In time, validated tools will be available, which will allow for accurate, ongoing evaluation and documentation of RDNs' NFPE skills.

XIV   CONCLUSION

The NFPE is part of a comprehensive approach to accurately diagnose malnutrition and identify specific nutrient deficiencies. The invaluable information obtained through the NFPE, patient interview, and keen observation of patient behavior and emotions cannot be replaced by laboratory tests or documented information in the electronic health record. The hands-on NFPE also allows the RDN to establish rapport with the patient, which otherwise may not be achievable with a more traditional brief patient encounter. RDNs can utilize this vital tool in all types of settings such as inpatient acute care, critical access, outpatient clinics, long-term care, and home care to appropriately diagnose macronutrient and micronutrient deficiencies, implement individualized nutrition treatment, and promote positive clinical outcomes for their patients.

REFERENCES

1. Litchford M. Putting the nutrition focused physical assessment into practice in long-term care settings. *Ann Longterm Care*. 2013;21(11):38–41.
2. Norman K, Pichard C, Lochs H, Pirlich M. Prognostic impact of disease-related malnutrition. *Clin Nutr*. 2008;27(1):5–15.
3. Tobert CM, Mott SL, Nepple KG. Malnutrition diagnosis during adult inpatient hospitalizations: analysis of a multi-institutional collaborative database of academic medical centers. *J Acad Nutr Diet*. 2018;118(1):125–131.
4. Jensen GL, Compher C, Sullivan DH, Mullin GE. Recognizing malnutrition in adults: definitions and characteristics, screening, assessment, and team approach. *JPEN J Parenter Enteral Nutr*. 2013;37(6):802–807.
5. Odelli C, Burgess D, Bateman L, et al. Nutrition support improves patient outcomes, treatment tolerance and admission characteristics in oesophageal cancer. *Clin Oncol (R Coll Radiol)*. 2005;17(8):639–645.
6. Persson M, Hytter-Landahl A, Brismar K, Cederholm T. Nutritional supplementation and dietary advice in geriatric patients at risk of malnutrition. *Clin Nutr*. 2007;26(2):216–224.
7. Babineau J, Villalon L, Laporte M, Payette H. Outcomes of screening and nutritional intervention among older adults in healthcare facilities. *Can J Diet Pract Res*. 2008;69(2):89–94.
8. Norman K, Kirchner H, Freudenreich M, Ockenga J, Lochs H, Pirlich M. Three month intervention with protein and energy rich supplements improve muscle function and quality of life in malnourished patients with non-neoplastic gastrointestinal disease – a randomized controlled trial. *Clin Nutr*. 2008;27(1):48–56.
9. White JV, Guenter P, Jensen G, Malone A, Schofield M. Consensus statement: Academy of Nutrition and Dietetics and American Society for Parenteral and Enteral Nutrition: characteristics recommended for the identification and documentation of adult malnutrition (undernutrition). *JPEN J Parenter Enteral Nutr*. 2012;36(3):275–83.
10. White JV, Guenter P, Jensen G, Malone A, Schofield M. Consensus statement of the Academy of Nutrition and Dietetics/American Society for Parenteral and Enteral Nutrition: characteristics recommended for the identification and documentation of adult malnutrition (undernutrition). *J Acad Nutr Diet*. 2012;112(5):730–738.

11. Esper DH. Utilization of nutrition-focused physical assessment in identifying micro-nutrient deficiencies. *Nutr Clin Pract*. 2015;30(2):194–202.

12. Litchford MD. *Nutrition Focused Physical Assessment: Making Clinical Connections*. Case Software & Books; 2015.

13. Fischer M, JeVenn A, Hipskind P. Evaluation of muscle and fat loss as diagnostic criteria for malnutrition. *Nutr Clin Pract*. 2015;30(2):239–448.

14. Bickley LS, Szilagyi PG, Hoffman RM. *Bates' Guide to Physical Examination and History Taking*. Wolters Kluwer; 2017.

15. Secker DJ, Jeejeebhoy KN. How to perform Subjective Global Nutritional assessment in children. *J Acad Nutr Diet*. 2012;112(3):424–431.e6.

16. Xiao J. *Muscle Atrophy*. Springer Singapore; 2018.

17. Powers SK, Lynch GS, Murphy KT, Reid MB, Zijdewind I. Disease-induced skeletal muscle atrophy and fatigue. *Med Sci Sports Exerc*. 2016;48(11):2307–2319.

18. Hermans G, Van den Berghe G. Clinical review: intensive care unit acquired weakness. *Crit Care*. 2015;19(1):274.

19. Fuhrman MP, Charney P, Mueller CM. Hepatic proteins and nutrition assessment. *J Am Diet Assoc*. 2004;104(8):1258–1264.

20. Morgan PT, Smeuninx B, Breen L. Exploring the impact of obesity on skeletal muscle function in older age. *Front Nutr*. 2020;7:569904. Published December 1, 2020.

21. Dhillon RJS, Hasni S. Pathogenesis and management of sarcopenia. *Clin Geriatr Med*. 2017;33(1):17–26.

22. Delmonico MJ, Harris TB, Lee JS, et al. Alternative definitions of sarcopenia, lower extremity performance, and functional impairment with aging in older men and women. *J Am Geriatr Soc*. 2007;55(5):769–774.

23. Sieber CC. Malnutrition and sarcopenia. *Aging Clin Exp Res*. 2019;31(6):793–798.

24. O'Shea K. *Staff Development Nursing Secrets*. Hanley & Belfus; 2002.

25. Zechariah S, Lehman L, Waller JL, De Leo G, Stallings J, Gess AJ. Item generation in the development of an Interactive Nutrition Specific Physical Exam Competency Tool (INSPECT): a qualitative study utilizing technology-based focus groups in the United States. *Healthcare*. 2021;9(5):576.

26. Whelan L. Competency assessment of nursing staff. *Orthop Nurs*. 2006;25(3):198–202.

27. MacQuillan EL, Ford J, Baird K. Clinical competence assessed using simulation: development of a standardized tool to assess nutrition-focused physical exam skill competence for Registered Dietitian Nutritionists. *J Nutr Educ Behav*. 2021;53(2):174–182.

7 Assessment – Nutrition-Focused Physical Exam to Detect Micronutrient Deficiencies

Angela Prinzo

CONTENTS

I INTRODUCTION

Performing a nutrition-focused physical exam (NFPE) to identify indicators of nutrition status supports best practice in patient care. In addition to providing evidence of energy and/or protein deficiency resulting in muscle and fat wasting (see Chapter 6), the NFPE can reveal critical clues to identify micronutrient deficiencies, which provides insight into nutrient intake, digestion, absorption, and metabolism.[1]

Micronutrient deficiencies, especially B vitamins, are often found in groups, rather than in isolation.[2] The oral cavity, specifically the mouth and tongue, can reflect signs of various vitamin B deficiencies. Multiple deficiencies are common in some disease states, such as malabsorptive conditions like inflammatory bowel disease (IBD), short bowel syndrome, celiac disease, and post bariatric surgery. Other conditions in which multiple deficiencies are common include alcoholism and end-stage renal disease.[2,3]

The NFPE process uses a "head to toe" approach, which starts with the hair and completes with the toes, and is a key component in diagnosing micronutrient deficiency. In addition to using visual cues to identify signs of malnutrition and micronutrient deficiencies, inspection and palpation are common exam techniques used to assess skin, nails, hair, eyes, and the oral cavity.

DOI: 10.1201/9781003177586-7

Prior to conducting the NFPE, the registered dietitian nutritionist (RDN) or other trained clinician should gather the appropriate tools, ask the patient permission to conduct the exam, explain the rationale, and provide a brief overview of the process. The clinician may need to ask open-ended questions during the physical assessment to gather additional information about potential micronutrient deficiencies. For example, if a patient's nails are covered with lacquer, the clinician should ask the patient about any recent changes (i.e. color, texture, frailty) to their nails or nail beds. Other information to gather includes the patient's diet history, details of which can suggest potential micronutrient deficiencies and guide the clinician to focus on specific areas while conducting the NFPE. For example, diets low in vitamin A may drive the clinician to carefully assess the eyes.

There are limitations to using NFPE findings to identify micronutrient deficiencies, as signs and symptoms may be non-specific.[1] For example, hair loss may be a result of inadequate protein intake, or a factor not related to a nutrient deficiency, such as a medical condition (e.g. alopecia areata), excessive chemical alterations, or aging. The clinician should use critical thinking skills to correlate physical findings with the patient's nutrition and social history, medical comorbidities, medications, and biochemical data.

Biochemical values can be used to assess for micronutrient deficiencies; however, they should be interpreted with caution as many factors influence serum levels, including inflammation, disease state, and medications. Additionally, serum levels may only reflect recent intake instead of actual nutrient stores. Laboratory tests can reveal trends that reflect the patient's micronutrient status, but are only one part of the assessment that must also include a diet history and NFPE.[1,2]

This chapter will review the use of the NFPE in assessing the skin, hair, orofacial region, and nails to detect nutrient deficiencies. Table 7.1 depicts potential nutrient deficiencies and non-nutrient causes of NFPE findings. Risk factors, diagnosis and treatment of micronutrient deficiencies are covered in detail in Chapters 9 and 10.

II HAIR

Hair follicles have a rapid cell turnover, much like that of nails.[4] Healthy hair is shiny and smooth. The clinician should palpate the scalp and gently pull hair to determine if it is resilient and not easily plucked. Poor hair quality observed during the NFPE can be associated with a variety of micronutrient deficiencies. It is important that the clinician asks detailed assessment questions to determine if visible changes are diet-driven vs. chemically altered (e.g. color treated).

Alopecia is a condition described as hair thinning or loss in which it often falls out in patches on the scalp, eyebrows, or extremities. Hair loss may be permanent or it may grow back slowly, depending on the cause. Potential nutrient deficiencies related to hair loss include protein, zinc, essential fatty acids (EFAs) and biotin. Possible non-nutrient causes are male-pattern baldness, hypopituitarism, hypothyroidism, cancer treatment, chemical alterations, infection, psoriasis, Cushing's disease and medications such as lithium, propranolol, heparin and valproic acid.[4-6]

TABLE 7.1
Physical Examination Micronutrient Chart[2-4]

Exam location	Physical signs	Possible nutrient deficiency	Possible non-nutrient causes
Hair	Alopecia	Protein, zinc, biotin, EFA	Male pattern baldness, hypopituitarism, hypothyroidism, cancer treatment, chemical alteration, infection, psoriasis, Cushing disease, medications
	Dull, thin, sparse, lackluster	Protein, zinc, iron, EFA	Aging, chemotherapy, chemical alteration
	Easily pluckable	Protein	Chemical alteration
	Lightened color	Copper, selenium, protein	Chemical alteration
	Flag sign (children)	Protein	Chemical alteration
Eyes	Pale conjunctivae	Iron, folate, vitamin B_{12}	Low cardiac output
	Bitot's spots	Vitamin A	Pinguecula, Gaucher disease, pterygium
	Angular palpebritis	Vitamins B_2, B_3, and B_6; iron	
	Conjunctival xerosis	Vitamin A	Chemical or environmental irritation
	Corneal xerosis	Vitamin A	
	Keratomalacia	Vitamin A	Hyperthyroidism
Oral cavity	Cheilosis	Vitamins B_2, B_3 and B_6; iron	Dehydration, herpes
	Angular stomatitis	Vitamins B_2, B_3, and B_6; iron	Irritation from ill-fitting dentures; chapping from harsh environments, herpes or other infectious disease
	Bleeding, spongy	Vitamin C	Gingivitis, amyloidosis, acute myeloid leukemia, drugs, periodontal disease
	Pale color	Iron	Low flow state
	Lesions	Zinc	Trauma, infections, graft vs host disease, cancer treatment, canker sores
	Glossitis	Vitamins B_2, B_3, B_6 and B_{12}; folate, iron	Crohn's disease, uremia, infection, malignancy, chemotherapy, trauma
	Atrophic filiform papillae	Vitamins B_2, B_3 and B_{12}; folate, iron	

(Continued)

TABLE 7.1 (Continued)
Physical Examination Micronutrient Chart[2-4]

Exam location	Physical signs	Possible nutrient deficiency	Possible non-nutrient causes
Skin	Petechiae	Vitamins C and K	Blood disorders, liver disease, anticoagulation overdose
	Purpura	Vitamins C and K	Injury, anticoagulation therapy, thrombocytopenia
	Dermatitis	Zinc, EFAs	Allergic or medication reactions, rashes, cellulitis, psoriasis
	Seborrheic dermatitis	Vitamins A, B_2 and B_6; zinc, EFAs, biotin	Nasal drainage
	Pellagrous dermatitis	Vitamin B_3, tryptophan	Burn, Addison's disease, psoriasis
	Nasolabial seborrhea	Vitamins B_2, B_3 and B_6; zinc	Tuberous sclerosis
	Pallor	Iron, folate, vitamin B_{12}	Blood loss, low perfusion states, sickle cell anemia, albinism, vitiligo
	Xerosis	EFAs, vitamin A	Dehydration, environmental factors, aging
	Poor/delayed wound healing	Vitamins C, A, D, E and K; iron, selenium, copper, zinc, protein	Peripheral vascular disease, diabetes mellitus, cellulitis
	Poor turgor		Dehydration
	Corkscrew hair	Vitamin C, copper	Chemical alteration
Nails	Koilonychia	Iron, with or without anemia	Hemochromatosis, diabetes, hereditary factors, Raynaud's disease, trauma
	Beau's transverse line	Protein	Chemotherapy, trauma, poor blood circulation
	Poor blanching, pale, mottled	Vitamins A and C	
	Flaky, dry, brittle, cracked	Vitamin C	Trauma
	Clubbing		Respiratory disorders, cardiovascular disease, cirrhosis
	Splinter hemorrhages	Vitamin C, hemochromatosis (elevated iron stores)	Septicemia, trauma, hemodialysis

Abbreviation: EFA = essential fatty acid.

The appearance of dull, thin, sparse, or lackluster hair may be a result of protein, zinc, iron or EFA deficiency. Possible non-nutrient causes include aging, chemotherapy and chemical alteration.[2,4] Easily pluckable hair is described as removal of hair strands with gentle pulling, and is most commonly associated with protein deficiency.

Lightened color is most commonly a result of chemical alterations; however, it can also be caused by nutrient deficiencies, which include copper, selenium and protein.[4] An in-depth patient interview is critical to determine underlying causes of hair color changes. Periods of inadequate protein intake in children, although rare, may result in alternating depigmented bands of hair, known as flag signs.[4]

III EYES

Examination of the eyes with the use of a penlight includes inspection for color variations and abnormalities in appearance. The clinician should have the patient look left then right, shining the light from the side of each eye. Some examples of eye abnormalities are reviewed below.

The sclera, a protective layer that surrounds the cornea, should be white and the conjunctiva, the membrane that lines the eyelid and covers the surface of the eye, should appear pink. Pallor or paleness of the sclera or conjunctiva can indicate potential iron, folate, or vitamin B_{12} deficiency (see Figure 7.1).[2,5,6] A potential non-nutrient cause of pale conjunctiva may be low cardiac output as seen in congestive heart failure and respiratory failure.[4]

Bitot's spots, which may be caused by vitamin A deficiency, appear as a white or gray spongy spot on the white of the eye (see Figure 7.2).[2,4,5] Possible non-nutrient causes include pinguecula (a benign growth that develops on the eye, commonly found in the elderly), Gaucher disease (rare, inherited metabolic disorder) and pterygium ("Surfer's eye") which is a raised fleshy growth filled with blood vessels that originates in the conjunctiva and spreads over the cornea.[4]

Angular palpebritis, which can be caused by deficiencies in niacin, riboflavin, iron and vitamin B_6, is characterized by redness and inflammation of the corners of the eyelids. Symptoms include burning, itching, swollen and crusty eyelids.[7]

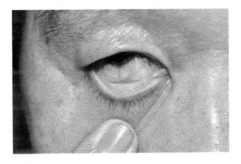

FIGURE 7.1   Pale conjunctiva.

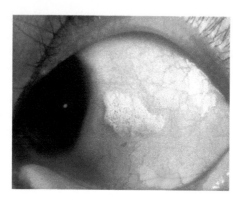

FIGURE 7.2   Bitot's spots.

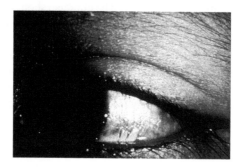

FIGURE 7.3   Corneal xerosis.

Vitamin A deficiency may also cause several other eye disorders that are identifiable by conducting an NFPE, including conjunctival xerosis, corneal xerosis
(Figure 7.3) and keratomalacia.[2,4] Conjunctival xerosis is characterized by severe
dryness to the eyes, specifically the conjunctiva, and occurs bilaterally. It can then
progress to dryness of the cornea, known as corneal xerosis, which appears as a dull,
opaque milky cornea. Keratomalacia, or "hazy cornea", characterized by drying and
clouding of the cornea, is progressive and results from untreated xerosis. A potential
non-nutrient cause of keratomalacia is hyperthyroidism.[4]

IV   ORAL CAVITY

Exam locations include the lips, gums, oral mucosa and tongue. The clinician should
inspect the lips for cracks, lesions, color, or texture changes, and with a penlight and
tongue depressor inspect the mouth for swelling, lesions, color and/or texture alterations. The clinician should instruct the patient to open the mouth and stick out their
tongue. It is important to be aware of other non-nutritional factors that promote alterations and or limitations of the oral exam. For example, poor oral health or inadequate
oral hygiene is a common cause of cracked lips and bleeding gums.

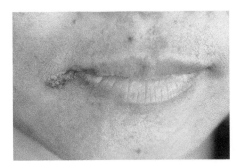

FIGURE 7.4   Cheilosis / angular stomatitis.

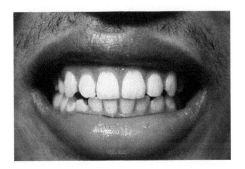

FIGURE 7.5   Spongy, bloody, receding gums.

A   LIPS

Common physical signs of micronutrient deficiencies exhibited on the lips include cheilosis, or angular stomatitis (Figure 7.4). Cheilosis is an inflammation of one or both corners of the mouth, and appears as fissures and sores on the lips, which may split and bleed. Potential micronutrient deficiencies associated with this condition include vitamins B_2, B_3 and B_6, as well as iron. Potential non-nutrient causes include dehydration, chapping from harsh climates, and herpes and/or other infectious diseases.[4,8]

B   GUMS

Healthy gums appear firm and pink. Changes in color, texture, appearance or presence of lesions can be indicators of potential nutrient deficiencies or disease. Pale gums can be caused by an iron deficiency or low flow state, characterized by reduced cardiac stroke volume.[4]

Vitamin C deficiency is a potential cause of spongy, bloody and receding gums (Figure 7.5). Possible non-nutrient causes include gingivitis, amyloidosis, acute myeloid leukemia, drugs (blood thinners, blood pressure medications and antidepressants) and periodontal disease.[4,8,9]

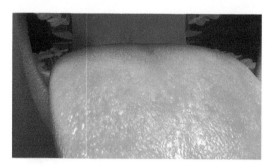

FIGURE 7.6   Glossitis.

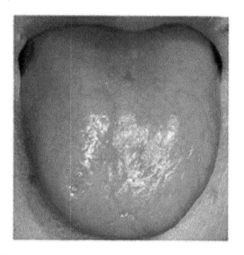

FIGURE 7.7   Atrophic glossitis.

The presence of gum lesions can indicate a possible zinc deficiency but most commonly they appear from trauma (e.g. rubbing from a sharp edge or object), infections, graft versus host disease, cancer treatment and aphthous ulcers (i.e. canker sores).[4,5,8] Lesions may form individually or multiple lesions may be present.

C Tongue

The tongue should appear moist and pink in color. Glossitis is an inflammation of the tongue which causes it to swell and become magenta in color (see Figure 7.6). Deficiencies in several micronutrients may lead to glossitis, including vitamins B_2, B_3, B_6, B_{12}, folate and/or iron.[4,8] Several non-nutrient causes include Crohn's disease, uremia, infection, malignancy, chemotherapy, or trauma.[5,6] In atrophic glossitis, caused by atrophied filiform papillae, the tongue has a glossy, smooth appearance with partial to complete absence of papillae (see Figure 7.7). Potential micronutrient deficiencies include vitamins B_{12}, B_2, B_3 and folate, as well as iron.[7]

V   SKIN

The skin is the largest organ of the body and is composed of three layers: the epidermis, dermis, and hypodermis. The main functions of the skin include temperature regulation (i.e. sweating and insulation), sensory perception, vitamin D synthesis, and providing a protective barrier from environmental factors. The skin should be smooth and uniform in color and appearance and feel cool to slightly warm. It can vary in thickness and color, which may be influenced by a variety of factors including ethnicity, gender, age, and skin type.[4,9]

Examination of the skin includes inspection for lesions, alterations in pigmentation, wounds, and palpation to evaluate temperature, turgor and texture. Challenges in assessing the skin include the presence of rashes, such as those caused by allergies or medications, as well as differences in pigmentation, which can mask signs of micronutrient deficiencies.

Some examples of skin abnormalities are reviewed below. These conditions may present in different locations; therefore, it is important to survey all areas of the skin while performing an NFPE.

Petechiae are small, hemorrhagic spots commonly found on the arms, legs and torso (see Figure 7.8). Potential micronutrient deficiencies include vitamin C and vitamin K. Possible non-nutrient causes include blood disorders, liver disease and anticoagulation overdose.[4]

Purpura, also called blood spots, are purple-colored spots and patches that are most recognizable on the skin but can also appear in mucous membranes, including the lining of the mouth. Potential micronutrient deficiencies include vitamin C and vitamin K. Purpura may also be caused by vitamin E toxicity, which has an anticoagulant effect on the blood. Possible non-nutrient causes include anticoagulation therapy, injury or thrombocytopenia.[7]

Dermatitis appears as swollen, reddened skin that may blister or ooze. Potential micronutrient deficiencies include EFAs or zinc. Possible non-nutrient causes include allergic or medication reactions, rashes, cellulitis and psoriasis.[4,9–11]

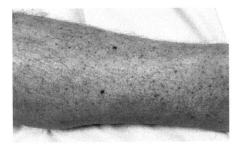

FIGURE 7.8   Petechiae.

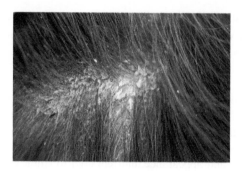

FIGURE 7.9   Seborrheic dermatitis.

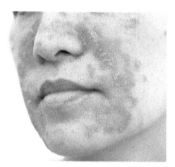

FIGURE 7.10   Nasolabial seborrhea.

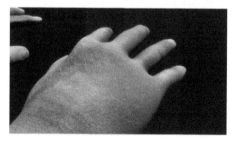

FIGURE 7.11   Pellagrous dermatitis.

Seborrheic dermatitis is a skin condition which causes scaly, crusty, red patches of skin which are mainly found on the scalp (see Figure 7.9). Potential micronutrient deficiencies include biotin, vitamin B_6, riboflavin, EFA and vitamin A.[7] Nasolabial seborrhea is characterized by redness and scaling around the nostrils (see Figure 7.10). Potential micronutrient deficiencies include vitamins B_2, B_3 and B_6. A possible non-nutrient cause is tuberous sclerosis, a genetic condition.[4]

Pellagrous dermatitis presents as hyperpigmentation of areas of the skin following exposure to sunlight or trauma (see Figure 7.11). A specific presentation of pellagrous

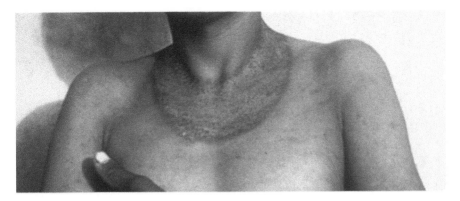

FIGURE 7.12   Casal's necklace.

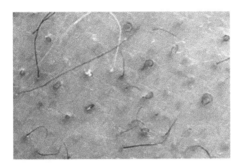

FIGURE 7.13   Corkscrew hairs.

dermatitis is Casal's necklace, a broad band or collar of hyperpigmentation around the neck (see Figure 7.12). Potential micronutrient deficiencies include vitamin B_3 or tryptophan. Possible non-nutrient causes include burns, Addison's disease or psoriasis.[4,10]

Pallor, or abnormally pale skin color, is commonly associated with anemia and may indicate an iron, folate or vitamin B_{12} deficiency.[4,10] Possible non-nutrient causes include a low perfusion state, shock, stress, sickle cell anemia, cancer, and genetic conditions which affect pigmentation, such as albinism and vitiligo.[4] An in-depth patient interview is recommended to differentiate between pallor and naturally pale skin. Pallor may be more challenging to identify in darker-skinned individuals; the appearance of the conjunctiva of the eye (see Figure 7.1), nail beds, and the oral mucosa can provide additional evidence of deficiency.

Corkscrew or coiled hairs (see Figure 7.13) are commonly found on the arms, legs, and torso and result from an excessive development of keratin in the hair follicles, known as follicular hyperkeratosis (see Figure 7.14), most notably a result of vitamin A deficiency. Corkscrew hairs may also be caused by copper deficiency, as well as chemical alteration. When conducting an NFPE, a common cutaneous sign of scurvy as a result of vitamin C deficiency is pinpoint bleeding around the hair follicle. At-risk

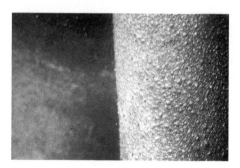

FIGURE 7.14   Follicular hyperkeratosis.

FIGURE 7.15   Xerosis.

individuals are those who have an overall poor diet lacking fruits and vegetables, and those over 65 years of age.[12]

Xerosis, characterized by dry, scaly, flaky skin, may be caused by EFA or vitamin A deficiency (see Figure 7.15). Possible non-nutrient causes include environmental factors, dehydration as well as aging.[4]

Skin integrity can be compromised by poor or delayed wound healing, which may be exacerbated by deficiencies of zinc, vitamins C, A, D, E and K, iron, selenium and/or copper.[3,4,10] In addition to contributing to delayed wound healing, poor nutritional status can increase the risk of developing pressure injuries, which result from prolonged pressure on the skin that covers bony areas of the body such as the heels, tailbone, ankles and hips.[13] In addition to poor intake and malnutrition, other risk factors for pressure injuries include medical conditions affecting blood flow such as peripheral vascular disease and diabetes, as well as immobility.

Skin turgor refers to the elasticity of the skin. To assess turgor, pinch the skin on the arm or hand to form a tent; it should spring back within one to two seconds. Poor skin turgor may be a sign of dehydration; however, skin loses elasticity with age, thus poor turgor in adults over 65 years of age may occur in the absence of dehydration. Therefore, a thorough diet history and in-depth assessment of hydration status should be conducted to correctly identify the underlying etiology.

VI NAILS

Nails are composed of a fibrous protein called keratin. The nail bed should be free of splints, feel smooth, and appear uniformly thick and symmetrical.[2] Healthy nails are translucent with a pink hue, and are flat or slightly convex. Changes to nails can be related to nutritional deficiencies or may suggest underlying systemic disease.[14]

Nails exhibiting koilonychia have a spoon-shaped appearance, which may be caused by iron deficiency with or without anemia (see Figure 7.16). Possible non-nutrient causes include hemochromatosis, diabetes mellitus, hereditary factors, Raynaud's disease and trauma.[2,4]

Beau's transverse lines appear as horizontal grooves along the nail bed and can be caused by inadequate protein intake or zinc deficiency (see Figure 7.17). Possible non-nutrient causes may include trauma, chemotherapy and/or poor blood circulation.[4]

Nails that present as flaky, dry, brittle and with cracked nail beds may be caused by vitamin C deficiency, while possible non-nutrient causes include trauma. Splinter hemorrhages appear as reddish-brown lines under the nail beds and can indicate scurvy or hemochromatosis (see Figure 7.18).[4,14]

Nails that have poor blanching are pale in color and mottled. Blanching is assessed by applying pressure to the nail bed for three seconds or less or until it turns white and then quickly releasing pressure. The blanched nail should return to its normal pink hue a few seconds after the discontinuation of pressure. Delayed return suggests impaired blood flow from poor circulation, a potential non-nutrient cause. Potential micronutrient deficiency includes vitamins A and C, as well as iron.[4,10]

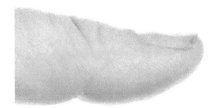

FIGURE 7.16   Koilonychia.

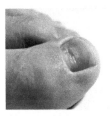

FIGURE 7.17   Beau's transverse lines.

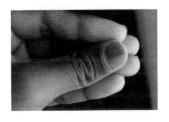

FIGURE 7.18   Splinter hemorrhages.

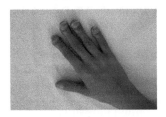

FIGURE 7.19   Nail clubbing.

Nail clubbing is a change in the structure of the fingernails or toenails (see Figure 7.19). Clubbing occurs when the tips of the fingers enlarge and the nails curve around the fingertips, which appear red and sponge-like.[9] There are no nutrient deficiencies associated with clubbing as it is often linked to medical conditions such as inflammatory bowel disease, pulmonary malignancy, chronic obstructive pulmonary disease, chronic bronchitis, cirrhosis, congenital heart disease, and endocarditis.[4,14]

VII CONCLUSION

Diagnosis of micronutrient deficiencies is a complex process requiring assessment of physical findings, nutritional intake and biochemical data. An initial NFPE establishes a baseline and allows the clinician to investigate for the presence of physical signs of micronutrient deficiencies, and combine these findings with the patient's history to complete a comprehensive evaluation. When findings are suggestive of micronutrient deficiencies the results should be reviewed with the medical team to determine etiology and establish effective intervention strategies. Treatment of micronutrient deficiencies is reviewed in Chapters 8 and 9.

REFERENCES

1. DeChicco R, Coughlin KL, Escuro A, Jezerski D, Dowak D, eds. *Nutrition Support Handbook.* 4th ed. Cleveland Clinic Foundation; 2020.
2. Esper DH. Utilization of nutrition-focused physical assessment in identifying micronutrient deficiencies. *Nutr Clin Pract.* 2015;30(2):194–202.
3. DiBaise M, Tarleton SM. Hair, nails and skin: differentiating cutaneous manifestations of micronutrient deficiencies. *Nutr Clin Pract.* 2019;34(4):490–503.
4. Hamilton C. *Nutrition-Focused Physical Exam: an Illustrated Handbook.* American Society for Parenteral and Enteral Nutrition; 2016.
5. Almohanna HM, Ahmed AA, Tsatalis JP, Tosti A. The role of vitamin and minerals in hair loss: a review. *Dermatol Ther.* 2018;9(1):51–70.
6. Shear N, Litt JZ. *Litt's Drug Eruption Reference Manual Including Drug Interactions.* 10th ed. CRC Press; 2004.
7. Mordarski B, Wolff J, eds. *Nutrition Focused Physical Exam Pocket Guide.* 2nd ed. Academy of Nutrition and Dietetics; 2018.
8. Radler DR, Lister T. Nutrient deficiencies associated with nutrition-focused physical findings of the oral cavity. *Nutr Clin Pract.* 2013;28(6):710–721.
9. Dabrowska AK, Spano F, Derler S, Adlhart C, Spencer ND, Rossi RM. The relationship between skin function, barrier properties, and body-dependent factors. *Skin Res Technol.* 2017;24(2):165–174.
10. McKeever L. Vitamins and Trace Elements. In: Mueller C, Lord LM, Marian M, McClave S, Miller SJ. *The ASPEN Adult Nutrition Support Core Curriculum.* 3rd ed. American Society for Parenteral and Enteral Nutrition; 2017.
11. Glutsch V, Hamm H, Goebeler M. Zinc and skin: an update. *J Dtsch Dermatol Ges.* 2019; 17(6):589–96.
12. Vogt KA, Lehman, JS. Corkscrew hairs. *Clevel Clin J Med.* 2015;82(4):216.

13. Pressure Injuries (Bedsores). Cleveland Clinic. Updated November 7, 2018. Accessed August 27, 2021. https://my.clevelandclinic.org/health/diseases/17823-pressure-injuries-bedsores.
14. Cashman MW, Sloan SB. Nutrition and nail disease. *Clin Dermatol.* 2010;28(4):420–425.

8 Assessment – Macronutrient Needs and Oral Intake

Laura D. Howenstine

CONTENTS

I BACKGROUND

The human body requires adequate energy, protein, and fluid to efficiently function and sustain life. Each individual's needs differ depending on metabolic rate, which in turn is influenced by a number of factors including age, sex, body composition, and the presence of acute illness/injury or chronic disease.[1] Regardless of the setting, the role of the nutrition professional is to assess each individual as a whole, identify factors that have an effect on metabolic rate, and determine appropriate macronutrient needs in order to develop an effective treatment plan.

An essential role of the nutrition professional is the proper identification, diagnosis, and treatment of malnutrition. Malnutrition is more often identified in the acute care setting; however, poor nutrition status is prevalent in a variety of patient populations.[2,3] Malnutrition can be precipitated by inadequate intake, increased nutrient needs, or impaired nutrient absorption and metabolism. Many etiologic factors can contribute to these challenges, including disease state, socioeconomic status, age, and environmental influences.[1] Clinicians should be well-versed in assessment and diagnosis of malnutrition, including identification of etiologic factors, in order to improve the nutrition status of their clients and patients. Malnutrition diagnosis and etiology are

DOI: 10.1201/9781003177586-8

covered in Chapters 2 and 3. This chapter briefly reviews macronutrient metabolism, then focuses on evaluation of macronutrient requirements and intake to help guide nutrition professionals in the assessment and treatment of populations that are malnourished or at risk of malnutrition.

II MACRONUTRIENT METABOLISM

In a healthy individual, macronutrients are broken down to their end products by action of gastrointestinal secretions containing enzymes. Carbohydrates are digested to monosaccharides and metabolized through glycolysis and the tricarboxylic acid (TCA) cycle to be utilized as energy. The body stores carbohydrate in the form of glycogen, mainly found in the liver and skeletal muscle. Liver glycogen can be catabolized to be used as glucose for the entire body whereas skeletal muscle glycogen specifically fuels the muscle cells. Metabolic pathways are regulated in a variety of ways, by directing insulin and glucagon produced by beta and alpha pancreatic cells, respectively. Dietary fat is digested into fatty acids, absorbed in micelles by way of bile salts, and stored as adipose tissue. Protein is digested into free amino acids and peptides by action of gastric acid and pancreatic enzyme hydrolysis. Among several other functions, amino acids are utilized to build and repair muscle, as well as restore damaged skin.[1]

Conversely, metabolism in a malnourished individual, or one at risk of malnutrition, may differ considerably from healthy individuals. Malnutrition can occur in states of chronic disease, starvation or acute inflammation, and macronutrient metabolism differs between these conditions. Although several diagnostic guidelines for malnutrition have been published, the most recent and widely accepted guidelines, from the American Society of Parenteral and Enteral Nutrition (ASPEN) / Academy of Nutrition and Dietetics (Academy) and the Global Leadership Initiative on Malnutrition, are etiology-based.[4,5] Etiology of malnutrition is generally categorized based on the degree and duration of inflammation. The exception is starvation-related malnutrition, in which inflammation does not play a role. Chronic disease-related malnutrition refers to a prolonged state of inflammation of mild to moderate degree that is caused by a chronic disease such as organ dysfunction or failure.[4] Chronic conditions are defined as those existing for three months or longer. Acute illness-related malnutrition is defined as a severe and more rapid-onset inflammation due to trauma or injury, such as that caused by burns or a head injury.[4] The body prioritizes macronutrient metabolism and preservation of lean body mass (LBM), depending on the level of inflammation and severity of disease.[4] The following sections describe metabolism in individuals in starvation states, and those with chronic and acute disease.

A Chronic Disease

Malnutrition in the setting of chronic disease is characterized by the presence of prolonged inflammation as a result of disease. Different than acute inflammation, chronic disease leads to a mild to moderate state of inflammation resulting in a loss of LBM and fat mass, and a decrease in functional status.[6,7] Decreased nutrient intake, coupled with the effects of chronic inflammation on metabolism, results in more long-term consequences.[6] The goals of nutrition therapy in this case are to both attain and maintain adequate levels of body fat and LBM.[7]

B   Starvation

The early stage of starvation is a fasted state, characterized by blood glucose levels returning to baseline prior to the next time food is consumed. By the action of pancreatic cells, insulin levels decrease while glucagon levels increase, signaling the initiation of glycogenolysis within two to three hours of fasting. Even when in short supply, certain tissues, particularly red blood cells and the brain, have a highly preferential requirement for a consistent influx of glucose. In periods of starvation, protein from muscle breakdown is the primary source of glucose for these tissues, as hepatic glycogen stores can be depleted in as little as 24 hours.

Four to six hours into a fast, gluconeogenesis from non-carbohydrate sources, such as glycerol, begins. In the case of adequate adipose tissue stores, the body oxidizes fatty acids, resulting in ketone body production. Within two days of fasting, the brain has changed its energy source from glucose to ketone bodies. The rate of metabolic processes is diminished as LBM decreases, leading to a reduction in resting energy expenditure. After approximately one week, the body begins to adapt to starvation, attempting to limit muscle breakdown by minimizing gluconeogenesis.[1] Malnutrition in the setting of starvation, such as anorexia nervosa, is not associated with inflammatory conditions.[6]

C   Acute Inflammation/Injury

Periods of acute inflammation, as seen in critical illness or trauma, dramatically alter macronutrient metabolism and nutrient requirements compared to normal populations. Preventing excess loss of LBM and supporting increased metabolic demand are the crucial focuses of nutrition therapy in critical care. Although loss of LBM is inevitable in acute illness, partially due to immobility, catabolism is further exacerbated in certain cases. Lean body mass is rapidly broken down to provide amino acids for immune function, acute-phase proteins, wound healing, and gluconeogenesis.[1] Negative nitrogen balance occurs when exogenous protein is inadequately supplied, and excess breakdown of LBM occurs.[1]

The degree of protein breakdown following sepsis, critical illness, or trauma is directly associated with the severity of illness. In periods of trauma or injury protein turnover is increased, leading to both increased synthesis and catabolism.[1] Metabolism in trauma and critical illness is characterized by a catabolic response leading to hyperglycemia, insulin resistance, negative nitrogen balance, and fatty acid oxidation. Because the clearance rate of circulating lipids is significantly reduced, hypertriglyceridemia and hepatic fat accumulation may occur. Similarly, LBM is catabolized as an energy source, thus increasing protein needs.[1] For this reason, carbohydrate is the preferred energy source for the critically ill population with adequate protein to preserve LBM. However, difficulty may arise because glucose oxidation is compromised and hyperglycemia commonly occurs, which has negative consequences including increased mortality and morbidity.[1]

III   MACRONUTRIENT REQUIREMENTS

A variety of factors affect metabolic rate, including disease state, body composition, age, and sex. Accurately assessing metabolic rate enables the clinician to determine energy, protein, and fluid needs in all stages of disease. There are multiple methods to estimate needs, including indirect measurement and predictive equations, as discussed below. Research is ongoing to determine the most precise methods for different disease states and care settings.[1]

A   ENERGY

Basal metabolic rate (BMR) and resting metabolic rate (RMR) are at times used interchangeably; however, these terms refer to different values. Both are measured in a fasted state; however, BMR refers to the metabolic rate measured immediately after waking in the morning or prior to any energy expenditure, whereas RMR is more practical as it allows some light movement (dressing or walking) prior to measurement.[1] BMR and RMR values are quite similar, although RMR tends to be slightly higher.[1] Several factors affect RMR including sex, age, body size, and body composition, leading to differences between populations. For example, RMR tends to be lower in both females and the elderly.[1] Because of the difficulty in measurement, most studies regarding macronutrient metabolism include data in a resting state rather than a basal state.[1]

Direct measurement is the most reliable method of determining RMR. The gold standard for measuring energy requirements is indirect calorimetry, which measures gas exchange (carbon dioxide and oxygen) as a reflection of metabolic rate. When the necessary calorimetry equipment is not available, predictive equations can be used. Over 200 predictive equations have been published, each unique to a specific population of patients.[1]

1   Calorimetry

Metabolism can be described as the combination of substrates and oxygen being converted in the body to heat, carbon dioxide, and water.[8] Substrates include carbohydrates, fat and protein, as well as micronutrients and trace elements. The body releases energy in the form of heat, as well as carbon dioxide through the respiratory system.[8] Metabolic rate is most accurately measured in a direct or indirect fashion.

Direct calorimetry is a measure of heat production by the body during metabolism. Most of the energy utilized by the body is eventually converted into heat, which is therefore a direct reflection of the metabolic rate.[1] Direct calorimetry is typically performed in a room large enough to accommodate heat generation during moderate activity, making the procedure more costly and cumbersome. Direct calorimetry also measures urine output to account for the minor chemical energy lost. This method typically takes several days to complete and requires a more controlled environment, such as a research or academic setting.[1] Direct calorimetry provides a more accurate estimation of energy needs; however, that level of precision is not necessary or practical for clinical care.

Indirect calorimetry (IC) quantifies metabolic rate by assessing gas exchange, in the form of oxygen consumption and carbon dioxide production, by measuring inspiratory and expiratory air flow. The test results include the volume of oxygen inspired (VO_2), volume of carbon dioxide expired (VCO_2), respiratory quotient, and resting energy expenditure (REE).[8] IC devices are much smaller and more portable than direct calorimetry, making this test more economical and easily performed in a less controlled setting.[1] The measurement typically takes about 30 minutes and can be completed on both ventilated and non-ventilated patients.[1] Chemical losses in urine excretion are negligible, therefore urine is not collected for IC studies.[1]

2   Predictive Equations

Predictive equations are the most common method of estimating RMR or energy needs in the clinical setting as they are less expensive and time-consuming to use. Numerous equations have been published; however, not all have been validated for use in a clinical setting or in all patient populations. Of those that have been tested for validity, only a handful are generally accepted as accurate enough to be of use. Even validated equations have some degree of error and may over- or underestimate needs compared to IC. Different equations use a variety of factors including weight, height, severity of illness, age, sex, activity, body temperature, respiratory rate, or heart rate.[1] Refer to Table 8.1 for a summary of the equations explained in this chapter.

a   Harris-Benedict

The Harris-Benedict equation (HBE) was first published in 1919, making it one of the oldest equations used to predict RMR.[1] Since its publication, several studies have demonstrated that the HBE tends to overestimate needs and other equations appear to be more reliable.[9] For this reason, use of the HBE alone has faded in recent years, although it is used as part of the Mifflin-St. Jeor equation.[9]

TABLE 8.1
Summary of Predictive Equations to Estimate Energy Needs[1,9,10]

Equation	Validated use
Harris-Benedict	Use has faded, only utilized as part of the Mifflin-St. Jeor equation
Mifflin-St. Jeor	Non-critically ill adults, regardless of BMI
Penn State 2003b	Non-obese critically ill adults *or* obese critically ill adults < 60 years of age
Penn State 2010	Obese, critically ill adults ≥ 60 years of age
Ireton-Jones	Not recommended for critical care due to low accuracy in mechanically ventilated patients

Abbreviation: BMI = body mass index.

b Mifflin-St. Jeor

In 1990, a new equation to predict RMR was published, the Mifflin-St. Jeor (MSJ). This equation is similar to the HBE in that both utilize body weight, height, age, and sex; however, the MSJ has been studied in both obese and non-obese subjects.[1] The MSJ is validated for both men and women, including those with a body mass index (BMI) above 42 kg/m^2, or the greatest BMI of subjects studied.[1] With an 87% and 75% accuracy rate for non-obese and obese adults, respectively, the Academy recommends this equation for non-critically ill adults, regardless of BMI.[1,10]

Mifflin-St. Jeor Equation:

Men: RMR = $(10 \times W) + (6.25 \times H) - (5 \times A) + 5$

Women: RMR = $(10 \times W) + (6.25 \times H) - (5 \times A) - 161$

RMR is expressed in kcal/d; W = weight (kg); H = height (cm); A = age (years)

c Penn State

The Penn State equation, first published in 1998, has been modified and subsequently validated for use in both non-obese and obese critically ill patients.[1] The authors of some studies are critical of the equation due to questionable accuracy; however, data from these studies should be interpreted cautiously because of study design flaws and limitations, including miscalculations and a retrospective approach.[1] The Penn State equation is widely accepted for use in mechanically ventilated patients, including the morbidly obese.[1] According to the Academy's Evidence Analysis Library, the Penn State 2003b equation is most appropriate for non-obese, critically ill adults, as well as critically ill obese adults under the age of 60 years, with an accuracy of approximately 70%.[10] The 2010 equation is a modified version with 74% accuracy in obese, critically ill adults ≥ 60 years of age.[10]

Penn State Equation (2003b)

$$\text{RMR} = (\text{Mifflin-St. Jeor} \times 0.96) + (V_E \times 31) + (T_{max} \times 167) - 6212$$

RMR and Mifflin-St. Jeor are measured in kcal/d; T_{max} = maximum body temperature in the previous 24 hours (degrees Celsius); and V_E = minute ventilation (L/min)

Penn State Equation (2010)

$$\text{RMR} = (\text{Mifflin-St. Jeor} \times 0.71) + (V_E \times 64) + (T_{max} \times 85) - 3085$$

RMR and Mifflin-St. Jeor are measured in kcal/d; T_{max} = maximum body temperature in the previous 24 hours (degrees Celsius); and V_E = minute ventilation (L/min) *d Ireton-Jones*

Predictive equations that account for hypermetabolism and changes in body temperature, conditions frequently found in mechanically ventilated or trauma patients, may be more reliable in the critically ill population. The Ireton-Jones equation includes more static values such as presence or absence of trauma or burns, with the limitation that it does not account for fluid changes in the critically ill.[1] Studies demonstrate that the Ireton-Jones equation, when compared to indirect calorimetry, appears accurate; however, it is not consistent in prediction by gender. The equation tends to overestimate REE for men while underestimating REE for women.[11] This equation is described in the Academy's Nutrition Care Manual but is not typically recommended for use in critical care because of relatively low accuracy in mechanically ventilated patients.[1,10]

3 Weight-Based

In the absence of indirect calorimetry, another commonly used method to estimate energy requirements is a simple weight-based equation. Energy needs are inversely associated with BMI and recommended ranges may differ depending on disease state, age, sex, and activity level.[12] Although this method is more commonly utilized, validation studies demonstrate weight-based ratios to be less than 50% accurate in the critically ill population.[1] This low accuracy is probably due to the fact that this method fails to account for changes in RMR due to age and sex, as well as acute physiological changes aside from those identified by clinical judgment.[1]

ASPEN and Society of Critical Care Medicine (SCCM) critical care guidelines do not promote the use of a specific predictive equation for critically ill adults but do suggest that obese patients receive a hypocaloric feeding regimen, defined as < 65–70% of estimated needs as determined by an equation or IC.[13] Alternatively, needs may be calculated by weight as described below.

- BMI < 30:   25–30 kcal/kg actual body weight
- BMI 30–50: 11–14 kcal/kg actual body weight
- BMI > 50:   22–25 kcal/kg ideal body weight

Energy needs may be higher in patients with significant wounds, trauma, or burns.[12] For non-obese hospitalized adults a range of 25–30 kcal/kg actual body weight can be used, although this range may be adjusted based on age, sex, disease state, presence of malnutrition, and goals of care.[13]

Although energy needs are generally higher for patients with malnutrition, the range may vary depending on etiology. Estimated energy needs can be increased to compensate for malabsorption or hypermetabolism seen with certain conditions such as gastrointestinal disorders, cancer, or acquired immune deficiency syndrome (AIDS).[14–16] Patients with malabsorption or decreased immune function are at an increased risk of both malnutrition and micronutrient deficiencies.[14] In the critical care setting, adequate energy should be provided without overfeeding to prevent hyperglycemia, refeeding, or hypercapnia.[17] Energy provision may be increased once the patient is out of the acute illness/inflammatory stage of critical illness.[17] Refer to

Chapters 11 and 12 for the treatment of patients with malnutrition in the context of acute and chronic illness.

B PROTEIN

There are several methods of measuring protein metabolism; however, only nitrogen balance studies are used in a clinical setting. Other methods, while more precise, are complex and expensive, thus only used in research. The most common method used to estimate protein needs in the clinical setting is a weight-based equation.

1 Nitrogen Balance

A nitrogen balance study uses a 24-h urine collection to measure urea excretion, based on the assumption that urea accounts for about 80% of nitrogen lost in the urine. Because a nitrogen balance study requires urine collection, accuracy may be compromised in cases of renal dysfunction. High-output ostomies, fistulas, wound drainage, or chyle leaks may also confound results as protein may be lost in output from these sources. The nitrogen balance equation accounts for the approximate 4 g/day loss of nitrogen from stool, skin, GI secretions, and other insensible losses without the need for measurement.[1,43] This study relies on carefully monitored protein intake, as well as daily urine output, and is most accurate when utilized in a controlled setting when enteral or parenteral nutrition is the sole source of protein intake. For this reason, this study is most often utilized in a critical care setting. A negative nitrogen balance suggests protein intake is insufficient to meet needs however does not accurately estimate the actual amount of protein needed to achieve a positive nitrogen balance.[43]

- Nitrogen balance = nitrogen intake − nitrogen output
- Nitrogen balance = (protein intake g/d / 6.25) − (urinary urea nitrogen g/d + 4 g/d)

2 Weight-Based

If nitrogen balance studies are not used, protein needs may be estimated by a weight-based equation (i.e. grams per kilogram). Protein needs in non-critically ill patients may vary considerably depending on disease state, including malnutrition. When estimating needs, it is important to consider age, as protein needs are higher in healthy older vs. younger adults (1–1.2 g/kg vs. 0.8–1 g/kg, respectively).[18] Protein needs are higher in patients with malnutrition, and, as in well-nourished patients, must be adjusted based on age and disease state. The European Society for Clinical Nutrition and Metabolism (ESPEN) recommends 1.2–1.5 g/kg protein for adults who are malnourished or at risk of malnutrition to maintain strength and support muscle anabolism.[18,19]

Protein needs in critically ill patients are higher than in their non-critically ill peers to account for increased protein catabolism and decreased protein synthesis during periods of acute illness.[12] ASPEN describes protein in the critically ill as the most vital macronutrient for preservation of LBM, supporting immune function, and healing wounds.[12] Protein requirements are based on BMI with the use of either actual or ideal body weight. Exceptions to this recommendation include patients with cirrhosis, hepatic failure, or other comorbidities leading to fluid retention; in these cases an estimated dry weight should be used to calculate protein needs.[12]

- BMI < 30: 1.2–2 g/kg actual body weight
- BMI 30–40: 2 g/kg ideal body weight
- BMI > 40: 2–2.5 g/kg ideal body weight

Regardless of the method used to estimate energy and protein needs, frequent monitoring is essential. In hospitalized patients, energy needs should be reevaluated at least once weekly, more often in the critical care setting.[13] Protein remains a vital macronutrient to support immune function, wound healing, and maintaining LBM in the acute care setting.[13] Therefore, adequacy of protein provision should be monitored on a regular basis.

C DIETARY REFERENCE INTAKES

The Dietary Reference Intakes (DRI) were developed through a collaboration between several research conglomerates, including the Institute of Medicine and the Food and Nutrition Board, with the goal of determining the Recommended Daily Allowance (RDA) or adequate intake (AI) of macro- and micronutrients for healthy adults and children. The RDA is estimated to meet the needs of 97% of a healthy population, while the estimated average requirement (EAR) is set to meet the needs of roughly 50% of the population within a certain gender or age group.[20] Similarly, AI represents the recommended amount of a particular substance required by all members of the population, and is utilized when there is insufficient evidence to determine the RDA for specific nutrients.[20] The tolerable upper level refers to the highest nutrient intake level that is not known to produce adverse effects. See Table 8.2 for a summary of the macronutrient DRIs for adults.

Also outlined by the DRI is a guideline of recommended macronutrient distribution for healthy populations, which suggests consumption of 45–65% of daily caloric intake in the form of carbohydrates, 10–35% protein, and 20–35% fat (5–10% *n*–6 polyunsaturated fatty acids and at least 0.6–1.2% *n*–3 polyunsaturated fatty acids).[20] It is important to remember that the DRIs are estimations for healthy individuals, and needs may be different for those with malnutrition and other diseases or conditions.

IV MACRONUTRIENT INTAKE

After estimating macronutrient needs, the clinician must assess intake to determine if needs are being met. Intake is usually inadequate in individuals with malnutrition, especially those in healthcare settings.

TABLE 8.2
Recommended Dietary Allowance (RDA) for Macronutrients in Adults[20]

Age (years)	Total water (L/d)	Carbohydrate (g/d)	Fiber (g/d)	Protein (g/d)
Males				
19–30	3.7	*130*	38	*56*
31–50	3.7	*130*	38	*56*
50–70	3.7	*130*	30	*56*
> 70	3.7	*130*	30	*56*
Females				
19–30	2.7	*130*	25	*46*
31–50	2.7	*130*	25	*46*
50–70	2.7	*130*	21	*46*
> 70	2.7	*130*	21	*46*

Note: Italicized = RDA; Not italicized = Adequate Intake.

A   INTAKE TRENDS IN HEALTHCARE SETTINGS

Regardless of ventilator status, intensive care patients have been shown to receive as little as 0.5 g/kg protein, well below estimated needs.[21] Elevated protein needs, coupled with inadequate protein intake, are problematic as critical care patients who do not meet energy, and more importantly protein, needs have more days on the ventilator, higher infection rates, and increased mortality.[22–24]

Once patients are transferred out of the intensive care unit, adequate protein and energy intake is still paramount to decrease the risk of malnutrition and/or developing other complications such as hospital-acquired pressure injuries. Close monitoring is recommended as non-critically ill patients on oral diets reportedly consume on average 68% of protein needs, which in turn increases the risk of developing complications and longer hospital length of stay.[25] A 10% increase in protein intake has been shown to be correlated with a 10% reduction in both of the aforementioned outcomes.[25] The same study demonstrated that an average energy intake of 79% of needs was adequate to prevent malnutrition.[25]

Weight loss, poor dietary intake, and low BMI are all prevalent findings in the long-term care (LTC) setting.[26] A plethora of factors contribute to poor nutrition status, including difficulty chewing or swallowing, reduced appetite, and decreased functional status.[26] Although the normal BMI range for adults is 18.5–24.9 kg/m^2, this range increases for older adults to 23–30 kg/m^2 due to increased mortality associated with sarcopenia.[27] Roughly two-thirds of LTC residents have a BMI < 24 kg/m^2, placing this population at risk of being underweight for age.[26] Patients with dementia are at a particularly high risk of nutrition-related issues, with approximately 80% of this population showing difficulty chewing or swallowing, and almost 50% fail to meet estimated energy and protein needs.[2]

B INTAKE ASSESSMENT TOOLS

A complete nutrition assessment includes anthropometric measurements, laboratory data, clinical findings, and dietary intake patterns. Along with an assessment of macronutrient intake, a thorough nutrition assessment should also include evaluation of fluid intake, use of supplements (e.g. protein, vitamin/minerals, botanicals, etc.), pharmaceuticals (e.g. appetite stimulants, bowel medications, enzymes, etc.), and physical activity. Fluid intake assessment should include consumption of sugar-sweetened and alcoholic beverages along with more commonly consumed fluids (e.g. water, milk, etc.) to obtain the most accurate and thorough information. The diet should be evaluated for adequacy of vitamins and minerals, including intake from supplements, since their use is common in the United States. In fact, 58% of American adults over the age of 20 report consuming dietary supplements, women more commonly than men.[28] Although herbal and botanical supplements may not contribute significantly to macro- or micronutrient intake, their consumption should still be assessed as their components may interact with pharmaceuticals or cause symptoms that can affect intake. Micronutrient requirements are discussed in detail in Chapters 9 and 10.

Several assessment tools have been validated to evaluate the adequacy of intake, measured against the gold standard weighed food journal.[29] Intake must then be analyzed by a registered dietitian nutritionist (RDN) to determine nutrition adequacy as compared to estimated needs. Although the majority of these tools were originally designed to be used in a weight management setting, they are also beneficial for assessment and diagnosis of malnutrition. Each tool is most advantageous when tailored to the healthcare setting and clients' or patients' needs. Refer to Table 8.3 for a summary of each method described.

1 Weighed Food Journal

A weighed food journal is considered the gold standard of tools to gather macronutrient intake data.[29] In comparison to other methods, this assessment does not rely on memory recall, instead requiring participants to weigh and document all foods and beverages consumed throughout the day. This approach also requires measuring food waste to obtain more accurate information.[29] The primary benefit of this method is a more accurate assessment of portion sizes and actual foods consumed. After data collection, the RDN compares the information to the estimated energy and protein needs to assess intake and malnutrition risk. Due to the necessary time and equipment requirements of this method, a weighed food journal is considerably more cumbersome than other tools and may result in decreased compliance. This method is typically utilized in a controlled situation, such as a research setting.

2 Food Diary/Journal

One of the more common dietary assessment tools used in practice is the food diary or journal, which requires participants to document the timing and preparation of foods consumed. This tool has not only been validated against a weighed food journal but is also significantly more cost-effective than the latter. In the context of weight management, consistent tracking of dietary intake is correlated with significant weight

TABLE 8.3
Summary of Intake Assessment Tools[29–32,34–37,39–42]

Method utilized	Setting/population	Benefits	Limitations
Weighed food journal	Controlled setting (e.g. research)	Does not rely on memory recall Results in more accurate data collection	Time-consuming, requires weighing of all foods consumed and food waste
Food diary/journal	Outpatient	More cost-effective Results in greater weight loss or slowed weight gain	Requires accurate documentation of food and beverages consumed including timing, portion sizes, and preparation methods
24-h diet recall	Inpatient	Less time-consuming Does not require cumbersome equipment	Requires a well-trained clinician to collect data Tends to underestimate macronutrient intake
Food frequency questionnaire	Large epidemiological studies	Provides broad information for large populations Culturally customizable Shortened versions available and effective	Less detailed Tends to overestimate fruit and vegetable intake and underestimate fat, sodium, and beverage intake
Technological approaches	Outpatient; low-literacy clients	When combined with counseling, results in greater alterations to macronutrient intake than counseling alone.	Requires the use of a smartphone, tablet, Internet access, or photo/video device

loss, probably due to heightened awareness of energy density of foods and appropriate portion sizes.[30] This approach has also been shown to slow weight gain when used consistently.[30] Clients should be instructed to provide detailed records of foods and beverages consumed, including preparation methods, portion sizes, and time of consumption. This tool is useful in the outpatient setting to allow the RDN to monitor changes in intake over time.

3   24-Hour Diet Recall

The 24-hour diet recall is a validated method to assess dietary intake; however, its use does present some challenges.[13] Although this method is less time-consuming than a weighed food record or food journal, it does require clinician training in order to obtain detailed and accurate information. The clinician must ask a series of detailed questions related to the client/patient's intake over the previous 24 hours. Multiple questions for each food item must be asked to obtain accurate and comprehensive information about meal timing, portion sizes, and preparation methods.[31] The 24-h diet recall does tend to underestimate macronutrient intake, therefore collecting at least three days of data is recommended.[31,32] This method is generally utilized in the inpatient setting due to its relative low cost and absence of cumbersome equipment.

Lastly, a 24-h recall can be performed using a web-based format, thereby providing a more cost-effective and accurate tool for clients.[33]

4 Food Frequency Questionnaire

The food frequency questionnaire (FFQ) is the most commonly utilized data collection tool in large epidemiological studies.[34] This method requires patients or study participants to record frequency of intake using a specific list of food items. A FFQ is less detailed than other collection tools, using the average or estimated macronutrient content of general food groups to assess dietary habits in large studies.[34] A shortened FFQ is available and presents a more cost-effective and less time-consuming option compared to other tools.[35,36] As with some other methods, a drawback of the FFQ is overestimation of fruit and vegetable intake and underestimation of beverage, fat, and sodium intake.[34] An FFQ can easily be customized to include culturally appropriate food items and is available in several languages.[37]

5 Technological Approaches

In recent years, written assessment tools have been upgraded to more modern versions such as audio-visual journaling or electronic diet records. The Academy describes telenutrition as an interactive experience that utilizes modern technology to implement the nutrition care process.[38] This approach may include using smartphone applications, photo logs, or audio-visual food journaling, among other options.[39] Research demonstrates that use of a technological approach such as a smartphone application, in addition to traditional counseling, results in more dramatic alterations to macronutrient intake than counseling alone.[39] Utilizing photo or audio-visual food journaling is comparable to a weighed food record and may be a more appropriate method for low-literacy clients.[40] Electronic diet records are not only validated against tangible food journals but also result in greater percentage of fat loss than written versions.[41,42]

V CONCLUSION

Properly assessing macronutrient requirements and intake is a key component of a comprehensive malnutrition assessment. The job of the nutrition professional is to assess each individual as a whole, keeping in mind their socioeconomic status, age, sex, body composition, and disease state in order to estimate macronutrient requirements. Nutrition status is a fluid condition, therefore should be monitored frequently, regardless of the setting.

REFERENCES

1. Mueller CM, ed. *The ASPEN Adult Nutrition Support Core Curriculum: 3rd Edition.* American Society of Parenteral and Enteral Nutrition; 2017.
2. Drisdelle C, Kestens Y, Hamelin AM, Mercille G. Disparities in access to healthy diets: how food security and food shopping behaviors relate to fruit and vegetable intake [published correction appears in *J Acad Nutr Diet.* 2021 Mar 17]. *J Acad Nutr Diet.* 2020;120(11):1847–1858.

3. Hanson LC, Ersek M, Lin FC, Carey TS. Outcomes of feeding problems in advanced dementia in a nursing home population. *J Am Geriatr Soc.* 2013;61(10): 1692–1697.

4. Jensen GL, Mirtallo J, Compher C, et al. Adult starvation and disease-related malnutrition: A proposal for etiology-based diagnosis in the clinical practice setting from the International Consensus Guideline Committee. *JPEN J Parenter Enteral Nutr.* 2010;34(2):156–159.

5. Cederholm T, Jensen GL, Correia MITD, et al. GLIM criteria for the diagnosis of malnutrition – a consensus report from the Global Clinical Nutrition Committee. *Clin Nutr.* 2018;38(1):P1–9.

6. Jensen GL, Mirtallo J, Compher C, et al. Adult starvation and disease-related malnutrition: a proposal for etiology-based diagnosis in the clinical practice setting from the International Consensus Guideline Committee. *JPEN J Parenter Enteral Nutr.* 2010; 34(2):156–159.

7. Hamilton C, Boyce VJ. Addressing malnutrition in hospitalized adults. *JPEN J Parenter Enteral Nutr.* 2013;37(6):808–815.

8. Mtaweh H, Tuira L, Floh AA, Parshuram CS. Indirect calorimetry: history, technology, and application. *Front Pediatr.* 2018;6:257.

9. Owen OE, Holup JL, D'Alessio DA, et al. A reappraisal of the caloric requirements of men. *Am J Clin Nutr.* 1987;46(6):875–85.

10. Nutrition Care Manual Calculators. Nutrition Care Manual website. Accessed May 8, 2021. www.nutritioncaremanual.org/calculators.

11. Choban P, Dickerson R, Malone A, et al. ASPEN clinical guidelines – nutrition support of hospitalized adult patients with obesity. *JPEN J Parenter Enteral Nutr.* 2013;37(6):714–744.

12. Kross EK, Sena M, Schmidt K, Stapleton RD. A comparison of predictive equations of energy expenditure and measured energy expenditure in critically ill patients. *J Crit Care.* 2012;27(3):321.e5–321.e12.

13. McClave SA, Taylor BE, Martindale RG, et al. Guidelines for the provision and assessment of nutrition support therapy in the adult critically ill patient. *JPEN J Parenter Enteral Nutr.* 2016;40(2):159–211.

14. The Academy of Nutrition and Dietetics. Practice paper of the Academy of Nutrition and Dietetics: nutrition intervention and human immunodeficiency virus infection. *J Acad Nutr Diet.* 2018;118(3):486–498.

15. Vigano AL, Tomasso JD, Kilgour RD, et al. The abridged patient-generated subjective global assessment is a useful tool for early detection and characterization of cancer cachexia. *J Acad Nutr Diet.* 2014;114(7):1088–1098.

16. Lin A, Micic D. Nutrition considerations in inflammatory bowel disease. *Nutr Clin Prac.* 2021;36(2):298–311.

17. Preiser JC, van Zanten AR, Berger MM, et al. Metabolic and nutritional support of critically ill patients: consensus and controversies. *Crit Care.* 2015;19(1):35.

18. Deutz NE, Bauer JM, Barazzoni R, et al. Protein intake and exercise for optimal muscle function with aging: recommendations from the ESPEN Expert Group. *Clin Nutr.* 2014;33(6):929–936.

19. Bauer J, Biolo G, Cederholm T, et al. Evidence-based recommendations for optimal dietary protein intake in older people: a position paper from the PROT-AGE Study Group. *J Am Med Dir Assoc.* 2013;14(8):542–559.

20. The National Academies Press. *Dietary Reference Intakes for Energy, Carbohydrate, Fiber, Fat, Fatty Acids, Cholesterol, Protein, and Amino Acids (2005).* National Academies Press; 2005.

21. Nicolo M, Heyland DK, Chittams J, Sommarco T, Compher C. Clinical outcomes related to protein delivery in a critically ill population: a multicenter, multinational observation study. *JPEN J Parenter Enteral Nutr*. 2016;40(1):45–51.

22. Heyland DK, Cahill N, Day AG. Optimal amount of calories for critically ill patients: depends on how you slice the cake! *Crit Care Med*. 2011;39(12):2619–2626.

23. Alberda C, Gramlich L, Jones NE, et al. The relationship between nutritional intake and clinical outcomes in critically ill patients: results of an international multicenter observation study. *Intensive Care Med*. 2009;35(10):1728–1737.

24. Heyland DK, Stephens KE, Day AG, McClave SA. The success of enteral nutrition and ICU-acquired infections: a multicenter observational study. *Clin Nutr*. 2011;30(2):148–155.

25. Dijxhoorn DN, IJmker-Hemink VE, Kievit W, Wanten GJA, van den Berg MGA. Protein intake at the first day of full-oral intake during hospitalization is associated with complications and hospital length of stay. *JPEN J Parenter Enteral Nutr*. 2020;10. Online ahead of print. doi:10.1002/jpen.2026.

26. Bell CL, Tamura BK, Masaki KH, Amella EJ. Prevalence and measures of nutritional compromise among nursing home patients: weight loss, low body mass index, malnutrition, and feeding dependency, a systematic review of the literature. *J Am Med Dir Assoc*. 2013;14(2):94–100.

27. Winter JE, MacInnis RJ, Wattanapenpaiboon N, Nowson CA. BMI and all-cause mortality in older adults: a meta-analysis. *Am J Clin Nutr*. 2014;99(4):875–890.

28. Mishra S, Stierman B, Gahche JJ, Potischman N. Dietary supplement use among adults: United States, 2017–2018. NCHS Data Brief, no 399. National Center for Health Statistics; 2021.

29. Weighed Food Record (WFR). International Dietary Data Expansion Project. Published 2015. Updated 2021. Accessed May 8, 2021. https://inddex.nutrition.tufts.edu/data4diets/data-source/weighed-food-record-wfr.

30. Ingels JS, Misra R, Stewart J, Lucke-Wold B, Shawley-Brzoska S. The effect of adherence to dietary tracking on weight loss: using HLM to model weight loss over time. *J Diabetes Res*. 2017;2017:6951495.

31. Yuan C, Spiegelman D, Rimm EB, et al. Relative validity of nutrient intakes assessed by questionnaire, 24-hour recalls, and diet records as compared with urinary recovery and plasma concentration biomarkers: findings for women. *Am J Epidemiol*. 2018;187(5):1051–1063.

32. Ma Y, Olendzki BC, Pagoto SL, et al. Number of 24-hour diet recalls needed to estimate energy intake. *Ann Epidemiol*. 2009;19(8):553–559.

33. Foster E, Lee C, Imamura F, et al. Validity and reliability of an online self-report 24-h dietary recall method (Intake24): a doubly labelled water study and repeated-measures analysis [published correction appears in J Nutr Sci. 2019 Dec 19;8:e41]. *J Nutr Sci*. 2019;8:e29.

34. Steinemann N, Grize L, Ziesemer K, Kauf P, Probst- Hensch N, Brombach C. Relative validation of a food frequency questionnaire to estimate food intake in an adult population. *Food Nutr Res*. 2017;61(1):1305193.

35. Sam CHY, Skidmore P, Skeaff S, Wall C, Bradbury KE, Parackal S. Relative validity and reproducibility of a short food frequency questionnaire to assess nutrient intakes of New Zealand adults. *Nutrients*. 2020;12(3):619.

36. Yokoyama Y, Takachi R, Ishihara J, et al. Validity of short and long self-administered food frequency questionnaires in ranking dietary intake in middle-aged and elderly Japanese in the Japan public health center-based prospective study for the next generation (JPHC-NEXT) Protocol Area. *J Epidemiol*. 2016;26(8):420–432.

37. Villano DM, Mata R, Coccia C. Development of a culturally appropriate food frequency questionnaire for midlife and older Mexican Americans. *J Acad Nutr Diet.* 2013;113(9)Supplement:A80.

38. Practicing Telehealth. Academy of Nutrition and Dietetics website. Updated 2021. Accessed May 8, 2021. www.eatrightpro.org/practice/practice-resources/telehealth/practicing-telehealth.

39. Recio-Rodriguez JI, Agudo Conde C, Calvo-Aponte MJ, et al. The effectiveness of a smartphone application on modifying the intakes of macro and micronutrients in primary care: a randomized controlled trial. The EVIDENT II Study. *Nutrients.* 2018;10(10):1473.

40. Jago E, Gauthier A, Pegoraro A, Dorman S. An assessment of the validity of an audio-video method of food journaling for dietary quantity and quality. *J Nutr Metab.* 2019; Article ID 9839320:1–8.

41. Raatz SK, Scheett AJ, Johnson LK, Jahns L. Validity of electronic diet recording nutrient estimates compared to dietitian analysis of diet records: randomized controlled trial. *J Med Internet Res.* 2015;17(1):e21.

42. Chung LM, Law QP, Fong SS, Chung JW. Teledietetics improves weight reduction by modifying eating behavior: a randomized controlled trial. *Telemed J E Health.* 2014;20(1):55–62.

43. Dickerson RN. Nitrogen balance and protein requirements for critically ill older patients. *Nutrients.* 2016;8(4):226.

9 Vitamin Deficiencies – Diagnosis and Treatment

Mary Kronik and Diane Nowak

CONTENTS

I INTRODUCTION

Vitamins are essential organic substances needed in small amounts for normal growth, metabolism, and cellular integrity. Thirteen vitamins plus the dietary component choline are considered essential. Vitamins are grouped into those that are fat-soluble (vitamins A, D, E, K) and those that are water-soluble (vitamin C, B vitamins and choline) to account for differences in absorption, transport and excretion.[1]

This chapter will review vitamin needs in adults, as well as risks, diagnosis and treatment of vitamin deficiencies. Physical signs of deficiency are more comprehensively reviewed in Chapter 7.

DOI: 10.1201/9781003177586-9

TABLE 9.1

Function, Needs and Sources of Fat-Soluble Vitamins[2,4,8,9]

Nutrient	Function	RDA	Sources
Vitamin A	Vision; wound healing; skin, bone and cellular health	Men – 900 RAE Women – 700 RAE Pregnant – 770 RAE Lactating – 1300 RAE	Liver, fortified milk, eggs, and dark-green, yellow-orange vegetables
Vitamin D	Maintain serum calcium and phosphorus levels, may be important in the management of multiple medical conditions (such as infections, cancer, cardiovascular disease)	Adults < 70 years – 600 IU Adults > 70 years – 800 IU	Sunlight, fish liver oils, fatty fish, fortified milk, breakfast cereals
Vitamin E	Cell wall integrity	All adults – 15 mg	Vegetable oils, wheat germ, asparagus, peanuts
Vitamin K	Blood clotting	Men – 120 µg Women – 90 µg	Liver, green leafy vegetables, broccoli, peas, green beans

Abbreviations: RDA = Recommended Daily Allowance; RAE = retinol activity equivalents; IU = international units; mg = milligrams; µg = micrograms.

II FAT-SOLUBLE VITAMINS

Fat-soluble vitamins are stored, primarily in fatty tissue and the liver. They are effectively absorbed with dietary fat, and because they are stored in fatty tissue, daily intake is not needed. Treatment for deficiency should be given cautiously, as fat-soluble vitamins can more easily reach toxic levels when supplemented.[1] Table 9.1 reviews the function, needs and sources of fat-soluble vitamins. Table 9.2 summarizes biochemical diagnostic tests and treatment of fat-soluble vitamin deficiencies.

A Vitamin A

1 Deficiency Risk Factors

Those most at risk of vitamin A deficiency have fat malabsorption disorders, cholestatic liver disease and decompensated cirrhosis; pregnant women are also at risk due to increased needs. Zinc deficiency can depress the synthesis of retinol-binding protein, which is required to transport vitamin A (retinol) from the liver to targeted tissues. Therefore zinc deficiency can impact vitamin A status due to its role in absorption, transport, and utilization.[1]

2 Diagnosis: Biochemical and Physical Signs

Vitamin A is the name of a group of fat-soluble retinoids, including retinol, retinal, and retinyl esters. Two forms of vitamin A are available in the human diet: preformed

TABLE 9.2

Diagnostic Tests and Treatment of Fat-Soluble Vitamin Deficiencies[1,10,13,16,19,21,30]

Nutrient	Biochemical test	Treatment
Vitamin A	Serum retinol • ≤ 0.35 µmol/L (10 µg/dL): low/depleted • ≥ 1.05–3.5 µmol/L (30-100 µg/dL): adequate • ≥ 3.5 µmol/L (100 µg/dL): toxic	Oral: 60,000 IU of vitamin A palmitate for two days, followed by 4500 IU/d IM: 100,000 IU/d for three days, followed by 50,000 IU/d for two weeks
Vitamin D	Serum 25-hydroxyvitamin D • ≥ 50 nmol/L (≥ 20 ng/mL): sufficient • 30 to < 50 nmol/L (12 to < 20 ng/mL): insufficient • < 30 nmol/L (≤ 12 ng/mL): deficient	Vitamin D_3 6000 IU/d or 50,000 IU/week for eight weeks followed by maintenance dose of 1000 to 2000 IU/d
Vitamin E	Serum vitamin E • < 0.5 mg/dL: deficient • 0.5-2.0 mg/dL: normal • > 2.0 mg/dL: toxicity	Oral: 200 to 2000 mg/d
Vitamin K	Plasma phylloquinone • 0.15–1.0 µg/L: reference values in healthy adults	Oral or IM: 2.5 to 10 mg twice weekly to daily

Abbreviations: µmol/L = micromole per liter; µg/dL = microgram per deciliter; IU = International Units; nmol/L = nanomole per liter; ng/mL = nanogram per mililiter; mg/dL = milligram per deciliter; mg/d = milligram per day; µg/L = microgram per liter; IM = intramuscular.

vitamin A (retinol and its esterified form, retinyl ester) and provitamin A carotenoids. The most important provitamin A carotenoid is beta-carotene, which is the main precursor of vitamin A and has many immune and antioxidant properties. Both retinyl esters and provitamin A carotenoids are converted to retinol. Retinol is the primary form of vitamin A in the human body, thus plasma retinol levels are useful for diagnosing vitamin A deficiency. However, their value for assessing marginal vitamin A status is limited because they do not decline until vitamin A levels in the liver are almost depleted.[2]

A blood test can measure the amount of retinol and can be interpreted as follows:[1]

- ≤ 0.35 µmol/L (10 µg/dL):   *Low/Depleted*
- ≥ 1.05 µmol/L (30 µg/dL) to 3.5 µmol/L (100 µg/dL):   *Adequate*
- ≥ 3.5 µmol/L (100 µg/dL):   *Toxic*

Physical signs of vitamin A deficiency can include conjunctival xerosis, night blindness, Bitot's spot, keratomalacia (hazy cornea), and impaired wound healing.

3 Treatment

Treatment of vitamin A deficiency can be undertaken with both oral and injectable forms, generally in the form of vitamin A palmitate. Depending on the severity of the deficiency, supplementation with 2000 to 200,000 international units (IU) may be warranted.[1] Vitamin A deficiency is traditionally treated orally with 60,000 IU/d of vitamin A palmitate for two days, followed by 4500 IU/d.[3] When oral administration is not feasible, an initial dose of 100,000 IU/d intramuscular (IM) for three days, followed by a maintenance dose of 50,000 IU/d IM for two weeks, can correct a deficiency.[3] In pregnant women, supplementation should be given cautiously as vitamin A toxicity may cause birth defects.

Specialized fat-soluble vitamin supplements specifically designed to meet the needs of people with difficulty absorbing fat are available. These specialized vitamins are in a water-miscible form and are taken daily with enzymes to help improve absorption.[1]

B VITAMIN D

1 Deficiency Risk Factors

Individuals with inadequate sun exposure, extensive skin damage such as burns, fat-malabsorptive disorders, and renal disease are all at risk of vitamin D deficiency. Older adults are also at risk, partly because the skin's ability to synthesize vitamin D declines with age. People with dark skin are at risk of deficiency due to greater amounts of the pigment melanin in the epidermal layer of the skin, which reduces the skin's ability to produce vitamin D from sunlight. Subcutaneous fat sequesters vitamin D, therefore obese populations may need greater intakes to achieve adequate levels.[4] Patients on long-term parenteral nutrition (PN) may also be at higher risk of vitamin D deficiency due to factors such as malabsorptive disorders and self-limiting behaviors related to outdoor activities (to avoid damaging intravenous (IV) catheters). Some medications such as laxatives, anti-diarrheals, anti-convulsants, and corticosteroids can reduce absorption, increase metabolism and decrease serum vitamin D levels.[1]

2 Diagnosis: Biochemical and Physical Signs

Vitamin D refers to both ergocalciferol (vitamin D_2) and cholecalciferol (vitamin D_3), which are either consumed in the diet or synthesized in the skin. Vitamin D must undergo two hydroxylations for activation. The first, which occurs in the liver, converts vitamin D to 25-hydroxyvitamin D, also known as calcidiol. The second hydroxylation occurs primarily in the kidney and forms the physiologically active 1,25-dihydroxyvitamin D, also known as calcitriol.[4]

Serum calcidiol is the primary biochemical indicator of vitamin D status. It reflects vitamin D obtained from foods and supplements, and has a fairly long circulating half-life of 15 days. In contrast to calcidiol, circulating calcitriol has a short half-life (less than 24 hours) and is therefore not a good indicator of vitamin D status. Serum calcitriol levels are tightly regulated by parathyroid hormone, calcium, and phosphate, and do not typically decrease until vitamin D deficiency is severe.[4]

Serum concentrations of calcidiol are reported in both nanomoles per liter (nmol/L) and nanograms per milliliter (ng/mL). Optimal serum levels of vitamin D remain a matter of some disagreement among various scientific groups who have proposed differing diagnostic criteria. However, the most commonly recognized interpretation of serum calcidiol levels are as follows:[4,5]

- ≥ 50 nmol/L (≥ 20 ng/mL):   *Sufficient*
- 30–< 50 nmol/L (12–< 20 ng/mL):   *Insufficient*
- < 30 nmol/L (≤ 12 ng/mL):   *Deficient*

Physical and clinical signs of vitamin D deficiency include osteomalacia, tetany (intermittent muscular spasms and overactive neurological reflexes) and hypocalcemia.[6]

3 Treatment

Vitamin D requirements depend largely on the degree of the deficiency and underlying risk factors. Initial supplementation with oral vitamin D_3, 6000 IU daily or 50,000 IU weekly for eight weeks, can be considered. Once the serum calcidiol level exceeds 30 ng/mL, a daily maintenance dose of 1000 to 2000 IU is recommended.[7] Vitamin D deficiency in high-risk adults may require a higher initial dose of 10,000 IU vitamin D_3 daily. Once serum calcidiol levels exceed 30 ng/mL, a maintenance dose of 3000 to 6000 IU/day is recommended.[7]

C Vitamin E

1 Deficiency Risk Factors

Patients who have fat-malabsorptive disorders such as Crohn's disease, cystic fibrosis, compromised biliary function, or extensive resection of the small intestine are at risk of vitamin E deficiency. Patients on PN for greater than three months without lipid emulsions or vitamin E supplementation are also at risk.[1]

2 Diagnosis: Biochemical and Physical Signs

Laboratory tests for vitamin E levels include plasma or serum vitamin E, which may be interpreted as follows:[1]

- < 0.5 mg/dL: *Deficient*
- 0.5 to 2.0 mg/dL: *Normal*
- > 2.0 mg/dL: *Toxicity*

Physical signs of deficiency of vitamin E include age spots, vision changes or loss, ophthalmoplegia (weakness of muscles responsible for eye movements), ptosis (drooping of the upper eyelid), dysarthria and ataxia. Other signs can include hemolytic anemia, increased platelet aggregation, and urinary creatinine wasting.[1]

3 Treatment

Without a history of inadequate intake or a predisposing condition, vitamin E deficiency is unlikely. In the event of deficiency, recommended doses of oral vitamin E range from 200 to 2000 mg/d; however, this is dependent on the underlying causative disease as follows:[1,8]

- Chronic cholestasis: 15–25 IU/kg per day
- Cystic fibrosis: 5–10 IU/kg per day
- Short-bowel syndrome: 200–3600 IU per day
- Isolated vitamin E deficiency: 800–3600 IU per day

D   VITAMIN K

1   Deficiency Risk Factors

Patients with fat malabsorption, inflammatory bowel disease and long-term PN without lipid emulsion are at increased risk of vitamin K deficiency. Long-term antibiotic therapy may also increase risk as certain antibiotics especially cephalosporins, can act as vitamin K antagonists and prevent absorption of the vitamin.[9]

2   Diagnosis: Biochemical and Physical Signs

Patients on anticoagulant therapy may require closer monitoring, as warfarin and vitamin K counteract each other. Anticoagulant doses are adjusted to achieve a therapeutic international normalized ratio (INR). INR is calculated based on prothrombin time (PT), which measures how long it takes for a clot to form in a blood sample. Once the goal INR is met, daily vitamin K intake should remain consistent. Without warfarin dose adjustments, increased vitamin K intake leads to an increased risk of blood clots, whereas decreased vitamin K intake could increase the risk of bleeding. The INR is the most common laboratory test used to monitor warfarin therapy and detect potential bleeding problems, while plasma phylloquinone is measured to assess vitamin K status. Normal fasting phylloquinone levels in healthy adults are 0.15 to 1.0 µg/L.[1]

Physical signs of vitamin K deficiency include bruising, prolonged bleeding, decreased bone density, and an increased PT.[1]

3   Treatment

There are no guidelines for treating vitamin K deficiency; however, supplementation of oral or IM vitamin K, 2.5 to 10 mg twice weekly to daily, is commonly prescribed.[1]

III   WATER-SOLUBLE VITAMINS

Unlike fat-soluble vitamins, water-soluble vitamins are not stored in the body because they dissolve in water. Therefore, frequent intake of these vitamins is needed because they become depleted more rapidly, and supplementation is less likely to result in toxicity. Table 9.3 reviews the function, needs and sources of the water-soluble vitamins. Table 9.4 summarizes biochemical diagnostic tests and treatment of water-soluble vitamin deficiencies.

A   THIAMIN (VITAMIN B$_1$)

1   Deficiency Risk Factors

Thiamin deficiency risk factors include alcohol use disorder (AUD), long-term PN or dialysis, recurrent vomiting, gastric bypass, refeeding syndrome, and malabsorption.

TABLE 9.3

Function, Needs and Sources of Water-Soluble Vitamins[2,4,8,9]

Nutrient	Function	RDA	Sources
Thiamin (vitamin B_1)	Energy metabolism, nerve function	Men – 1.2 mg Women – 1.1 mg Pregnant – 1.4 mg Lactating – 1.5mg	Enriched or fortified whole grain, pork, legumes, sunflower seeds, wheat germ
Riboflavin (vitamin B_2)	Energy production; cellular function, growth, and development; metabolism of fats, drugs, and steroids	Men – 1.3 mg Women – 1.1 mg	Organ meats, milk, bread, fortified cereals
Niacin (vitamin B_3)	Metabolism of amino acids, fatty acids and carbohydrates	Men – 16 mg Women – 14 mg Pregnant – 18 mg Lactating – 17 mg	Meat, fish, poultry, enriched and fortified breads and cereals
Pantothenic acid (vitamin B_5)	Energy release from fat, carbohydrates and ketogenic amino acids; gluconeogenesis; heme and sterol synthesis; acetylation reactions; synthesis of bile salts, cholesterol, steroid hormones and fatty acids; transportation of long-chain fatty acids into the mitochondria	AI: Men and women – 5 mg Pregnant – 6 mg Lactating – 7 mg	Sunflower seeds, beef liver, mushrooms, peanuts, eggs, broccoli, milk
Pyridoxine (vitamin B_6)	Formation of enzyme needed for protein metabolism, red blood cell production	Men and women ≤ 50 yr – 1.3 mg Men > 50 yr – 1.7 mg Women > 50 yr – 1.9 mg Pregnant – 1.9 mg Lactating – 2 mg	Fortified cereals, organ meats, whole grains
Biotin (vitamin B_7)	Genetic expression of more than 2000 enzymes, cofactor for conversion of CO_2 to various substrates needed in many metabolic pathways	AI: Men and women – 30 µg Pregnant – 35 µg	Liver, with smaller amounts found in other cuts of meat, fruits
Folic acid	DNA and new cell production	Men and women – 400 DFE Pregnant – 600 DFE Lactating – 500 DFE	Enriched grain, dark green leafy vegetables, fortified cereals
Vitamin B_{12}	Part of an enzyme needed for making new cells, nerve function	Men and women – 2.4 µg Pregnant – 2.6 µg Lactating – 2.8 µg	Fortified cereals, meat, fish, poultry, eggs

(*Continued*)

TABLE 9.3 (Continued)

Function, Needs and Sources of Water-Soluble Vitamins[2,4,8,9]

Nutrient	Function	RDA	Sources
Vitamin C	Part of an enzyme needed for protein metabolism, immune system health, aids in iron absorption	Men – 90 mg Women – 75 mg Pregnant – 100 mg Lactating – 120 mg	Citrus fruits, vegetables in the cabbage family, cantaloupe, strawberries, peppers, tomatoes, potatoes, lettuce, papayas, mangoes, kiwi fruit

Abbreviations: RDA = Recommended Daily Allowance; mg = milligrams; yr = year; CO_2 = carbon dioxide; AI = adequate intakes; µg = micrograms; DNA = deoxyribonucleic acid; DFE = dietary folate equivalent.

Thiamin deficiency may also occur in populations whose diet consists mostly of refined carbohydrates. According to the 2003–2006 National Health and Nutrition Examination Survey, only 6% of the US population has a thiamin intake below the estimated average requirement.[10]

2   Diagnosis: Biochemical and Physical Signs

Measurement of erythrocyte transketolase activity is the preferred method for assessing thiamin status, but 24-hour urinary thiamin excretion can also be measured.[1,11] A urinary thiamin excretion of less than 100 µg/day in adults suggests insufficient intake, and less than 40 µg/day indicates extremely low intake.[10]

Early physical signs of thiamin deficiency, or beriberi, are non-specific and include negative effects on the central nervous system such as fatigue, irritability, poor memory, sleep disturbances, sharp stabbing chest pain, anorexia, and abdominal discomfort. Deficiency can also manifest itself in three distinct ways, each with unique symptoms. Dry beriberi refers to peripheral neurological deficits which primarily affect the lower extremities. Muscle wasting can also occur. Cardiovascular, or wet, beriberi is a myocardial disease whose signs include vasodilation, tachycardia, a wide pulse pressure, sweating, warm skin, and lactic acidosis. Left untreated, this can result in heart failure.[11]

Wernicke-Korsakoff's syndrome includes Wernicke's encephalopathy and Korsakoff's syndrome, which are distinct disorders but often occur together in patients with AUD who do not consume adequate amounts of thiamin-fortified foods. Wernicke's encephalopathy is characterized by psychomotor slowing, nystagmus, ataxia, ophthalmoplegia (paralysis or weakness of eye muscles), and impaired consciousness. Korsakoff's syndrome is characterized by memory deficits. If left untreated Wernicke-Korsakoff's syndrome will lead to coma and death.[11]

Diagnosis of thiamin deficiency is often based on a favorable response to thiamin replacement in patients who exhibit signs or symptoms of deficiency. However, thiamin-deficient patients with hypomagnesemia may not respond to replacement as magnesium is a necessary cofactor in thiamin-dependent metabolism.

TABLE 9.4

Biochemical Diagnostic Tests and Treatment of Water-Soluble Vitamin Deficiencies[1,10,13,16,19,21,30]

Nutrient	Biochemical test	Treatment
Thiamin	Erythrocyte transketolase • 0–15%: normal • 16–24%: marginally deficient • > 25%: deficient • 24-h urinary thiamin excretion • < 100 µg/d: insufficient intake • < 40 µg/d: extremely low intake	100 mg IV when deficiency suspected Wernicke's encephalopathy or Wernicke-Korsakoff's syndrome: 100–200 mg IV three times daily for 3 to 5 days, followed by 10 mg oral three times daily for 1 to 2 weeks, and then 10 mg/d oral thereafter. (If a diagnosis of Wernicke's encephalopathy or Wernicke-Korsakoff's syndrome is confirmed, the initial dose should be increased to 200–500 mg IV or IM three times daily for 5 to 7 days before switching to oral replacement.)
Riboflavin	EGRAC • < 1.2: adequate • 1.2–1.4: marginal deficiency • > 1.4: deficiency	10 to 20 mg daily
Niacin	Urine NMN • < 5.8 µmol/d: deficient	Rare in the United States due to many foods fortified with niacin. Niacin can be supplemented to treat dyslipidemia regardless of deficiency. Pellagra: IM injections of 50–100 mg nicotinic acid three times daily for 3 to 4 days, followed by 250 to 500 mg/d oral nicotinamide
Pantothenic acid	24-h urinary excretion • < 1 mg/d: deficient	Dose has not been established
Pyridoxine	Plasma PLP • 20 nmol/L: adequate	100 mg/d oral
Biotin	Serum biotin • 200 pg/mL: deficient • 24-h urinary biotin excretion • < 6 µg/d: deficient	3–20 mg/d oral
Folic acid	Serum folate • < 2 ng/mL: deficient • 2–4 ng/mL: inadequate – check MMA and homocysteine • MMA normal, elevated homocysteine: folate deficient	1–5 mg/d oral
Vitamin B_{12}	Serum B_{12} • < 200 pg/mL: deficient • 200–300 pg/mL: borderline low • MMA elevated: B_{12} deficient	1000–2000 µg/d oral 100–1000 µg IM at one-month intervals until corrected for severe deficiency

(Continued)

TABLE 9.4 (Continued)

Biochemical Diagnostic Tests and Treatment of Water-Soluble Vitamin Deficiencies[1,10,13,16,19,21,30]

Nutrient	Biochemical test	Treatment
Vitamin C	Plasma ascorbic acid • > 23 mg/dL: sufficient • 12–23 mg/dL: low • ≤ 11 mg/dL: deficient	100 mg oral three times daily Initial IV dose 60–100 mg 100–200 mg/d to aid in wound healing

Abbreviations: μg/d = microgram per day; IV = intravenous; IM = intramuscular; EGRAC = erythrocyte glutathione reductase activity coefficient; mg = milligram; NNM = *N*-methylnicotinamide; μmol/d = micromole per day; US = United States; mg/d = milligram per day; PLP = plasma pyridoxal 5-phosphate; nmol/L = nanomole per liter; ng/mL = nanogram per milliliter; pg/mL = picogram per milliliter; μg = microgram; mg/dL = milligram per deciliter.

Cardiovascular beriberi in particular may be difficult to differentiate from other disorders that can cause heart failure, but a trial of thiamin supplementation could be considered.[11]

3   Treatment

Thiamin deficiency symptoms may worsen with glucose infusions because thiamin is needed for glucose metabolism. IV thiamin supplementation of 100 mg should be given prior to glucose infusions when a deficiency is suspected. Treatment for Wernicke's encephalopathy or Wernicke-Korsakoff's syndrome is 100–200 mg IV or IM thiamin three times daily before high-carbohydrate meals for 3 to 5 days, followed by 10 mg oral thiamin three times daily for 1 to 2 weeks, and then 10 mg oral thiamin once daily thereafter. If a diagnosis of Wernicke's encephalopathy or Wernicke-Korsakoff's syndrome is confirmed, the initial thiamin dose should be increased to 200–500 mg IV or IM three times daily for 5 to 7 days before switching to oral replacement. Thiamin supplementation is only effective if magnesium is repleted, as magnesium is a necessary cofactor in thiamin-dependent metabolism.[11]

Patients with chronic AUD, who often have poor food intake, are at greater risk of developing thiamin deficiency. Ethanol reduces gastrointestinal absorption of thiamin, thiamin stores in the liver, and thiamin phosphorylation. In the United States patients with AUD are traditionally prescribed 100 mg of IV or IM thiamin for 3 to 7 days, followed by oral thiamin indefinitely as long as the patient continues to consume alcohol.[12]

B   RIBOFLAVIN (VITAMIN B$_2$)

1   Deficiency Risk Factors

Individuals with AUD may be at risk of riboflavin deficiency due to limited intake and absorption. Those with thyroid disorders are also at risk as a result of altered riboflavin metabolism. Individuals with type 2 diabetes, trauma, or extreme stress are at higher risk of deficiency due to increased urinary riboflavin excretion. Patients with chronic malabsorption are also at risk.[1]

2   Diagnosis: Biochemical and Physical Signs

More than 90% of dietary riboflavin is in the form of flavin adenine dinucleotide (FAD) or flavin mononucleotide (FMN), while the remaining 10% is composed of the free form and riboflavin glycosides or esters. Although not routinely measured in healthy people, a stable and sensitive measure of riboflavin deficiency is the erythrocyte glutathione reductase activity coefficient (EGRAC). The most appropriate EGRAC thresholds to assess riboflavin status are uncertain. An EGRAC of 1.2 or less is usually used to indicate adequate riboflavin status, 1.2–1.4 to indicate marginal deficiency, and greater than 1.4 to indicate deficiency. However, it is important to note that a higher EGRAC does not necessarily correlate with the degree of riboflavin deficiency. In addition, the EGRAC cannot be used in people with glucose-6-phosphate dehydrogenase deficiency, which is present in about 10% of Black people.[13]

Physical signs of deficiency include seborrheic dermatitis of the face and scrotum, hyperemia (reddening and edema of the mouth and throat due to increased blood flow), angular stomatitis (lesions at the corners of the mouth), cheilosis (swollen, cracked lips), hair loss, reproductive problems, sore throat, itchy and red eyes, and degeneration of the liver and nervous system.[13]

3   Treatment

Deficiency is rare in the US population, but if inadequate riboflavin status is suspected or diagnosed, daily supplementation of 10 to 20 mg of riboflavin should be given until the deficiency is resolved.[1]

C   NIACIN (VITAMIN B₃)

1   Deficiency Risk Factors

Risk factors for niacin deficiency include malabsorptive disorders and AUD. Patients on isoniazid are also at risk of deficiency because isoniazid inhibits tryptophan metabolism, which reduces niacin production. Mercaptopurine may also increase risk of deficiency, because it interferes with the conversion of niacin to its active form, nicotinamide adenine dinucleotide (NAD).[1]

2   Diagnosis: Biochemical and Physical Signs

A niacin deficiency is defined as urinary levels of N-methylnicotinamide (NMN) less than 5.8 μmol/d. The measurement of plasma levels of 2-pyridone or NMN may also be used to assess niacin status. Decreased concentrations of NAD in red blood cells coupled with low plasma tryptophan levels may also suggest niacin deficiency.[1]

Physical signs of niacin deficiency include dermatitis, sun sensitivity causing symmetrical pigmented rash, glossitis, dementia, peripheral neuritis and extremity paralysis. Pellagra is the classic niacin-deficiency disease and is most commonly seen in less developed nations. It can affect the GI tract, nervous system, and skin, thus presents as the "three Ds": diarrhea, dementia, and dermatitis.[1]

3 Treatment

In the United States, deficiency is extremely rare because many food products are fortified with niacin. Advanced stages of pellagra are treated via IM injections of 50–100 mg nicotinic acid three times daily for 3 to 4 days, followed by oral therapy of 250 to 500 mg/day nicotinamide.[14] Combined with other agents, niacin has been known to be an effective treatment for dyslipidemia, thus may be taken not for deficiency but to reach serum lipid targets.[15]

D Pantothenic Acid (Vitamin B$_5$)

1 Deficiency Risk Factors

Vitamin B$_5$ is widely available in many foods, thus deficiency is rare except in people with severe malnutrition.[15] Patients with inflammatory bowel disease or AUD are at increased risk of deficiency because the mechanism for absorption is impaired. Consumption of large amounts of alcohol may also increase requirements. Often a vitamin B$_5$ deficiency occurs along with multiple other nutrient deficiencies, especially other B vitamins.[1]

2 Diagnosis: Biochemical and Physical Signs

Vitamin B$_5$ whole blood assays and urinary excretion can be measured to assess for deficiency, although assessment for deficiency in healthy people is rare.[16] Whole blood pantothenic acid may be measured, but this requires enzyme pretreatment to release free pantothenic acid from coenzyme A. Further, plasma levels of pantothenic acid do not correlate well with changes in intake or status. The urinary analysis is the more reliable marker of a deficiency as it is closely related to dietary intake.[16] Urinary analysis is the easiest test to perform and interpret, although 24-hour urine collection is required. A level of < 1 mg/d is considered deficient.[1]

Physical signs of deficiency include poor wound healing, neuromuscular disturbances, numbness, parethesias, staggering gait, mental depression, listlessness, irritability, restlessness, malaise, sleep disturbances, muscle cramps, fatigue, nausea, abdominal cramps, vomiting, diarrhea, hypoglycemia, increased insulin sensitivity, compromised immune function and diminished engraftment after transplants.[1]

3 Treatment

An optimal dose of vitamin B$_5$ for treatment of deficiency has not been established, but diarrhea has been reported with supplementation that exceeds 10 g per day.[1]

E Pyridoxine (Vitamin B$_6$)

1 Deficiency Risk Factors

A secondary vitamin B$_6$ deficiency can occur in patients with AUD, undernutrition, chronic dialysis or receiving medications that inhibit vitamin activity such as anti-seizure medications, corticosteroids and chelating agents. Older adults are also at increased risk of deficiency due to decreased absorption, increased catabolism and impaired phosphorylation.[17] Deficiency is rare but can occur because extensive processing can deplete foods of vitamin B_6. Deficiency can be caused by inborn errors of pyridoxine metabolism, although these conditions are rare.[18]

2 Diagnosis: Biochemical and Physical Signs

To ascertain a deficiency a combination of three tests is recommended: plasma pyridoxal 5-phosphate (PLP), 24-hour excretion of 4-pyridoxic acid, and activation of erythrocyte aspartate aminotransferase and erythrocyte alanine aminotransferase by PLP. PLP is the active coenzyme form of vitamin B_6, and has a role in amino acid one-carbon units, carbohydrate, and lipid metabolism. Plasma PLP is the most common measure of vitamin B_6 status; 20 nmol/L is considered adequate. Vitamin B_6 deficiency is more commonly assessed based on clinical presentation, especially in patients having seizures, those who are on anti-seizure medications, and those with other vitamin B deficiencies, as may be seen with AUD or undernutrition.[18]

Nasolabial seborrhea (scaling around nostrils), cheilosis, angular stomatitis (bilateral cracks and redness of lips), glossitis (inflammation resulting in a swollen, red and smooth tongue) and magenta-colored tongue are all signs of vitamin B_6 deficiency.[6]

3 Treatment

Treatment for deficiency is 100 mg/d of oral vitamin B_6. Patients receiving isoniazid may be given 25–50 mg/d as a prophylactic treatment.[1]

F Biotin (Vitamin B_7)

1 Deficiency Risk Factors

Biotin deficiency is rare. Risks include long-term PN, AUD, partial or total gastrectomy, and anticonvulsant therapy. Plasma and breastmilk concentrations of biotin decrease in pregnant and lactating women, even in those with adequate intakes. Plasma biotin decreases in one-third of pregnant women.[19] More research is needed to understand the clinical significance of this occurrence.

2 Diagnosis: Biochemical and Physical Signs

The most common biochemical measures indicative of biotin deficiency are serum concentration of less than 200 pg/mL and 24-hour biotin urinary excretion less than 6 μg/d.[1] Whole blood and serum biotin concentrations are not as reliable as urinary analysis, thus the most valid measurement is abnormally decreased urinary excretion of biotin and an abnormally increased urinary excretion of 3-hydroxyisovaleric acid greater than 3.3 mmol/mol creatinine.[19]

The most common physical signs of deficiency include pallor, erythematous seborrheic dermatitis and alopecia. Others include vision problems, glossitis, cheilosis, nervous instability, dementia, hallucinations, paresthesia in extremities, depression, hypotonia (decreased muscle tone), anorexia, nausea, vomiting, lethargy, muscle pain, ketolactic acidosis, and elevated cholesterol.[1,19]

3   Treatment

A deficiency is treated by giving 3–20 mg/day of oral biotin. No evidence of toxicity has been reported, even in patients with a biotin-responsive inborn error of metabolism or acquired biotin deficiency treated with 200 mg of biotin orally or 20 mg IV.[1]

G   Folic Acid

1   Deficiency Risk Factors

Alcohol use disorder increases the risk of folic acid deficiency because of decreased intake and absorption. Pregnant women are also at risk due to the increased demand for DNA synthesis necessary for fetal development, as well as periconceptual and premenopausal women. Drugs such as methotrexate, phenytoin, and sulfasalazine can antagonize folate utilization, and inhibit its absorption or conversion to its active form, resulting in folate deficiency.[20]

2   Diagnosis: Biochemical and Physical Signs

An elevated mean corpuscular volume (MCV) indicates macrocytic anemia and warrants investigation for both folate and vitamin B_{12} deficiency. Serum folate levels less than 2 ng/mL are considered deficient, while levels greater than 4 ng/mL are considered normal. Serum folate levels between 2 and 4 ng/mL warrant further confirmation for folate deficiency by measurement of methylmalonic acid (MMA) and homocysteine levels. Folate deficiency can be confirmed with a normal B_{12}, normal MMA level and elevated homocysteine levels.[20]

Patients being evaluated for folic acid deficiency should also be assessed for vitamin B_{12} deficiency. The body uses both folic acid and vitamin B_{12} similarly and therefore symptoms of deficiency, such as macrocytic anemia, can be the same. Vitamin B_{12} deficiency may thus go undetected, so vitamin B_{12} levels should also be checked.[20]

Physical signs of folate deficiency include cheilosis, glossitis, nervous instability, dementia, and meagaloblastic or macrocytic anemia.[1]

3   Treatment

Treatment of folate deficiency is 1 to 5 mg oral folate daily. Excessive amounts of folic acid (100 times the RDA) may result in seizures in individuals taking phenytoin. Prophylactic treatment for chronic AUD is 1 mg oral folate daily.[1]

H   Cyanocobalamin (Vitamin B_{12})

1   Deficiency Risk Factors

Most people in the United States consume adequate amounts of vitamin B_{12}.[21] Vitamin B_{12} deficiency results from insufficient intake, inadequate absorption, decreased utilization due to enzyme deficiencies, liver disorders (related to transport protein abnormality), and use of certain drugs. Malabsorption may occur due to surgical or medical conditions, as well as an autoimmune condition in which the body produces antibodies to intrinsic factor, resulting in a condition known as pernicious anemia. In addition to those with malabsorption syndromes, others at increased risk of deficiency include people with low gastric acid secretion (commonly seen in older adults, those with *Helicobacter pylori* infection, gastrectomy, and antacid use), metformin therapy, and repeated exposure to nitrous oxide, which reduces vitamin B_{12} absorption. Vegetarian and vegan populations, especially those who are breastfeeding, are also at risk of B_{12} deficiency due to insufficient intake.[22,23]

2   Diagnosis: Biochemical and Physical Signs

Most commonly a complete blood count (CBC), serum vitamin B_{12} and folate levels are obtained to assess for deficiency.[22] Tissue B_{12} and macrocytic indexes are typically affected before anemia occurs, thus a high MCV should trigger investigation of vitamin deficiency even if hemoglobin is not low. Folate supplementation may alleviate macrocytic anemia; however, it will mask a vitamin B_{12} deficiency (and vice versa). Therefore, it is important that levels of both be checked to help differentiate the etiology. A vitamin B_{12} level of 200 to 300 pg/mL is considered borderline low, and < 200 pg/mL (< 145 pmol/L) indicates a deficiency.[22,23]

To further assist in etiologic differentiation, serum methylmalonic acid (MMA) can be checked, as an elevated MMA occurs with B_{12} deficiency, but not folate deficiency. It is important to note that an elevated MMA level may also be due to renal failure. Elevated homocysteine concentrations may also occur; however, this effect is seen in both B_{12} and folate deficiency and therefore is not a specific indicator of B_{12} deficiency.[22]

A measure called the Schilling test was developed to diagnose pernicious anemia; however, it is no longer in use as the radiolabeled cobalamine used in the test can no longer be obtained.[24]

Vitamin B_{12} is stored primarily in the liver, and elevated serum vitamin B_{12} levels occur in acute hepatitis, severe alcoholic liver disease, cirrhosis, hepatocellular carcinoma and metastatic liver disease.[25] This is predominantly caused by vitamin B_{12} release during hepatic cytolysis and/or decreased vitamin B_{12} clearance by the affected liver.[26]

Physical signs of vitamin B_{12} deficiency include bone marrow changes, bone fractures, glossitis (though uncommon), mental status changes, pallor, and pale conjunctivae.[6] Neurological symptoms will develop independently from and often without hematological abnormalities.[22] Demyelinating or axonal peripheral neuropathies, degenerative changes that mostly affect brain and spinal cord white matter, may occur. A deficiency also results in megaloblastic anemia more severe than its symptoms indicate because it has a slow evolution that allows for physiological adaptation.[22]

3   Treatment

Supplementation of oral 1000 to 2000 μg/d vitamin B_{12} should be given to patients who do not have severe deficiency or neurological signs or symptoms. For more severe forms of deficiency, treatment includes IM injections of 100–1000 μg vitamin B_{12} at one-month intervals until corrected. Injections can initially be dosed more frequently with symptomatic deficiency, and then reduced to monthly.[22]

Nasal gel preparations of vitamin B_{12} are also available, but are more costly than oral forms. The nasal gel appears to be effective in raising vitamin B_{12} blood levels in adults and children.[27] Large oral doses of vitamin B_{12} can be absorbed even when intrinsic factor is absent.[22]

Adult vegans and strict vegetarians with normal B_{12} absorption may take a standard multivitamin and/or consume foods that are fortified with vitamin B_{12}, such as fortified nutritional yeasts, which can reduce the risk of deficiency.[28]

I Vitamin C

1 Deficiency Risk Factors

A vitamin C deficiency can occur due to general undernutrition, but a severe deficiency that results in scurvy is uncommon.[29] Those at increased risk of vitamin C deficiency include older adults, people on dialysis, smokers, and patients with malabsorptive disorders or poor diets combined with AUD. Increased vitamin C turnover may increase risk of deficiency, and can be seen in patients with type 2 DM and certain types of cancer.[1] Other causes of vitamin C deficiency are recent surgeries, febrile illnesses, inflammatory disorders especially diarrheal, smoking, hyperthyroidism, iron deficiency, cold or heat stress, protein deficiency and burns.[29]

2 Diagnosis: Biochemical and Physical Signs

Plasma ascorbic acid is used to evaluate the status of vitamin C with interpretation as follows:[30]

- > 23 mg/dL: *Sufficient*
- 12–23 mg/dL: *Low*
- ≤ 11 mg/dL: *Deficient*

Physical signs of deficiency include petechiae, non-healing wounds, pale nail beds, spongy bloody gums and corkscrew hair.[6]

3 Treatment

A dose of 100 mg oral vitamin C three times daily is recommended to treat deficiency, but may initially be treated with an IV dose of 60–100 mg. For those with wounds, including pressure injuries, supplementation of 100–200 mg/day of vitamin C is common. The major function of vitamin C is to assist in the formation of collagen, which is the most important protein of connective tissue.[31] Individuals who smoke require 35 mg/day more vitamin C than nonsmokers.[30]

Individuals with renal failure, kidney stones or iron overload disease and patients receiving heparin or warfarin therapy should avoid large vitamin C doses. In patients with chronic kidney disease, high doses of vitamin C (100 – 500 mg/d) can result in increased serum oxalate levels, which can precipitate oxalate crystal formation in soft tissues, therefore increasing the risk of kidney stones and further renal function compromise.[1] However, patients on dialysis can also have low vitamin C levels, so should be supplemented with a lower dose of 60–100 mg/d of vitamin C.[32]

IV   CONCLUSION

Compared to macronutrients, only small quantities of vitamins are needed; however, they are still considered essential nutrients because they cannot be synthesized in amounts sufficient to meet the body's needs and must be obtained from the diet or a synthetic source. The functions of vitamins are of a catalytic or regulatory nature, where they aid in chemical reactions in the body's cells. Vitamin deficiencies may develop if intake is insufficient, absorption or metabolism is impaired, or excretion is increased.[1] Clinicians need to perform a comprehensive physical exam to assess for micronutrient deficiencies while considering disease states, intake and biochemical markers to assess adequacy.

REFERENCES

1. McKeever L. *Vitamins and Trace Elements*. The ASPEN Adult Nutrition Support Core Curriculum, 3rd ed. 2017:141–160.
2. National Institutes of Health, Office of Dietary Supplements. Vitamin A Fact Sheet for Health Professionals. Updated March 26, 2021. Accessed February 9, 2022. https://ods.od.nih.gov/factsheets/VitaminA-HealthProfessional/.
3. Johnson LE. Vitamin A Deficiency. Merck Manual Professional Version. Updated November 2020. Accessed February 9, 2022. www.merckmanuals.com/professional/nutritional-disorders/vitamin-deficiency,-dependency,-and-toxicity/vitamin-a-deficiency?query=vitamin%20A.
4. National Institutes of Health, Office of Dietary Supplements. Vitamin D Fact Sheet for Health Professionals. Updated August 17, 2021. Accessed February 9, 2022. https://ods.od.nih.gov/factsheets/VitaminD-HealthProfessional/.
5. Stoffers A, Weber D, Levine M. An update on vitamin d deficiency in the twenty-first century: nature and nurture. *Curr Opin Endocrinol Diabetes Obes*. 2022;29(1):36–43.
6. Hamilton C, ed. *Nutrition-Focused Physical Exam: An Illustrated Handbook*. 2nd ed. American Society for Parenteral and Enteral Nutrition and the Cleveland Clinic; 2022.
7. Sizar O, Khare S, Goyal A, et al. Vitamin D deficiency. In: StatPearls [Internet]. Updated July 21, 2021. Accessed February 9, 2022. www.ncbi.nlm.nih.gov/books/NBK532266/.
8. National Institutes of Health, Office of Dietary Supplements. Vitamin E Fact Sheet for Health Professionals. Updated March 26, 2021. Accessed February 9, 2022. https://ods.od.nih.gov/factsheets/VitaminE-HealthProfessional/.
9. National Institutes of Health, Office of Dietary Supplements. Vitamin K Fact Sheet for Health Professionals. Updated March 29, 2021. Accessed February 9, 2022. https://ods.od.nih.gov/factsheets/vitaminK-HealthProfessional/.
10. National Institutes of Health, Office of Dietary Supplements. Thiamin Fact Sheet for Health Professionals. Updated March 26, 2021. Accessed February 9, 2022. https://ods.od.nih.gov/factsheets/Thiamin-HealthProfessional/.

11. Johnson LE. Thiamin Deficiency. Merck Manual Professional Version. Updated November 2020. Accessed February 9, 2022. www.merckmanuals.com/professional/nutritional-disorders/vitamin-deficiency,-dependency,-and-toxicity/thiamin-deficiency?query=thiamin.

12. Xiong GL, Bienenfeld D, ed. Wernicke-Korsakoff Syndrome Treatment & Management. Medscape. Updated: May 16, 2018.

13. National Institutes of Health, Office of Dietary Supplements. Riboflavin Fact Sheet for Health Professionals. Updated March 26, 2021. Accessed February 9, 2022. https://ods.od.nih.gov/factsheets/Riboflavin-HealthProfessional/.

14. Redzic S, Gupta V. Niacin deficiency. In: StatPearls [Internet]. Updated November 29, 2021. Accessed February 9, 2022. www.ncbi.nlm.nih.gov/books/NBK557728/?report=printable.

15. Miller M. Niacin as a component of combination therapy for dyslipidemia. *Mayo Clin Proc.* 2003;78(6):735–742.

16. National Institutes of Health, Office of Dietary Supplements. Pantothenic Acid Fact Sheet for Health Professionals. Updated March 26, 2021. Accessed February 9, 2022. https://ods.od.nih.gov/factsheets/PantothenicAcid-HealthProfessional/.

17. Kjeldby IK, Fosnes GS, Ligaarden SC, Farup PG. Vitamin B6 deficiency and diseases in elderly people – a study in nursing homes. *BMC Geriatr.* 2013;13:13.

18. Johnson LE. Pyridoxine Deficiency and Dependence. Merck Manual Professional Version. Updated November 2020. Accessed February 9, 2022. www.merckmanuals.com/professional/nutritional-disorders/vitamin-deficiency,-dependency,-and-toxicity/vitamin-b6-deficiency-and-dependency?query=pyridoxine.

19. National Institutes of Health, Office of Dietary Supplements. Biotin Fact Sheet for Health Professionals. Updated January 10, 2022. Accessed February 9, 2022. https://ods.od.nih.gov/factsheets/Biotin-HealthProfessional/.

20. Khan KM, Jialal I. Folic acid deficiency. In: StatPearls [Internet]. Updated September 28, 2021. Accessed February 9, 2022. www.ncbi.nlm.nih.gov/books/NBK535377/.

21. National Institutes of Health, Office of Dietary Supplements. Vitamin B_{12} Fact Sheet for Health Professionals. Updated April 6, 2021. Accessed February 9, 2022. https://ods.od.nih.gov/factsheets/VitaminB12-HealthProfessional/.

22. Johnson LE. Vitamin B12 Deficiency. Merck Manual Professional Version. Updated November 2020. Accessed February 9, 2022. www.merckmanuals.com/professional/nutritional-disorders/vitamin-deficiency,-dependency,-and-toxicity/vitamin-b12-deficiency?query=vitamin%20b12.

23. Ankar A, Kumar A. Vitamin B12 deficiency. In: StatPearls [Internet]. Updated June 7, 2021. Accessed February 9, 2022. www.ncbi.nlm.nih.gov/books/NBK441923/.

24. Ramphul K, Mejias SG. Schilling Test. In: StatPearls [Internet]. Updated October 4, 2021. Accessed February 9, 2022. www.ncbi.nlm.nih.gov/books/NBK507784/.

25. Sugihara T, Koda M, Okamoto T, et al. Falsely elevated serum vitamin B12 levels were associated with the severity and prognosis of chronic viral liver disease. *Yonago Acta Med.* 2017;60(1):31–39.

26. Ermens AAM, Vlasveld LT, Lindemans J. Significance of elevated cobalamin (vitamin B12) levels in blood. *Clin Biochem.* 2003;36(8):585–590.

27. Slot WB, Merkus FW, Van Deventer SJ, Tytgat GN. Normalization of plasma vitamin B12 concentration by intranasal hydroxocobalamin in vitamin B12-deficient patients. *Gastroenterology.* 1997;113(2):430–433.

28. Pawlak R, Lester SE, Babatunde T. The prevalence of cobalamin deficiency among vegetarians assessed by serum vitamin B12: A review of literature. *Eur J Clin Nutr.* 2014;68(5):541–548.

29. Johnson LE. Vitamin C Deficiency. Merck Manual Professional Version. Updated November 2020. Accessed February 9, 2022. www.merckmanuals.com/professional/ nutritional-disorders/vitamin-deficiency,-dependency,-and-toxicity/vitamin-c-deficie ncy?query=vitamin%20c.

30. National Institutes of Health, Office of Dietary Supplements. Vitamin C Fact Sheet for Health Professionals. Updated March 26, 2021. Accessed February 9, 2022. https:// ods.od.nih.gov/factsheets/VitaminC-HealthProfessional/.

31. Moores J. Vitamin C: a wound healing perspective. *Br J Community Nurs.* 2013;18(S12):S6,S8–S11.

32. Handelman GJ. Vitamin C deficiency in dialysis patients—are we perceiving the tip of an iceberg? *Nephrol Dial Transplant.* 2007;22(2):328–331.

10 Trace Mineral Deficiencies – Diagnosis and Treatment

Kavitha Krishnan and Julianne Werner

CONTENTS

I   INTRODUCTION

Minerals are essential to all forms of metabolism, and include both electrolytes and trace elements (or trace minerals), which are usually defined as minerals that are required for adults in amounts of 1 to 100 mg/day.[1] Increased demand, reduced intake, reduced absorption or altered metabolism may cause trace element deficiencies.[2] Minerals are found naturally in multiple food sources, listed in Table 10.1. See Table 10.2 for the Recommended Daily Allowance (RDA) or Dietary Reference Intake (DRI) for select trace elements.

This chapter will review risk factors, diagnosis, and treatment of deficiencies for iron, zinc, iodine, selenium, copper and manganese. Tables 10.3–10.5 summarize these topics. See Chapter 7 for more details on physical signs and symptoms of deficiency.

II   IRON

Iron is required for the synthesis of oxygen-transport proteins, in particular hemoglobin and myoglobin, and for the formation of heme and other iron-containing enzymes involved in electron transfer and oxidation-reductions.[11,12] Iron is predominantly bound to these hemo proteins, heme enzymes, or non-heme compounds such as

DOI: 10.1201/9781003177586-10

TABLE 10.1
Trace Mineral Functions and Dietary Sources[2-10]

Mineral	Function	Sources
Iron	Oxidative metabolism, cellular immune response, erythropoietic function; component of numerous proteins	Meat, beans, lentils, seafood, broccoli, peas, bran, enriched bread, tofu, cashews, dark leafy greens
Zinc	Helps with immune function, lipid peroxidation, wound healing, neuromodulation, and metabolism; involved with gene expression, cell growth, and insulin synthesis; supports growth in pregnancy and adolescence	Seafood, meats, nuts, beans, whole grains, dairy products, dark leafy greens
Iodine	Key component of thyroid hormones which regulate many biochemical reactions, including protein synthesis and enzymatic activity, and metabolic activity	Seafood, iodized salt
Selenium	Cofactor in the metabolism of glutathione peroxidase, thyroid hormone, and iodine; involved in reproduction, DNA production; protection from infection and cell damage	Fish, organ meats, brazil nuts, eggs, milk, cereals, grains, dairy products
Copper	Needed for enzymes involved in aerobic metabolism, adequate growth, cardiovascular health, lung function, neuroendocrine function, and iron metabolism; involved in neovascularization, neuropeptide activation, neurotransmitter synthesis, gene expression, immune function, brain development, cholesterol and glucose metabolism, and melatonin production	Shellfish, seeds and nuts, organ meats, wheat-bran cereals, whole-grain products, beans, dried fruits, chocolate
Manganese	Involved in amino acid, lipid, and carbohydrate metabolism; essential for bone formation; activates glycosyltransferases, phosphoenolpyruvate, carboxylase, and glutamine synthetase	Nuts, oats, whole grains, clams, oysters, mussels, legumes, coffee, tea, dark leafy greens

TABLE 10.2
Trace Minerals RDA and DRI for Adults[2]

Mineral	RDA Male (per day)	RDA Female (per day)
Iron	8 mg	18 mg
Zinc	11 mg	8 mg
Iodine	150 µg	150 µg
Selenium	55 µg	55 µg
Copper	900 µg	900 µg
Manganese	2.3 mg	1.8 mg

Abbreviations: RDA = Recommended Daily Allowance; DRI = Dietary Reference Intake.

flavin-iron enzymes, transferrin, and ferritin. The amount of iron present in the body depends on age, sex, weight, and nutritional status.[13]

A DEFICIENCY RISK FACTORS

According to the World Health Organization (WHO), anemia affects about 25% of the world's population, and 50% of cases are due to iron deficiency.[14] It is the most common nutrient deficiency worldwide.[14] Iron deficiency can result from inadequate iron intake in the diet, increased requirements such as in pregnancy, blood loss from heavy menstruation, gastrointestinal (GI) ulcers, hemodialysis, or surgery, and malabsorption from conditions such as inflammatory bowel disease (IBD), short bowel syndrome (SBS), bariatric surgery, and total or subtotal gastrectomy. Certain medications that decrease gastric acid production, such as antacids, H2 antagonists, and proton-pump inhibitors may result in decreased iron absorption.[2] A diet high in phytic acid or oxalic acid can also reduce iron absorption by forming insoluble iron complexes in the GI tract.[2,15]

B BIOCHEMICAL ASSESSMENT

A bone marrow biopsy is considered the gold standard to diagnose iron deficiency but is not used due to cost and patient discomfort. Serum ferritin is the preferred biochemical marker of iron stores. Iron deficiency occurs when iron stores are depleted, indicated by a serum ferritin level of 20 µg/L or less.[16] However, serum ferritin is a positive acute-phase protein, and as such during inflammation it may be elevated and not accurately depict deficiency states.[15] The average ferritin values for adult men and women are 100 µg/L and 30 µg/L, respectively.[17]

The major iron-transport protein in the blood is transferrin. During iron deficiency the ratio between iron and transferrin decreases because there is less iron to transport. Transferrin saturation is calculated by the formula: (serum iron × 100)/ total iron binding capacity (TIBC). TIBC is a marker for circulating transferrin. Transferrin saturation less than 18% indicates iron deficiency with a normal range from 18% to 50%. Mean corpuscular volume (MCV) is a measure of the size and volume of red blood cells. A low MCV defined as 80 fL or less may indicate iron deficiency; however, other causative factors, such as blood loss, should be ruled out.[16]

C PHYSICAL SIGNS AND SYMPTOMS

Iron deficiency may present as fatigue, sleepiness, headache, loss of appetite, and nausea.[18] Additional physical characteristics may include pallor, glossitis, koilonychia, pale conjunctivae, and pale gum color.[2,19] Patients can also exhibit extreme sensitivity to cold temperatures, increased susceptibility to infections and even an increase in lead absorption.[2,18] Iron deficiency can also cause restless leg syndrome.[20]

D TREATMENT

Treatment for iron deficiency may start with increasing intake of iron-rich foods. Heme and non-heme iron are the two main forms of dietary iron.[21] Plants and iron-fortified foods contain non-heme iron only, whereas both heme and non-heme iron are present in meat, seafood, and poultry.[22] In many countries, grain flours are fortified with iron,[23] and in the United States about half of dietary iron comes from grain products.[22,24] Heme iron has higher bioavailability than non-heme iron, and other dietary components have less effect on the bioavailability of heme than non-heme iron.[5,6]

Treating iron deficiency with oral iron supplements is both effective and inexpensive. A dosage of 150–200 mg/d of elemental iron for three months is recommended to treat iron deficiency.[25] Iron is most commonly available in the form of ferrous sulfate, ferrous gluconate and ferrous fumarate. Although fumarate is most easily absorbed, sulfate and gluconate forms are preferred since they are inexpensive, and are also bioavailable.[2] The amount of elemental iron in each iron salt varies, hence the type of the supplement will determine the dosage. Ferrous sulfate is 20% elemental iron, ferrous fumarate 33%, and ferrous gluconate 12%.[26]

Ascorbic acid facilitates the absorption of iron, thus iron supplements should be taken with foods high in vitamin C.[27] Tea tannins, phytates and certain medications such as antacids should be avoided since they may hinder the absorption of iron.[2] Taking iron supplements on an empty stomach increases absorption, as a lower gastric pH keeps the iron in a soluble form, thereby making it available for absorption.[28] Constipation and nausea are common side effects of iron supplements; delayed-release forms may be better tolerated in these cases, although they may not be absorbed as well as other forms.[2] Prolonged iron supplementation may also cause a mild copper deficiency.[29]

Intravenous (IV) iron is another treatment option. Indications include persistent GI side effects from oral supplements, gastric surgeries and intestinal disorders such as IBD which cause inefficient absorption, and the need for immediate improvement in iron levels as seen with severe anemia or bleeding.[30] It is important to note that iron is a growth factor for pathogens so IV iron is contraindicated in individuals with infections.[30]

III ZINC

Zinc is an important trace mineral present in all types of cells and is involved in cell growth, development, and differentiation.[35] Zinc also plays a vital role in both cell-mediated and humoral immunity.[36]

A DEFICIENCY RISK FACTORS

The prevalence of zinc deficiency worldwide is estimated to be greater than 20%.[35-37] Zinc deficiency can be caused by inadequate intake, decreased absorption, increased losses and increased demand.[38] Inadequate intake can result from zinc-deficient diets and inadequately supplemented parenteral nutrition (PN).[2]

TABLE 10.3
Trace Mineral Deficiency: Risk Factors and Signs/Symptoms[2–7,31–34]

Mineral	Risk factors	Signs/symptoms
Iron	Women of childbearing age, blood loss, malabsorption (e.g. SBS, celiac disease, Crohn's disease, bariatric surgery)	Anemia, fatigue, pallor, weaker immune system, tachycardia, glossitis, nausea
Zinc	Burns, surgical wounds, cirrhosis, malabsorption (e.g. intestinal bypass, bariatric surgery), renal disease	Anorexia, weight loss, impaired wound healing, diarrhea, decreased sense of taste/smell, impaired immune function, exfoliative dermatitis
Iodine	Pregnancy, no consumption of iodized salt, vegan diet, areas with iodine-deficient soil	Stunted growth and intellectual disability in children, fibrocystic breast disease, goiter, muscle weakness, tachycardia
Selenium	Areas with selenium-deficient soil, HIV/AIDS, dialysis	Cardiomyopathy (Keshan's disease), muscle pain or weakness, arrhythmias, altered thyroid hormone metabolism
Copper	Celiac disease, Menke's disease, excess zinc supplementation	Hypochromic, normocytic anemia; neutropenia, leukopenia, sensory ataxia, paresthesias in extremities, hypercholesterolemia, osteoporosis
Manganese	Manganese-free PN	Impaired insulin production, abnormal growth factor production, congenital abnormalities in reproduction, abnormal lipid and carbohydrate metabolism

Abbreviations: SBS = short bowel syndrome; HIV = human immunodeficiency virus; AIDS = acquired immune deficiency syndrome; PN = parenteral nutrition.

Zinc malabsorption can be caused by GI conditions like Crohn's disease, jejunoileal bypass, post bariatric surgery, small bowel resection, and acrodermatitis enteropathica. Pancreatic dysfunction, as seen in alcoholic pancreatitis and cystic fibrosis, diets rich in phytates or sodium polyphosphate, and chelating agents may also reduce zinc absorption.[2] Zinc losses can occur via the GI tract, skin, and urine. Increased GI losses may occur in IBD, diarrhea, steatorrhea, enterostomy, fistula, and chyle leaks.[39]

Zinc loss from urine occurs in patients with trauma, sepsis, renal disease, and alcohol use disorder (AUD), as well as in patients taking some medications (e.g. thiazides, penicillamine, diethylenetriamine pentacetate, valproate, angiotensin-converting enzyme inhibitors, angiotensin-receptor blockers, EDTA-containing propofol and chelating agents, cysteine, cisplatin).[13,38,40,41] Research has shown that patients with diabetes had a mean serum zinc level lower than non-diabetic patients, and the urinary zinc to creatinine ratio was significantly higher as compared to healthy subjects. The decrease in zinc was attributed to the increased urinary albumin excretion by microvascular damage.[42] Zinc can also be lost through burns.[43]

TABLE 10.4
Biochemical Assessment of Trace Minerals[2–7,32,33]

Mineral	Lab	Normal value
Iron	Serum iron*	60–170 µg/dL [50–170 men, 30–160 women]
	Ferritin+	< 20 µg/L = deficient [30–350 men, 18–340 women]
	Transferrin saturation	18–50%
	MCV	80–100
Zinc	Serum	70–120 µg/dL
Iodine	Urine	100–199 µg/L
	Serum	40–92 µg/L
Selenium	Serum selenium	70–150 µg/L
	Urine selenium	150–241 µg/L
	Erythrocyte glutathione peroxidase	≥ 10.5 U/mL
Copper	Serum	0.75–1.45 µg/mL
Manganese	Whole blood	4.7–18.3 µg/L
	Serum	0.0–2 µg/L

* Low with inflammation.
\+ High with inflammation.

B   BIOCHEMICAL ASSESSMENT

Plasma (or serum) zinc is the most widely used biomarker to determine zinc status; less than 70 µg/dL is considered low.[13,44] However, it is important to note that identifying zinc deficiency is difficult in patients during the acute inflammatory phase response as typically occurs in critical illness, stress or trauma. Serum zinc will decrease to half of its normal level as zinc is redistributed from the serum to the liver[45] and remain so until inflammation resolves.[46] In a non-inflammatory starvation state, tissue catabolism releases zinc into the blood circulation, causing a temporary increase in zinc levels.[44]

C   PHYSICAL SIGNS AND SYMPTOMS

Zinc deficiency may lead to anorexia, weight loss, taste and smell alterations, diarrhea, and alopecia. Skin manifestations include impaired epithelialization and wound healing, acrodermatitis enteropathica, and mouth lesions. The dermatitis appears as a vesicular or pustular rash on the perioral, perineal and peripheral body parts like fingers and toes. Zinc deficiency causes growth retardation in children.[2,19,47]

D   TREATMENT

The recommended dosage for correcting a deficiency is 220 mg of zinc sulfate twice a day.[48] This dosage is also commonly prescribed to promote wound healing; however, research showing benefits of zinc supplementation in patients who do not have a zinc deficiency is lacking. More research is warranted to support this practice.[49] Additional zinc supplementation is required in patients with extensive burns and excessive GI losses; however, prolonged zinc supplementation can induce copper deficiency.[2] Zinc should be supplemented to account for small bowel and ileostomy losses, dosed at 12 mg/L and 17 mg/L of zinc sulfate, respectively.[31]

IV IODINE

Iodine is essential for the synthesis of thyroid hormones, triodothyronine (T_3) and thyroxine (T_4). These hormones are important for metabolism, growth, and many other body functions.

A DEFICIENCY RISK FACTORS

Worldwide, about two billion people are iodine-deficient and 2.5% of this population have clinical manifestations of iodine deficiency.[50] Iodine deficiency most commonly occurs as a result of consuming a diet insufficient in iodine. The iodine content of plant foods is influenced by the iodine concentration of the soil in which the food is grown. Bread, milk, saltwater fish, and seafood are dietary sources of iodine;[51] however, the primary source in many countries is iodized salt.[12,52] People who do not consume iodized salt and live in regions with poor soil iodine concentration, as well as those who follow a vegan diet, are at an increased risk of iodine deficiency.[51] Consumption of goitrogenic foods, such as soy, cassava, and cruciferous vegetables, also increases the risk for iodine deficiency.[53] Use of anti-thyroid medications and other changes in thyroid hormone metabolism can also increase deficiency risk.[2,54] For example, iron and selenium deficiency may increase risk as these minerals are necessary for the production of thyroid hormone.[55] Pregnant and lactating women may produce anti-thyroid autoantibodies, and have increased glomerular filtration which increases urinary iodine excretion.[55]

B BIOCHEMICAL ASSESSMENT

To diagnose iodine deficiency, urine and serum values are reliable markers. Normal urine values are 100–199 μg/L and serum values are 40–92 μg/L. Urinary iodine is a good indicator of recent iodine intake since greater than 90% of iodine is excreted in the urine.[56] Twenty-four-hour urine samples should be repeated for 3 or 4 consecutive days as day-to-day dietary intake can vary. Iodine deficiency causes abnormal thyroid hormone production. If T_3 levels are greater than 24 ng/dL for those aged 20–50 years, and greater than 181 ng/dL for those older than 50 years, this indicates an iodine deficiency state.[2]

C PHYSICAL SIGNS AND SYMPTOMS

Goiter or thyroid enlargement can occur at any age. When deficient, if iodine is repleted too quickly it can cause iodine-induced hyperthyroidism, known as the Jon-Basedow phenomenon. Signs and symptoms of this syndrome include tachycardia, diarrhea, restlessness, heat intolerance, increased sweating, and insomnia.[57] Other signs and symptoms of iodine deficiency in adults include tachycardia, weight loss, muscle weakness, and skin warmth.[2,58]

D TREATMENT

Salt iodization for high-risk populations is an effective way to minimize iodine deficiency.[51] The American Thyroid Association recommends that women receive 150 μg of iodine supplements daily during pregnancy and lactation, and that all prenatal vitamin/mineral preparations contain 150 μg of iodine.[59]

V SELENIUM

Selenium is an essential trace element needed for growth and thyroid function, and is a component of the enzyme glutathione peroxidase.[60] Selenium protects cells from free-radical damage through its antioxidant properties. Free-radical concentrations are higher in numerous disease states associated with oxidative stress; selenium may help eliminate these reactive oxygen species.[61]

A DEFICIENCY RISK FACTORS

Primary causes of selenium deficiency include inadequate dietary intake, PN formulations without selenium, and AUD. Dietary sources of selenium are called

TABLE 10.5
Treatment of Trace Mineral Deficiencies[2–7,31]

Mineral	Type of supplement	Supplemental dose	Dose for deficiency
Iron	Oral ferrous sulfate, ferrous gluconate, or polysaccharide complex; IV iron dextran	65 mg ferrous sulfate, 38 mg ferrous gluconate, 150 mg polysaccharide complex	100–200 mg elemental iron with food divided amongst 3 dose/day, IV replacement
Zinc	Oral zinc gluconate, zinc sulfate, zinc acetate	Over 30 mg/d should be monitor by a physician	50 mg elemental zinc
Iodine	Oral	50–1000 μg/d	
Selenium	Selenomethionine, sodium selenite, high-selenium yeast	500–1000 μg/d	200 μg/d
Copper	Copper gluconate, copper citrate, cocoa powder	Copper gluconate 2–8 mg daily or every other day, cocoa powder 4 tsp pure powder	Little evidence other than case reports exists on amounts needed
Manganese	Oral manganese sulfate or aspartate	< 10 mg/day	—

Abbreviations: IV = intravenous; tsp = teaspoon.

selenoproteins as selenium is bound to the amino acids methionine and cysteine.[2,62] The amount of selenium in food is affected by the concentration of selenium in the soil, which varies greatly throughout the world, but is noted to be lower in China compared to other countries.[62] The Chinese population also has higher rates of some cancers, suggesting that selenium supplementation or consumption may have a protective effect; however, evidence directly relating selenium intake and cancer is lacking. Patients with surgical resection of the duodenum and proximal jejunum are also at risk of selenium deficiency as these are the primary locations of selenium absorption.[31,62]

B   BIOCHEMICAL ASSESSMENT

Biomarkers for deficiency include plasma and urine selenium concentrations, and erythrocyte glutathione peroxidase levels. Plasma selenium levels reflect recent intake; less than 70 µg/L is considered deficient.[13] Elevated urine selenium indicates a higher proportion of absorbed selenium is excreted; normal urine selenium values are 150–241 µg/L. Erythrocyte glutathione peroxidase reflects long-term selenium status; normal levels are greater than 10.5 U/mL.[2]

C   PHYSICAL SIGNS AND SYMPTOMS

Deficiency signs include Keshan's disease (a form of congestive cardiomyopathy), poor nail plate health, and impaired thyroid hormone metabolism.[2,64] Other signs of deficiency include male infertility and a type of osteoarthropathy called Kashin-Beck disease (KBD). KBD causes stiffened joints and shortened limbs, and is most prevalent in Korea, China, Siberia, and Tibet.[7]

D   TREATMENT

Adequate selenium intake is approximately 55 µg/day for adults.[13] More evidence is needed to determine an appropriate dose of selenium to correct deficiency.[7] Ultimately, consuming a balanced diet is the best way to prevent a selenium deficiency.

VI   COPPER

Copper is the third most abundant trace element after iron and zinc. It is bound to proteins and is an essential mineral that functions as a cofactor for several enzymes involved in oxidation-reduction and electron-transfer reactions, and is needed to produce red and white blood cells.[65] The body is able to regulate its copper well, so both deficiency and toxicity are quite rare.[65]

A   DEFICIENCY RISK FACTORS

Risk factors for copper deficiency include dietary deficiency, PN without copper, burns, losses from fistulas and ostomies, and malabsorption states such as SBS, celiac disease, and gastric surgery (e.g. gastric bypass and total or subtotal gastrectomy).[2,4,66] Prolonged zinc supplementation of 25–150 mg/d and high vitamin C intake greater than 1500 mg/d can impair copper absorption.[2,18,67,68] Copper absorption occurs in the small intestine and varies depending on serum copper levels. During lower dietary intake, copper is actively transported to aid in absorption, while during higher copper intake, passive diffusion is activated.[2] Copper deficiency is uncommon, but can result from decreased absorption or intake, or increased GI losses.

B   BIOCHEMICAL ASSESSMENT

The most reliable biomarker for determining copper status is serum copper. The normal range is 0.75–1.45 µg/mL. Serum copper levels respond to supplementation of copper in both deficient and non-deficient individuals.[2]

C   PHYSICAL SIGNS AND SYMPTOMS

Neurological effects of copper deficiency include paresthesias in extremities, spasticity, sensory ataxia, uncoordinated gait, and myeloneuropathy. Physical signs include lightened hair color and corkscrew hair.[2]

D   TREATMENT

Copper deficiency can be treated with 2 mg of copper chloride two to three times a day.[51] Since copper is excreted via the liver, people with hepatic dysfunction need to be cautious when taking copper to avoid toxicity.[2]

VII   MANGANESE

Manganese is an essential mineral found in numerous foods and is available as a supplement. It is best known to be involved in enzyme activation, bone formation, reproduction, blood clotting, and immune response.[5]

A   DEFICIENCY RISK FACTORS

Manganese deficiency is very rare and is most commonly caused by inadequate manganese in the diet. Absorption is only 1–5% of dietary intake, and can be inhibited by iron supplementation as both compete for binding sites during the absorption process.[2,52]

B   BIOCHEMICAL ASSESSMENT

There are no dependable biomarkers for determining manganese status; however, whole blood and serum levels are more frequently used. A normal range for whole blood is 4.7–18.3 µg/L and serum is 0.0–2 µg/L. Serum manganese levels indicate dietary manganese intake; however, they reflect only large deviations in intake. Urinary excretion reflects only severe deficiency.[2,69]

Manganese toxicity can be accessed via magnetic resonance imaging of the brain because manganese has paramagnetic properties. In toxicity, manganese can be seen in the globus pallidus of the basal ganglia in the center of the brain.[70] However, this method is expensive, thus whole blood and serum levels are more commonly used to monitor for toxicity. People prone to manganese toxicity include those on long-term PN, and those with a biliary duct obstruction, as manganese is mainly excreted via the hepatobiliary system.[2]

C   PHYSICAL SIGNS AND SYMPTOMS

Symptoms of manganese deficiency include growth retardation, alterations in lipid and carbohydrate metabolism such as changes in circulating HDL cholesterol and glucose levels, reproductive failure, bone deformities, and ataxia.[2]

D   TREATMENT

Manganese deficiency is very rare. Treatment depends upon the severity of deficiency; more research is needed in this area since deficiency is rarely seen in the human population.[7] Deficiency should be treated cautiously, as toxicity is a concern when manganese is supplemented.

VIII   TRACE ELEMENTS AND PARENTERAL NUTRITION

Attention to micronutrient status is important for people who rely solely on long-term PN for their nutritional needs, thus it is important to monitor lab values and assess for other signs of micronutrient deficiencies or toxicities. Periodic shortages of IV micronutrients may occur. ASPEN has published guidelines on how to allocate micronutrients to patients reliant on PN.[71] Prolonged elimination or reduction of micronutrient doses can lead to deficiency and should be monitored.

Toxicity of copper and manganese can also occur in PN patients with cholestasis, impaired biliary excretion, and hepatobiliary disease.[2] Further, many experts believe manganese doses are too high in some manufacturers' IV trace element products, and advocate for a reduction of the manganese dose to 55 µg/d.[72,73] Manganese may also be a contaminant of some IV solutions used for PN, which can further increase the risk of toxicity.[73]

It is recommended that zinc, copper, manganese, and selenium be added to PN daily and monitored every 6 months.[74]

IX   CONCLUSION

Trace elements are essential for the synthesis of body proteins, enzymes and coenzymes. Identifying trace mineral deficiencies can assist in diagnosing malnutrition. Although these deficiencies don't equate to a malnutrition diagnosis, they may point to poor oral intake and malabsorption issues, which could lead to malnutrition. When assessing nutritional status, it is important to be observant of any signs and symptoms of micronutrient deficiencies, and to understand the implications of and appropriate treatment for trace mineral deficiencies.

REFERENCES

1. Tako E. Dietary trace minerals. *Nutrients.* 2019;11(11):2823.
2. Clark S. Vitamins and trace elements. In: Mueller C, ed. *The ASPEN Adult Nutrition Support Core Curriculum.* 2nd ed. American Society of Parenteral and Enteral Nutrition; 2012:121–151.
3. Iodine. Fact Sheet for Health Professionals. National Institutes of Health. Office of Dietary Supplements. Updated March 29, 2021. Accessed September 6, 2021. https://ods.od.nih.gov/factsheets/Iodine-HealthProfessional/.
4. Copper. Fact Sheet for Health Professionals. National Institutes of Health. Office of Dietary Supplements. Updated March 29, 2021. Accessed September 6, 2021. https://ods.od.nih.gov/factsheets/Copper-HealthProfessional/.
5. Manganese. Fact Sheet for Health Professionals. National Institutes of Health. Office of Dietary Supplements. Updated March 29, 2021. Accessed September 6, 2021. https://ods.od.nih.gov/factsheets/Manganese-HealthProfessional/.
6. Zinc. Fact Sheet for Health Professionals. National Institutes of Health. Office of Dietary Supplements. Updated March 29, 2021. Accessed September 6, 2021. https://ods.od.nih.gov/factsheets/Zinc-HealthProfessional/.
7. Selenium. Fact Sheet for Health Professionals. National Institutes of Health. Office of Dietary Supplements. Updated March 29, 2021. Accessed September 6, 2021. https://ods.od.nih.gov/factsheets/Selenium-HealthProfessional./
8. Kaufman C. Foods to fight iron deficiency. Academy of Nutrition and Dietetics. Published January 23, 2020. Accessed September 6, 2021. www.eatright.org/health/wellness/preventing-illness/iron-deficiency/.
9. Muñoz M, García-Erce JA, Remacha AF. Disorders of iron metabolism. Part 1: molecular basis of iron homoeostasis. *J Clin Pathol.* 2011;64(4):281–286.
10. Ross AC, Manson JE, Abrams SA, et al. The 2011 Dietary Reference Intakes for Calcium and Vitamin D: what dietetics practitioners need to know. *J Am Diet Assoc.* 2011;111(4):524–527.
11. Hurrell RF. Bioavailability of iron. *Eur J Clin Nutr.* 1997;51(S1):S4–8.
12. McDowell LR. *Minerals in Animal and Human Nutrition.* 2nd ed. Elsevier Science; 2003:660.
13. Mueller CM, ed. *The ASPEN Adult Nutrition Support Core Curriculum.* 3rd ed. American Society for Parenteral and Enteral Nutrition; 2017.
14. McLean E, Cogswell M, Egli I, Wojdyla D, de Benoist B. World prevalence of anaemia, WHO vitamin and mineral nutrition information system, 1993–2005. *Pub Health Nutr.* 2009;12(4):444–454.
15. Wood RJ, Ronnenberg AG. Iron. In: Shils ME, Shike M, Ross AC, Caballero B, Cousins RJ, eds. *Modern Nutrition in Health and Disease.* 10th ed. Lippincott Williams & Wilkins; 2006:248–270.
16. Worwood M. Indicators of the iron status of populations: ferritin. In: *Assessing the Iron Status of Populations: Including Literature Reviews: Report of a Joint World Health*

Organization/Centers for Disease Control and Prevention Technical Consultation on the Assessment of Iron Status at the Population Level. 2nd ed. WHO; 2004.

17. Beutler E, Fairbanks VF. Iron deficiency. In: Lichtman MA, Beutler E, Kipps TJ, et al., eds. *Williams Hematology.* 9th ed. McGraw-Hill Medical; 2010.

18. Clark SF. Iron deficiency anemia. *Nutr Clin Pract.* 2011;23(2):128–141.

19. Hipskind P, Galang M, Jevenn A, Pogatschnik C. Assessment of micronutrient status. In: Hamilton C, ed. *Nutrition Focused Physical Exam an Illustrated Handbook.* Cleveland Clinic; 2016:44–50.

20. Allen RP, Auerbach S, Bahrain H, Auerbach M, Earley CJ. The prevalence and impact of restless legs syndrome on patients with iron deficiency anemia. *Am J Hematol.* 2013;88(4):261–264.

21. Wessling-Resnick M. Iron. In: Ross AC, Caballero B, Cousins RJ, eds. *Modern Nutrition in Health and Disease.* 11th ed. Lippincott Williams & Wilkins; 2014:176–188.

22. Aggett PJ. Iron. In: Erdman JW, Macdonald IA, Zeisel SH, eds. *Present Knowledge in Nutrition.* 10th ed. Wiley-Blackwell; 2012:506–520.

23. Whittaker P, Tufaro PR, Rader JI. Iron and folate in fortified cereals. *J Am Coll Nutr.* 2001;20(3):247–254.

24. Murray-Kolbe LE, Beard J. Iron. In: Coates PM, Betz JM, Blackman MR, et al., eds. *Encyclopedia of Dietary Supplements.* 2nd ed. Informa Healthcare; 2010:432–438.

25. Iron Deficiency Anaemia: Assessment, Prevention, and Control: A Guide for Programme Managers. United Nations Children's Fund, United Nations University, World Health Organization; 2001.

26. Rockey DC. Treatment of iron deficiency. *Gastroenterology.* 2006;30(4):1367–1368.

27. Lynch SR, Cook JD. Interaction of vitamin C and iron. *Ann N Y Acad Sci.* 1980;355:32–44.

28. Anderson GJ, Frazer DM. Current understanding of iron homeostasis. *Am J Clin Nutr.* 2017;106(Suppl 6):1559S–1566S.

29. Klevay LM. Iron overload can induce mild copper deficiency. *J Trace Elem Med Biol.* 2001;14(4):237–240.

30. Camaschella C. Iron deficiency. *Blood.* 2019;133(1):30–39.

31. Sriram K. Micronutrient and antioxidant therapy in adult critically ill patients. In: Cresci G, ed. *Nutrition Support for the Critically Ill Patient: A Guide to Practice.* 2nd ed. CRC Press; 2015:15–32.

32. Parrish CR, O'Donnell K. Copper deficiency: like a bad penny. Nutrition Issues in Gastroenterology, Series #200. July 2020.

33. Serum iron test. Revised February 6, 2020. Accessed October 18, 2021. www.mountsinai.org/health-library/tests/serum-iron-test.

34. Whitney E, Rolfes SR, eds. The trace minerals. In: *Understanding Nutrition.* 10th ed. Wadsworth Publishing; 2004:436–459.

35. Kawamura T, Ogawa Y, Nakamura Y, et al. Severe dermatitis with loss of epidermal Langerhans cells in human and mouse zinc deficiency. *J Clin Invest.* 2012;122(2):722–732.

36. Tuerk MJ, Fazel N. Zinc deficiency. *Curr Opin Gastroenterol.* 2009;25(2):136–143.

37. Wuehler SE, Peerson JM, Brown KH. Use of national food balance data to estimate the adequacy of zinc in national food supplies: methodology and regional estimates. *Public Health Nutr.* 2005;8(7):812–819.

38. Livingstone C. Zinc: physiology, deficiency, and parenteral nutrition. *Nutr Clin Pract.* 2015;30(3):371–382.

39. Thompson CW. Laboratory assessment. In: Charney P, Malone AM, eds. *ADA Pocket Guide to Nutrition Assessment*. 2nd ed. American Dietetic Association; 2009:129–130.

40. Suliburska J, Skrypnik K, Szulińska M, Kupsz J, Markuszewski L, Bogdański P. Diuretics, Ca-antagonists, and angiotensin-converting enzyme inhibitors affect zinc status in hypertensive patients on monotherapy: a randomized trial. *Nutrients*. 2018;10(9):1284.

41. Yanagisawa H. Clinical aspects of zinc deficiency. *Japan Med Assoc J*. 2002;127(2):261–268.

42. Al-Timimi DJ, Sulieman DM, Hussen KR. Zinc status in type 2 diabetic patients: relation to the progression of diabetic nephropathy. *J Clin Diagn Res*. 2014;8(11):CC04–CC8.

43. Berger MM, Cavadini C, Bart A, et al. Cutaneous copper and zinc losses in burns. *Burns*. 1992;18(5):373–380.

44. Lowe NM, Fekete K, Decsi T. Methods of assessment of zinc status in humans: a systematic review. *Am J Clin Nutr*. 2009;89(6):2040S–2051s.

45. Alker W, Haase H. Zinc and sepsis. *Nutrients*. 2018;10(8):976.

46. McClave SA, Martindale RG, Vanek VW, et al. Guidelines for the provision and assessment of nutrition support therapy in the adult critically ill patient: Society of Critical Care Medicine (SCCM) and American Society for Parenteral and Enteral Nutrition (ASPEN). *JPEN J Parenter Enteral Nutr*. 2009;33(3):277–316.

47. Esper DH. Utilization of nutrition-focused physical assessment in identifying micronutrient deficiencies. *Nutr Clin Pract*. 2015;30(2):194–202.

48. Stechmiller JK, Cowan L, Logan KM. Nutrition support for wound healing. *Support Line*. 2009;31:2–7.

49. Lin PH, Sermersheim M, Li H, Lee PHU, Steinberg SM, Ma J. Zinc in wound healing modulation. *Nutrients*. 2017;10(1):16.

50. Lazarus JH. The importance of iodine in public health. *Environ Geochem Health*. 2015;37:605–618.

51. Pearce EN, Lazarus JH, Moreno-Reyes R, Zimmermann MB. Consequences of iodine deficiency and excess in pregnant women: an overview of current knowns and unknowns. *Am J Clin Nutr*. 2016;104(Suppl 3):918S–923S.

52. Aschner JL, Aschner M. Nutritional aspects of manganese homeostasis. *Mol Aspects Med*. 2005;26(4–5):353–362.

53. *Dietary Reference Intakes for vitamin A, vitamin K, arsenic, boron, chromium, copper, iodine, iron, manganese, molybdenum, nickel, silicon, vanadium, and zinc*. Institute of Medicine, Food and Nutrition Board. National Academies Press; 2001.

54. Glinoer D. The importance of iodine nutrition during pregnancy. *Public Health Nutr*. 2007;10(12A):1542–1546.

55. Zimmermann MB, Köhrle J. The impact of iron and selenium deficiencies on iodine and thyroid metabolism: biochemistry and relevance to public health. *Thyroid*. 2002;12(10):867–878.

56. Zimmermann, M. Methods to assess iron and iodine status. *Br J Nutr*. 2008;99(S3):S2–S9.

57. Rose HR, Zulfiqar H. *Jod Basedow Syndrome*. StatPearls Publishing; 2021.

58. Zimmermann MB, Boelaert K. Iodine deficiency and thyroid disorders. *Lancet Diabetes Endocrinol*. 2015;3(4):286–295.

59. Zimmermann MB. Iodine deficiency. *Endocr Rev*. 2009;30(4):376–408.

60. Talbott SM, Hµghes K, eds. *The Health Professional's Guide to Dietary Supplements*. Lippincott Williams and Wilkins; 2007:272–320.

61. Tani LSK, Dennouni-Medjati N, Toubhans B, Charlet L. Selenium deficiency – from soil to thyroid cancer. *Appl Sci*. 2020;10(15):5368.

62. US Department of Health and Human Services, Centers for Disease Control and Prevention. Trace elements: selenium. In: National Report of Biochemical Indicators of Diet and Nutrition in the US Population 1999–2002. Published July, 2008. Accessed April 23, 2021. www.cdc.gov/nutritionreport/pdf/nr_ch4b.pdf.

63. Mayo Clinic Laboratories. Test Catalog. Accessed September 6, 2021. www.mayocliniclabs.com/test-catalog/.

64. Brown KM, Arthur JR. Selenium, selenoproteins and human health: a review. *Public Health Nutr*. 2001;4(2B):593–599.

65. Bhattacharya PT, Misra SR, Hussain M. Nutritional aspects of essential trace elements in oral health and disease: an extensive review. *Scientifica (Cairo)*. 2016;2016:5464373.

66. Fessler TA. Nutrition support 360: copper deficiency. *Today's Dietitian*. 2017;19(4):16.

67. Braunschweig C. Minerals and Trace Elements. In: Matarese LE, Gottschlich MM, eds. *Contemporary Nutrition Support Practice: A Clinical Guide*. Elsevier – Health Sciences Division; 1998:163–173.

68. Baldari S, Di Rocco G, Toietta G. Current biomedical use of copper chelation therapy. *Int J Mol Sci*. 2020;21(3):1069.

69. Delvin E, Levy E. Trace elements: functions and assessment of status through laboratory testing. In: Clarke W, Marzinke MA, eds. *Contemporary Practice in Clinical Chemistry*. 4th ed. Academic Press; 2020:851–864.

70. Lucchini R, Albini E, Placidi D, et al. Brain magnetic resonance imaging and manganese exposure. *Neurotoxicology*. 2000;21(5):769–775.

71. Parenteral Nutrition Trace Element Product Shortage Considerations. American Society for Parenteral and Enteral Nutrition. Accessed September 6, 2021. www.nutritioncare.org/News/Product_Shortages/Parenteral_Nutrition_Trace_Element_Product_Shortage_Considerations/.

72. Vanek VW, Borum P, Buchman A, et al. ASPEN position paper: recommendations for changes in commercially available parenteral multivitamin and multi-trace element products. *Nutr Clin Pract*. 2012;27(4):440–449.

73. Jin J, Mulesa L, Carrilero Rouillet M. Trace elements in parenteral nutrition: considerations for the prescribing clinician. *Nutrients*. 2017;9(5):440.

74. Ratliff A, Jaroch L, Nishnick A. Parenteral nutrition. In: DeChicco R, Coughlin K L, Escuro A, Jezerski D, Nowak D, eds. *Nutrition Support Handbook*. 4th ed. Cleveland Clinic; 2020:88–99.

11 Treatment – Acute Illness-Related Malnutrition

Christan Bury

CONTENTS

I INTRODUCTION

The treatment for malnutrition is dependent on the current etiology specific to the patient, which includes the extent of the inflammatory process. Acute illness or injury is associated with a significant inflammatory response, the extent and degree of which can predispose one to malnutrition, worsen existing malnutrition, and thwart intended treatments for malnutrition.[1-4] In acute illness-related malnutrition, immediate treatment should be based on nutrition guidelines for acute or critical illness, regardless of the etiology of the malnutrition that may be present on admission. It is therefore important that the registered dietitian nutritionist (RDN) thoroughly assess patients in order to identify the cause(s) of malnutrition, which will guide treatment and monitoring. See Chapter 12 for treatment for chronic illness-related malnutrition and Chapter 13 for treatment for social/environmental or starvation-related malnutrition.

This chapter reviews interventions for the prevention, treatment and monitoring of acute illness-related malnutrition.

DOI: 10.1201/9781003177586-11

II   NUTRITION THERAPY: TIMING AND MODALITY

In acute illness-related malnutrition, the majority of patients are considered critically ill and receive care in the intensive care unit (ICU). Some patients are able to take nutrition orally, in which case oral nutrition supplements and diet modifications can be made to optimize energy and protein intake. Strategies to promote oral intake are reviewed in Chapter 12 and can be used with acute illness-related malnutrition when appropriate. However, many critically ill patients are unable to receive nutrition via the oral route and thus require nutrition support – enteral nutrition (EN) or parenteral nutrition (PN).

It is well known that feeding patients adequately and preferably via the oral/enteral route improves ICU outcomes, such as mortality and length of stay (LOS), as well as improved gastrointestinal (GI) integrity. In malnourished medical patients, early nutrition support is associated with improved survival in non-elective hospital readmission rates[5] as well as reduced malnutrition severity at discharge.[6] However, evidence for the ideal route, amount, and specific breakdown of macronutrient content remains less definitive in the literature.

Malnutrition risk and status play a key role in the timing of nutrition interventions. In patients with low nutritional risk and low disease severity, specialized nutrition therapy/support is not required in the first week of an ICU stay.[7] However, in critically ill patients with high nutritional risk, or in those who are already malnourished, nutrition support should be initiated as soon as possible. If volitional intake cannot be maintained within 24–48 hours, medical nutrition therapy and/or EN should be considered in all patients, regardless of nutrition status or risk.[7,8]

A   ENTERAL NUTRITION

If oral intake is inadequate, and the GI tract is functional, EN should be initiated within 24–48 hours of the onset of acute illness, once the patient is fully resuscitated and/or stable.[7,8] EN should be withheld in patients with nausea, vomiting, or significant abdominal distention; however, absence of bowel sounds, a bowel movement, or flatus is not a contraindication to EN initiation.[7] EN can also be initiated in patients placed in the prone position.[9]

The aim of feeding is to meet > 80% of energy and protein needs within 48–72 hours of ICU admission, then increase to goal over the first week.[7] The goal of EN support in the ICU is to maintain gut integrity,[10] modulate the immune response,[11] and attenuate the metabolic response to stress[12].

For the majority of ICU patients, a standard polymeric isotonic or near isotonic formula is appropriate.[7] Specialized EN formulas may be beneficial for a subset of ICU patients, which is discussed in a future section. Most critically ill patients can be enterally fed into the stomach, with no difference in clinical outcomes including LOS, incidence of pneumonia, or mortality, compared to those fed into the small bowel.[13] Post-pyloric EN infusion is encouraged in patients at risk of aspiration and those intolerant of gastric EN.[7]

Whichever route or EN formula is chosen, it is prudent to ensure adequate infusion, and efforts to optimize this may include promotility agents for GI tolerance, or even rate-based adjustments to account for interruptions. Gastric residual volume

(GRV) should not routinely be monitored as it does not reflect EN tolerance nor does it correlate with incidence of pneumonia,[14,15] emesis, or aspiration.[16] More appropriate steps to monitor EN tolerance include daily bedside assessments as well as evaluation of radiological films and aspiration risks.[7]

B   PARENTERAL NUTRITION

When use of the GI tract is not feasible, PN is recommended. In patients who are low nutritional risk, PN should not be started in the first seven days of critical illness,[7] as the use of PN in previously well-nourished patients provides little benefit over this time frame.[17] However, if it is anticipated that EN or an oral diet will not be started within a week (e.g. permanent or prolonged PN-dependence, as with short bowel syndrome, or bowel discontinuity that will require additional surgery) then the clinician should not wait to start PN. For critically ill patients who are high nutritional risk or who are severely malnourished, PN should be started as soon as medically possible,[7] as the use of PN in this population is associated with fewer complications[18] when compared to withholding PN. Furthermore, withholding PN in malnourished patients unable to receive or tolerate EN is associated with a significantly higher risk of mortality as well as a trend toward higher infection rates.[19] Even in patients where EN is tolerated but not meeting > 60% of needs, supplemental PN (SPN) should be considered to increase energy and protein provision starting between days seven and ten of critical illness, but not before.[7] Early SPN provides little benefit compared to hypocaloric EN alone,[19] whereas later initiation of SPN is associated with shorter LOS, fewer infections, and a greater average reduction of healthcare costs.[20]

Once PN is started in any capacity, careful monitoring is imperative, including the use of protocols and nutrition-support teams, individualized dosing of macronutrients, micronutrients, and trace elements based on severity of illness and other clinical factors, as well as appropriate blood glucose control. Table 11.1 describes best practices for implementing nutrition therapy/support (oral, EN and PN) in the critically ill.

TABLE 11.1
Nutrition Therapy Interventions for the Critically Ill[7,8]

Malnutrition status	Feeding route	Timing
Low-risk / no malnutrition	Oral	ASAP
	EN	By ICU day 7
	PN	By ICU day 7 when EN not feasible
		By ICU day 7–10 when EN < 60% of energy and protein needs
High-risk / severe malnutrition	Oral	As able
	EN	Within 24–48 h of onset of critical illness
	PN	ASAP when EN not feasible

Abbreviations: ASAP = as soon as possible; EN = enteral nutrition; ICU = intensive care unit; PN = parenteral nutrition.

III ESTIMATING NUTRIENT NEEDS

Estimating energy and protein needs in the critically ill can be challenging due to many variables including body habitus, limitations of the ICU environment, as well as conditions that frequently change, including body temperature, ventilator settings and clinical condition. Whichever method is used to determine needs, it is imperative for the clinician to practice clinical judgment and closely monitor tolerance and progression of nutrition therapies.

A ENERGY

The gold standard for estimating energy needs is indirect calorimetry (IC), which evaluates the gas exchange of mechanically ventilated patients to precisely calculate energy needs and substrate utilization. The use of IC may be limited at most institutions due to cost, equipment and staff availability, and ICU variables including the use of certain inspiratory gasses, increased ventilator settings, the presence of air leak in chest tubes, or being on extra-corporal membrane oxygenation.[21]

In lieu of IC, predictive equations and/or weight-based equations are often used. Many predictive equations have been published, such as the Penn State, Ireton Jones, Harris-Benedict and Mifflin St. Jeor, with varying ranges of accuracy, and to date there is no single predictive equation universally accepted in the critically ill.[22–27] Weight-based equations are acceptable, practical, and efficient for use in the ICU patient, with the intent to use the most up-to-date dry weight possible, or ideal body weight in the case of an elevated body mass index (BMI). See Table 11.2 for ASPEN recommendations on when to use ideal vs. actual weight in calculating energy and protein needs. Over-feeding (particularly energy) any critically ill patient is not recommended, as it is associated with increased morbidity and mortality.[7,27,28] See Chapter 8 for further information on assessment of macronutrient needs.

B PROTEIN

Protein provision in the critically ill may be more important than total energy intake,[29] as higher protein intake is associated with improved wound healing and immune

---

TABLE 11.2
Estimation of Energy and Protein Needs in the Critically Ill[7]

BMI	Calories	Protein
BMI < 30	25–30/35 kcal/kg actual BW	1.2–2 g pro/kg actual BW
All classes of obesity	Do not exceed 65–70% REE	1.2–2 g pro/kg IBW
BMI 30–50	11–14 kcal/kg actual BW	2 g pro/kg IBW
BMI > 50	22–25 kcal/kg IBW	> 2.5 g pro/kg IBW

Abbreviations: BMI = body mass index; BW = body weight; REE = resting energy expenditure; IBW = ideal body weight.

function, maintenance of lean body mass[7] and overall improved ICU outcomes, such as LOS and mortality.[29–32] In fact, one study demonstrated that mechanically ventilated patients who received intended protein (1.3 g pro/kg) and energy delivery had a 50% reduction in 28-day mortality, while no decrease in mortality was seen in those patients who met energy targets alone.[29] For hospitalized patients taking oral nutrition, early administration of specialized, nutrient-dense oral nutritional supplements with high protein and hydroxymethylbutyrate has been associated with decreased post-discharge mortality and improved nutritional status.[33] Furthermore, a recent meta-analysis showed that early oral feeding of protein in the post-op period resulted in a statistically significant reduction in mortality, surgical-site infections, postop nausea and vomiting, and serious post-op complications, as well as significant improvement in outcomes.[34]

Critically ill patients will inevitably lose muscle mass during the ICU stay,[35,36] due in part to inflammation and immobility, and unfortunately muscle loss cannot be completely prevented with nutrition support.[37] The goal of nutrition therapy in this population is to mitigate protein losses and preserve muscle function. In fact, Fetterplace et al. demonstrated that muscle loss was attenuated in ICU patients receiving an average of 25 kcal/kg/d and 1.2 g pro/kg/d compared to those who received 18 kcal/kg/d and 0.75 g pro/kg/d at the time of ICU discharge.[6] The specific method of delivering protein has recently been questioned, as some research has shown intermittent bolus feeding of protein (and energy), as opposed to continuous infusion, has potential benefits including preservation of muscle, intestinal and hepatic tissue, as well as improved glycemic control.[38] More research is needed, as there are no guidelines at this time recommending bolus over continuous feeding in the critically ill patient. While muscle catabolism will inherently happen in critical illness, early mobilization with the use of physical therapy (PT) and adequate provision of protein has been shown to mitigate muscle loss.[39]

IV INDIVIDUALIZED APPROACH TO FEEDING THE CRITICALLY ILL

Critically ill patients are a heterogeneous population, with each individual displaying unique needs. The nutrition intervention is dependent on the clinical situation and nutrition status, and an individualized nutritional support regimen improves outcomes[40] and can improve mortality.[41] The following sections highlight common clinical conditions encountered in the ICU setting.

A SEPSIS

A wealth of evidence supports feeding critically ill patients early, ideally once they are hemodynamically stable, as delayed feeding can worsen malnutrition. Patients who are septic have a dramatically increased metabolic demand. Klaude et al. showed that in sepsis protein synthesis is unchanged while simultaneously protein degradation is dramatically increased.[42] Data regarding feeding patients with septic shock are conflicting, with some guidelines supporting early trophic/hypocaloric or early full EN, while conversely other guidelines suggest withholding EN until the patient is fully resuscitated.[7,43] Furthermore, the European Society for Clinical Nutrition and Metabolism (ESPEN) suggests that no evidenced-based answer can be proposed at this time given the lack of interventional studies.[8] In a recent review of the outcomes and safety of providing early EN in shock, the authors concluded that current evidence suggests early low-dose EN (i.e. trickle rate) is well tolerated and associated with preserved splenic blood flow and improved clinical outcomes.[44] Incidentally, both the American Society for Parenteral and Enteral Nutrition and the Society for Critical Care Medicine (ASPEN/SCCM), as well as the ESPEN guidelines, do not recommend the use of early PN in severe sepsis or septic shock regardless of nutrition risk or status.[7,8]

B SURGERY

Specific EN interventions in surgical ICU (SICU) patients differ from that of medical (MICU). In MICU and some SICU patients, a standard polymeric EN formula is recommended, as specialty disease-specific formulas (e.g. diabetic, pulmonary, renal or hepatic, elemental and immune-modulating) offer no clear benefit (although there is also no evidence that specialty formulas cause harm).[7] However, in acute postoperative SICU patients, an immune-modulating EN (IMEN) formula containing fish oils and arginine is recommended, as its use has been associated with reduced infection rates and hospital LOS.[7,45] SICU patients have increased energy and protein needs in the immediate post-operative period compared to the pre-operative period[46] due to the alterations associated with the physiological stress of surgery. During postoperative recovery, muscle loss may be hastened by malnutrition prior to surgery, as critically ill SICU patients deemed moderately or severely malnourished[47] have been shown to lose significantly more quadriceps muscle per day during a 10-day ICU stay compared with patients without malnutrition.[36] For all critically ill patients, infection, fevers, wounds, and other clinical challenges can also increase metabolic demand, thus it is important for the clinician to monitor the patient's clinical status closely to adjust medical nutrition therapy interventions accordingly.

C OBESITY

Estimating calorie and protein needs in obese critically ill patients can be challenging. BMI is used to define obesity; however, it does not account for body composition, so nutritional needs may vary considerably between patients with the same BMI. Permissive underfeeding, generally defined as providing approximately 70% of estimated calorie needs, has been shown in some studies to be more beneficial than full feeding in obese patients. However, it should be noted that permissive underfeeding refers to energy only; protein needs are high in critical illness and should be met even while underfeeding calories.[7] Table 11.2 provides more detail on calorie and protein recommendations for obese patients.

V MONITORING AND EVALUATION

Monitoring and evaluating patients with acute illness-related malnutrition can be difficult, as edema may mask muscle and fat losses. Objective laboratory values such as albumin, prealbumin and transferrin have long been suggested for use in the setting of critical illness; however, they are negative acute-phase proteins and indicative of severity of inflammation rather than nutrition status or adequacy of nutrient delivery.[7,50] More appropriate objective measures for monitoring body mass and malnutrition are emerging, including computed tomography scans and the use of bedside ultrasound. These novel methods show promise in improving the RDNs' evaluation of our most vulnerable patients (see Chapter 5). Finally, more practical ways to monitor progress of the critically ill include evaluating the clinical picture/ICU course such as time and duration of physical therapy sessions, time on mechanical ventilation, and an overall progression towards independence from ICU care.

Despite the application of best practices outlined in established guidelines for nutrition support in the critically ill, the inflammatory process still may prove difficult to overcome, leading to undesirable outcomes such as increased ICU and hospital LOS, longer time on mechanical ventilation, and increased mortality. For instance, Merker et al. showed that patients with significant inflammation (defined by the authors as a C-reactive protein (CRP) > 10 mg/dL) did not benefit from nutritional support in regard to 30-day mortality, whereas patients with a low or moderate inflammatory process (CRP < 10 mg/dL), experienced a significant reduction in 30-day mortality.[4]

Using clinical judgment, practitioners should apply established practice guidelines, individualize nutrition interventions, and closely monitor the efficacy of those interventions in an effort to give a patient the best chance of leaving the ICU with maximal function intact.

VI   BEYOND THE ICU

Critical illness does not resolve easily or abruptly. Inflammation can decrease gradually, and organ dysfunction caused or exacerbated by acute illness may resolve slowly or not at all, gradually shifting many patients to a state of chronic illness. Similarly, acute illness-related malnutrition may gradually develop into chronic disease-related malnutrition, in which inflammation is low or absent. This is a continuum, and individual to each person, thus patients should be monitored closely to reassess nutritional needs and reevaluate the malnutrition etiology in order to provide appropriate treatments. Failure to do so, such as continuing to permissively underfeed a patient longer than recommended, can significantly worsen malnutrition and clinical outcomes.

VII   CONCLUSION

In critically ill patients, primary recommendations from both research and clinical expertise include protocol-based nutrition support, and the appreciation of the inherent heterogeneity of patients in the ICU in order to create a specialized, evidence-based nutrition support regimen to best meet the needs of the individual to optimize post-ICU outcomes.[7] Insufficient nutrition treatment in critical illness is associated with poor outcomes, and can cause or worsen malnutrition.[7]

REFERENCES

1. Jensen GL. Inflammation as the key interface of the medical and nutrition universes: a provocative examination of the future of clinical nutrition and medicine. *JPEN J Parenter Enteral Nutr.* 2006;30(5):453–463.

2. Jensen GL, Bistrian B, Roubenoff R, Heimburger DC. Malnutrition syndromes: a conundrum vs continuum. *JPEN J Parenter Enteral Nutr.* 2009;33(6):710–716.

3. Jensen GL, Mirtallo J, Compher C, et al. Adult starvation and disease-related malnutrition: a proposal for etiology-based diagnosis in the clinical practice setting from the International Consensus Guideline Committee. *JPEN J Parenter Enteral Nutr.* 2010;34(2):156–159.

4. Merker M, Felder M, Gueissaz L, et al. Association of baseline inflammation with effectiveness of nutritional support among patients with disease-related malnutrition: a secondary analysis of a randomized clinical trial. *JAMA Netw Open.* 2020;3(3):e200663.

5. Gomes F, Baumgartner A, Bounoure L, et al. Association of nutritional support with clinical outcomes among medical inpatients who are malnourished or at nutritional risk: an updated systematic review and meta-analysis. *JAMA Netw Open.* 2019;2(11):e1915138.

6. Fetterplace K, Deane AM, Tierney A, et al. Targeted full energy and protein delivery in critically ill patients: a pilot randomized controlled trial (FEED Trial). *JPEN J Parenter Enteral Nutr.* 2018;42(8):1252–1262.

7. McClave SA, Taylor BE, Martindale RG, et al. Guidelines for the provision and assessment of nutrition support therapy in the adult critically ill patient: Society of Critical Care Medicine (SCCM) and American Society for Parenteral and Enteral Nutrition (ASPEN). *JPEN J Parenter Enteral Nutr.* 2016;40(2):159–211.

8. Singer P, Blaser AR, Berger MM, et al. ESPEN guideline on clinical nutrition in the intensive care unit. *Clin Nutr.* 2019;38(1):48–79.

9. Handu D, Moloney L, Rozga M, Cheng F. Malnutrition care during the COVID-19 pandemic: considerations for Registered Dietitian Nutritionists. *J Acad Nutr Diet.* 2021;121(5):979–987.

10. Kang W, Kudsk KA. Is there evidence that the gut contributes to mucosal immunity in humans? *JPEN J Parenter Enteral Nutr.* 2007;31(3):246–258.

11. Windsor AC, Kanwar S, Li AG, et al. Compared with parenteral nutrition, enteral feeding attenuates the acute phase response and improves disease severity in acute pancreatitis. *Gut.* 1998;42(3):431–435.

12. Ammori BJ. Importance of the early increase in intestinal permeability in critically ill patients. *Eur J Surg.* 2002;168(11):660–661; author reply 662.

13. Davies AR, Morrison SS, Bailey MJ, et al. A multicenter, randomized controlled trial comparing early nasojejunal with nasogastric nutrition in critical illness. *Crit Care Med.* 2012;40(8):2342–2348.

14. Montejo JC, Minambres E, Bordeje L, et al. Gastric residual volume during enteral nutrition in ICU patients: the REGANE study. *Intensive Care Med.* 2010;36(8):1386–1393.

15. Pinilla JC, Samphire J, Arnold C, Liu L, Thiessen B. Comparison of gastrointestinal tolerance to two enteral feeding protocols in critically ill patients: a prospective, randomized controlled trial. *JPEN J Parenter Enteral Nutr.* 2001;25(2):81–86.

16. McClave SA, Snider HL. Clinical use of gastric residual volumes as a monitor for patients on enteral tube feeding. *JPEN J Parenter Enteral Nutr.* 2002;26(6 Suppl):S43–48; discussion S49–50.

17. Heyland DK, MacDonald S, Keefe L, Drover JW. Total parenteral nutrition in the critically ill patient: a meta-analysis. *JAMA*. 1998;280(23):2013–2019.

18. Braunschweig CL, Levy P, Sheean PM, Wang X. Enteral compared with parenteral nutrition: a meta-analysis. *Am J Clin Nutr*. 2001;74(4):534–542.

19. Jonker MA, Hermsen JL, Sano Y, Heneghan AF, Lan J, Kudsk KA. Small intestine mucosal immune system response to injury and the impact of parenteral nutrition. *Surgery*. 2012;151(2):278–286.

20. Casaer MP, Mesotten D, Hermans G, et al. Early versus late parenteral nutrition in critically ill adults. *N Engl J Med*. 2011;365(6):506–517.

21. Schlein KM, Coulter SP. Best practices for determining resting energy expenditure in critically ill adults. *Nutr Clin Pract*. 2014;29(1):44–55.

22. Faisy C, Guerot E, Diehl JL, Labrousse J, Fagon JY. Assessment of resting energy expenditure in mechanically ventilated patients. *Am J Clin Nutr*. 2003;78(2):241–249.

23. Frankenfield DC, Coleman A, Alam S, Cooney RN. Analysis of estimation methods for resting metabolic rate in critically ill adults. *JPEN J Parenter Enteral Nutr*. 2009;33(1):27–36.

24. Ireton-Jones C, Jones JD. Improved equations for predicting energy expenditure in patients: the Ireton-Jones Equations. *Nutr Clin Pract*. 2002;17(1):29–31.

25. Mifflin MD, St Jeor ST, Hill LA, Scott BJ, Daugherty SA, Koh YO. A new predictive equation for resting energy expenditure in healthy individuals. *Am J Clin Nutr*. 1990;51(2):241–247.

26. Stucky CC, Moncure M, Hise M, Gossage CM, Northrop D. How accurate are resting energy expenditure prediction equations in obese trauma and burn patients? *JPEN J Parenter Enteral Nutr*. 2008;32(4):420–426.

27. Neelemaat F, van Bokhorst-de van der Schueren MA, Thijs A, Seidell JC, Weijs PJ. Resting energy expenditure in malnourished older patients at hospital admission and three months after discharge: predictive equations versus measurements. *Clin Nutr*. 2012;31(6):958–966.

28. Klein CJ, Stanek GS, Wiles CE, 3rd. Overfeeding macronutrients to critically ill adults: metabolic complications. *J Am Diet Assoc*. 1998;98(7):795–806.

29. Weijs PJ, Stapel SN, de Groot SD, et al. Optimal protein and energy nutrition decreases mortality in mechanically ventilated, critically ill patients: a prospective observational cohort study. *JPEN J Parenter Enteral Nutr*. 2012;36(1):60–68.

30. Alberda C, Gramlich L, Jones N, et al. The relationship between nutritional intake and clinical outcomes in critically ill patients: results of an international multicenter observational study. *Intensive Care Med*. 2009;35(10):1728–1737.

31. Elke G, Wang M, Weiler N, Day AG, Heyland DK. Close to recommended caloric and protein intake by enteral nutrition is associated with better clinical outcome of critically ill septic patients: secondary analysis of a large international nutrition database. *Crit Care*. 2014;18(1):R29.

32. Allingstrup MJ, Esmailzadeh N, Wilkens Knudsen A, et al. Provision of protein and energy in relation to measured requirements in intensive care patients. *Clin Nutr*. 2012;31(4):462–468.

33. Deutz NE, Matheson EM, Matarese LE, et al. Readmission and mortality in malnourished, older, hospitalized adults treated with a specialized oral nutritional supplement: A randomized clinical trial. *Clin Nutr*. 2016;35(1):18–26.

34. Pu H, Heighes PT, Simpson F, et al. Early oral protein-containing diets following elective lower gastrointestinal tract surgery in adults: a meta-analysis of randomized clinical trials. *Perioper Med (Lond)*. 2021;10(1):10.

35. Puthucheary ZA, Rawal J, McPhail M, et al. Acute skeletal muscle wasting in critical illness. *JAMA.* 2013;310(15):1591–1600.

36. Bury C, DeChicco R, Nowak D, et al. Use of bedside ultrasound to assess muscle changes in the critically ill surgical patient. *JPEN J Parenter Enteral Nutr.* 2021;45(2):394–402.

37. Ishibashi N, Plank LD, Sando K, Hill GL. Optimal protein requirements during the first 2 weeks after the onset of critical illness. *Crit Care Med.* 1998;26(9):1529–1535.

38. Hooper MH, Marik PE. Controversies and misconceptions in intensive care unit nutrition. *Clin Chest Med.* 2015;36(3):409–418.

39. McKendry J, Thomas ACQ, Phillips SM. muscle mass loss in the older critically ill population: potential therapeutic strategies. *Nutr Clin Pract.* 2020;35(4):607–616.

40. Schuetz P, Fehr R, Baechli V, et al. Individualised nutritional support in medical inpatients at nutritional risk: a randomised clinical trial. *Lancet.* 2019;393(10188): 2312–2321.

41. Baumgartner A, Hasenboehler F, Cantone J, et al. Effect of nutritional support in patients with lower respiratory tract infection: Secondary analysis of a randomized clinical trial. *Clin Nutr.* 2021;40(4):1843–1850.

42. Klaude M, Mori M, Tjader I, Gustafsson T, Wernerman J, Rooyackers O. Protein metabolism and gene expression in skeletal muscle of critically ill patients with sepsis. *Clin Sci (Lond).* 2012;122(3):133–142.

43. Rhodes A, Evans LE, Alhazzani W, et al. Surviving sepsis campaign: international guidelines for management of sepsis and septic shock: 2016. *Intensive Care Med.* 2017;43(3):304–377.

44. Patel JJ, Rice T, Heyland DK. Safety and outcomes of early enteral nutrition in circulatory shock. *JPEN J Parenter Enteral Nutr.* 2020;44(5):779–784.

45. Drover JW, Dhaliwal R, Weitzel L, Wischmeyer PE, Ochoa JB, Heyland DK. Perioperative use of arginine-supplemented diets: a systematic review of the evidence. *J Am Coll Surg.* 2011;212(3):385–399.

46. Long CL, Schaffel N, Geiger JW, Schiller WR, Blakemore WS. Metabolic response to injury and illness: estimation of energy and protein needs from indirect calorimetry and nitrogen balance. *JPEN J Parenter Enteral Nutr.* 1979;3(6):452–456.

47. White JV, Guenter P, Jensen G, et al. Consensus statement: Academy of Nutrition and Dietetics and American Society for Parenteral and Enteral Nutrition: characteristics recommended for the identification and documentation of adult malnutrition (undernutrition). *JPEN J Parenter Enteral Nutr.* 2012;36(3):275–283.

48. Makarenkova VP, Bansal V, Matta BM, Perez LA, Ochoa JB. CD11b+/Gr-1+ myeloid suppressor cells cause T cell dysfunction after traumatic stress. *J Immunol.* 2006;176(4):2085–2094.

49. Marik PE, Flemmer M. The immune response to surgery and trauma: Implications for treatment. *J Trauma Acute Care Surg.* 2012;73(4):801–808.

50. Evans DC, Corkins MR, Malone A, et al. The use of visceral proteins as nutrition markers: an ASPEN position paper. *Nutr Clin Pract.* 2021;36(1):22–28.

12 Treatment – Chronic Illness-Related Malnutrition

Jennifer Doley and Michelle Bratton

CONTENTS

I   INTRODUCTION

The definition of chronic illness-related malnutrition varies depending on the criteria used; however, it is generally characterized by low levels of inflammation (continuous or recurrent) and illness of a duration greater than three months.[1,2] Chronic illness-related malnutrition may also result from disease-related symptoms, but without the presence of inflammation.[1] See Chapter 2 for further detail on diagnosis. Disease- and treatment-related symptoms that contribute to malnutrition include those that result in inadequate oral intake, altered nutrient metabolism, and impaired nutrient absorption.

Because chronic illness-related malnutrition encompasses a wide variety of causes and disease states, the breadth of treatments is greater than those used to address acute illness-related malnutrition. In order to develop a comprehensive and effective treatment plan, clinicians must recognize that many factors contribute to malnutrition in chronic illness. This chapter describes medical nutrition therapy (MNT) strategies to address these etiologies, including modifications to oral intake, enteral nutrition (EN), parenteral nutrition (PN) and nutrition counseling.

DOI: 10.1201/9781003177586-12

II   ETIOLOGY

Many symptoms, such as poor appetite and nausea, can result in inadequate oral intake; these symptoms may arise from the illness itself or as a result of treatments such as medications, and surgeries or other procedures. Metabolic derangements such as hypermetabolism, altered nutrient utilization, and impaired nutrient absorption can also contribute to chronic illness-related malnutrition.

A   INADEQUATE ORAL INTAKE

Inadequate oral intake is usually multifactorial, as many issues that adversely influence intake are interrelated.

1   Anorexia

Perhaps the most common symptom that precipitates inadequate intake in chronic illness is anorexia. Appetite is a complex process regulated by neuropeptides, neurotransmitters, hormones, and a number of sensory inputs such as smell and taste. Any alterations to these factors can contribute to anorexia, which is associated with many chronic conditions, including cancer, acquired immune deficiency syndrome (AIDS), chronic kidney disease, chronic obstructive pulmonary disease (COPD), and chronic liver disease.[3] A common metabolic cause of anorexia is increased cytokine production as seen in cancer, AIDS, COPD, and some inflammatory and autoimmune conditions.[4]

It is widely recognized that patients with cancer in particular often exhibit anorexia, with a reported incidence of 50% in newly diagnosed patients and 27 to 58% in those with advanced disease.[5] Additionally, many antineoplastic therapies, especially chemotherapy, include anorexia among their nutrition-related side effects. Anorexia is further complicated by the fact that it is often associated with symptoms such as nausea, early satiety and other gastrointestinal (GI) side effects.[4]

2   Dyspnea and Fatigue

The presence of dyspnea when eating often leaves patients describing that they feel as if they can either breathe or eat, but doing both simultaneously is a challenge.[6] Similarly, patients with chronic heart failure often report limitations in eating and food preparation due to fatigue and an increased effort to breathe. Fatigue is also a well-known side effect of cancer and its treatment, with 30% to 60% of patients reporting this symptom.[7] Fatigue and dyspnea can impede a person's ability to shop for and prepare food, and patients may miss meals because they are resting.

3   Dysphagia

Dysphagia is also a risk factor for inadequate intake, and occurs in 30 to 50% of patients in the acute stage of a stroke. These patients can also exhibit facial and upper body weakness that makes self-feeding difficult.[8] Swallowing dysfunction is also frequently seen in patients with head/neck or esophageal cancer, amyotrophic lateral sclerosis, and Parkinson's disease, with resulting unintentional weight loss.[9] Normal aging can also cause a decline in swallowing ability.[10]

4 Difficulty Chewing

Issues with the mouth and teeth, including poor dentition, mouth sores or pain, xerostomia, and taste changes, can directly contribute to inadequate intake. Poor dentition, such as tooth loss, tooth pain or poorly fitting dentures, can result in difficulty chewing. This limits the types of foods an individual is able to consume, such as some raw fruits and vegetables, meats, and nuts, many of which are high in energy, protein, and phytonutrients. Mouth sores or pain are most commonly associated with cancer treatments such as chemotherapeutic agents and radiation to the head or neck; however, they are also side effects of some micronutrient deficiencies and infectious agents such as herpes simplex and candida.

5 Other Gastrointestinal Symptoms

Many GI symptoms may contribute to inadequate oral intake, including nausea, vomiting, diarrhea, and constipation. These symptoms may be transient when caused by temporary issues such as food-borne illness, emotional distress or short-term use of some medications. However, if prolonged, these GI symptoms can significantly impair oral intake and contribute to malnutrition. Myriad diseases or conditions, GI or otherwise, as well as their treatments can precipitate these symptoms.

Effective treatment for inadequate intake is highly individualized. Ultimately, the ideal treatment is management of the underlying disease or symptoms that inhibit intake, but often this is not a feasible option. In these cases, MNT plays a critical role in maximizing nutritional intake in order to prevent or treat malnutrition. Tables 12.1–12.3 list common causes of oral, GI and constitutional symptoms that may result in inadequate intake.

TABLE 12.1
Etiology of Oral Symptoms That May Impair Intake[11–14]

Problem	Common causes
Mouth sores or pain / difficulty chewing	• Head/neck radiation • Oral infections, e.g. herpes simplex or candida • Medications including chemotherapy, aspirin, penicillin, phenytoin, streptomycin • Micronutrient deficiencies (especially B vitamins) • Ill-fitting dentures, poor dentition / oral hygiene
Xerostomia / thick saliva	• Dehydration • Head/neck radiation • Medical conditions including DM, PD, viral infections, RA, Sjogren's syndrome, scleroderma, primary biliary cirrhosis, SLE • Increasing age • Medications including antiemetics, anti-Parkinson's, antihistamines, beta-blockers, calcium channel blockers, antidepressants, antipsychotics, diuretics • Polypharmacy

(Continued)

TABLE 12.1 (Continued)
Etiology of Oral Symptoms That May Impair Intake[11-14]

Problem	Common causes
Altered taste perception	• Head/neck radiation • Zinc deficiency • Medications including chemotherapy, antibiotics, antifungals, antipsychotics, corticosteroids, glipizide, diuretics, phenytoin
Difficulty swallowing	• Medical conditions including stroke, TBI, PD, MS, ALS; oral, pharyngeal, or esophageal tumors or surgery; dementia or other cognitive impairment; prolonged oro-tracheal intubation • Xerostomia • Increasing age, especially in those with frailty or sarcopenia • Head/neck radiation

Abbreviations: DM = diabetes mellitus; PD = Parkinson's disease; RA = rheumatoid arthritis; SLE = systemic lupus erythematosus; TBI = traumatic brain injury; MS = multiple sclerosis; ALS = amyotrophic lateral sclerosis.

TABLE 12.2
Etiology of GI Symptoms That May Impair Intake[15-17]

Problem	Common causes
Early satiety	• Gastroparesis • Surgical alterations to stomach (e.g. gastrectomy or gastric bypass) • Ascites or abdominal tumor compression of the stomach • Gastric outlet obstruction • Polypharmacy
Nausea	• Medical conditions including gastroparesis, cancer, gastritis, SBO, IBD, IBS, cyclic vomiting syndrome, functional dyspepsia, hepatobiliary disease, pancreatitis, scleroderma, SLE, renal disease, esophageal disorders, PD, CHF • Head/neck radiation • Medications including chemotherapy, antibiotics, opioids, anti-arrhythmics, anticonvulsants, NSAIDs, anticholinergics • Polypharmacy
Diarrhea	• Malabsorption (see Table 12.5) • GI infections (bacterial, viral, parasitic) • Medical conditions including IBD, diverticulitis, colon cancer, radiation colitis, hyperthyroidism, AUD, GI surgery (e.g. resection, gastric bypass, vagotomy), celiac disease, SBBO, IBS, lymphoma • Medications including laxatives, antacids, sugar alcohols, antibiotics, propranolol, hydralazine, ACE inhibitors, NSAIDs, metoclopramide, proton pump inhibitors

TABLE 12.2 (Continued)
Etiology of GI Symptoms That May Impair Intake[15–17]

Problem	Common causes
Constipation	• Dehydration, inadequate fluid intake • Low-fiber diet • Medical conditions including IBS, hypothyroidism, MS, PD, stroke, spinal cord injury, spina bifida, scleroderma, amyloidosis • Medications including opioids, NSAIDs, antihistamines, iron supplements, anti-Parkinson's, diuretics, anticonvulsants, antipsychotics, antacids • Sedentary lifestyle / limited mobility

Abbreviations: SBO = small bowel obstruction; IBD = inflammatory bowel disease; IBS = irritable bowel syndrome; SLE = systemic lupus erythematosus; PD = Parkinson's disease; CHF = congestive heart failure; NSAIDs = non-steroidal anti-inflammatory drugs; GI = gastrointestinal; AUD = alcohol use disorder; SBBO = small bowel bacterial overgrowth; ACE = angiotensin converting enzyme; MS = multiple sclerosis.

TABLE 12.3
Etiology of Constitutional Symptoms That May Impair Intake[18–20]

Problem	Common causes
Anorexia	• Alterations in taste or smell perception • Poor dentition / oral hygiene • Pain • GI symptoms including constipation, xerostomia, delayed gastric emptying, mouth pain, diarrhea • Medical conditions including cancer, COPD, CKD, chronic liver disease, RA, AIDS and other infectious diseases • Acute illness, especially infection • Psychological factors including depression and anxiety • Increasing age • Medications including chemotherapy, antibiotics, antifungals, antivirals, antipsychotics, tricyclic antidepressants
Fatigue	• Medical conditions including cancer, neurological disorders (e.g. stroke, TBI, PD, ALS, MS), inflammatory conditions (e.g. IBD, RA, SLE), chronic fatigue syndrome, end-stage disease / organ failure (e.g. hepatic, renal, cardiac, respiratory), sleep disorders, mental disorders (e.g. depression, stress, anxiety), acute and chronic infection, anemia, chronic pain • Malnutrition, iron deficiency • Medications including benzodiazepines, neuroleptics, antispastics, antiepileptic, antihistamines, narcotics/opioids

(*Continued*)

TABLE 12.3 (Continued)
Etiology of Constitutional Symptoms That May Impair Intake[18–20]

Problem	Common causes
Shortness of breath	• Conditions including acute respiratory illness or infection (e.g. pneumonia, flu, COVID-19), chronic respiratory illness (e.g. COPD, pulmonary fibrosis, asthma, lung cancer), obesity, cardiac conditions (e.g. cardiomyopathy, heart failure, aortic insufficiency, mitral valve stenosis), anxiety, iron deficiency / anemia, ALS

Abbreviations: GI = gastrointestinal; COPD = chronic obstructive pulmonary disease; CKD = chronic kidney disease; RA = rheumatoid arthritis; AIDS = acquired immune deficiency syndrome; TBI = traumatic brain injury; PD = Parkinson's disease; ALS = amyotrophic lateral sclerosis; MS = multiple sclerosis; IBD = inflammatory bowel disease; SLE = systemic lupus erythematosus; COVID-19 = coronavirus disease of 2019.

B   Metabolic Changes

In addition to the metabolic effects that contribute to anorexia, many diseases can alter metabolism, resulting in increased nutrient utilization, degradation, or losses. Metabolic changes are more difficult to mitigate than symptoms which reduce intake, as they are caused by chronic disease and thus may be prolonged or recurring. Effective management of the underlying disease to address metabolic changes is crucial; however, this may not be fully or even partially effective due to the degenerative nature of the condition, lack of treatment options, or inability to follow treatment regimens. Therefore, MNT plays a critical role in helping patients improve intake to meet increased nutrient demands.

C   Nutrient Absorption

Malabsorption can result from decreased GI absorptive surface area due to surgical resection (e.g. gastric bypass, intestinal resection), injury or inflammation of the GI mucosa (e.g. Crohn's disease, celiac disease), or insufficient enzyme production (e.g. chronic pancreatitis, pancreatic resection). Any macro- and/or micronutrients may be poorly absorbed depending on the underlying condition, the section of the GI tract affected or resected, and the severity of damage.

Treatment for malabsorption disorders, like other conditions that can lead to chronic malnutrition, is best addressed by treating the underlying cause. Malabsorption is more challenging in that it is generally not inherently curative, thus is best addressed by appropriate disease management. Treatment may include medications to increase GI absorptive capacity, disease management to reduce exacerbation of inflammation, and pancreatic enzyme replacement. However, MNT is one (or in some cases the only) treatment for chronic disease-related malnutrition caused by malabsorption. Successful MNT strategies depend on the condition and should be individualized to the patient, as symptoms and food intolerances can vary widely. Interventions may include avoidance of offending nutrients or foods, diet changes to reduce inflammation,

TABLE 12.4
Malabsorption: Common Causes, Diagnostic Tests and Treatment[21]

Cause	• Surgical resection
	◦ Gastric bypass
	◦ Gastrectomy
	◦ Small intestinal resections / SBS
	• GI inflammation
	◦ Celiac disease
	◦ Inflammatory bowel disease
	• Insufficient enzyme production
	◦ Chronic pancreatitis
	◦ Cystic fibrosis
	◦ Pancreatic resection
	◦ Lactose intolerance
Diagnosis	• Tests
	◦ Fat: 72 hour fecal fat test, fecal elastase test
	◦ Carbohydrate: hydrogen breath tests (lactose and fructose)
	• Signs/symptoms
	◦ Diarrhea
	◦ Post prandial urgency of defecation
	◦ Dyspepsia
	◦ Steatorrhea (bulky, pale, frothy or oily stools)
Treatment	• Individualize diet, keep food diary to identify offending foods
	• Eat small frequent meals
	• Increase calorie/protein intake to replace nutrient losses
	• Avoid sugar alcohols
	• Consider low FODMAP diet
	• Restrict fat if malabsorbed
	• Monitor for vitamin and mineral deficiencies, supplement as needed (water-miscible forms available if fat malabsorbed)
	• Supplement intake with MCTs (however, generally unpalatable and do not contain EFA)
	• Maintain hydration, consider oral rehydration solutions
	• Manage medication regimens, especially enzyme replacement (coordinate dose and timing with food intake)

Abbreviations: SBS = short bowel syndrome; GI = gastrointestinal; FODMAP = fermentable oligosaccharides, disaccharides, monosaccharides and polyols; MCT = medium chain triglycerides; EFA = essential fatty acids.

and increasing overall intake to compensate for GI losses. See Table 12.4 for common causes, diagnostic tests and treatment for malabsorption.

III MEDICAL NUTRITION THERAPY

As with any type of malnutrition, MNT intervention should start with an estimation of energy and protein needs and intake, in addition to any micronutrients that were identified during the nutrition assessment as deficient or at risk of deficiency.

Clinicians can more easily determine the most appropriate therapies when current intake is compared to estimated needs in order to assess the degree of intake deficiency. See Chapter 8 for assessing oral intake and estimating macronutrient needs.

MNT for chronic illness-related malnutrition may include changes to nutrient delivery, nutrition education or counseling, and coordination of care. These strategies must be individualized to the patient or client, in consideration of their symptoms, disease state, healthcare setting, and personal values and preferences.

A   NUTRIENT DELIVERY

Nutrient delivery encompasses oral intake from food and oral nutrition supplements (ONS), EN, or PN. Alterations to oral intake are generally preferred as the initial MNT intervention, as these treatments are most cost-effective and non-invasive. However, in patients who cannot safely consume food orally, or who have or are expected to have profound inadequate oral intake, initiation of nutrition support should not be delayed. Delays in the provision of adequate nutrition will increase the risk of, or worsen, malnutrition.

1   Food

Changes to food intake encompass the addition or elimination of certain foods in the diet, alterations in food texture and beverage consistency, or changes in the timing and/or portion sizes of meals or snacks. Tables 12.5–12.7 provide strategies to mitigate oral, GI and constitutional symptoms related to poor oral intake. Whenever possible, therapeutic diets that restrict intake of certain foods or nutrients in order to manage chronic disease should be avoided in malnourished patients.

Therapeutic diets are commonly prescribed for chronic disease management; however, restrictive diets reduce food intake which contributes to or exacerbates malnutrition. Liberalized diets are recommended in older adults in the long-term care setting to prevent malnutrition.[23] MNT for chronic disease management should be individualized, and unnecessary restrictions avoided when possible. However, the risk for malnutrition must be weighed against the risks associated with poor disease control. For example, a patient with diabetes mellitus who has esophageal cancer may become malnourished due to inadequate intake related to anorexia, nausea and difficulty swallowing. If blood glucose control is poor, is consumption of a consistent carbohydrate diet still recommended? Or is diabetes management via medications a better option, in order to allow the patient to consume a liberalized diet to promote adequate oral intake to more effectively treat malnutrition? These decisions should be made in conjunction with the medical team and aligned with the goals for disease management. Medication regimens such as diuretics to reduce edema or insulin to manage blood glucose, as well as other treatments such as dialysis to control electrolytes, may be implemented or modified to offset the consequences of a less restrictive diet.

2   Oral Nutrition Supplements

Oral nutrition supplements are defined as commercially prepared foods or beverages that are intended to provide additional nutrients, but are not meant to be a sole source of nutrition.[23] The effect of ONS consumption on malnutrition is difficult to

TABLE 12.5
Strategies to Mitigate Oral Symptoms That May Impair Oral Intake[11–14]

Problem	Intervention
Mouth sores or pain/difficulty chewing	• Avoid acidic and coarse foods, vinegar, hot peppers, caffeine, temperature extremes, and alcohol • Modify food consistency as needed • Moisten foods with gravies or sauces • Use straws with liquids • Use oral mouth rinses, lidocaine, artificial saliva, or saliva-stimulating medications • Maintain good oral hygiene
Xerostomia / thick saliva	• Consume fluids with meals and frequently throughout the day • Stimulate saliva production by chewing gum, sucking on hard candies, and eating tart foods • Avoid foods that are dry (e.g. crackers, toast) or sticky (e.g. peanut butter) • Consume beverages that thin secretions (e.g. club soda, seltzer water, papaya nectar) • Maintain adequate hydration • Use a humidifier in dry environments • Use oral mouth rinses, artificial saliva, or saliva-stimulating medications • Maintain good oral hygiene
Altered taste perception	• Rinse mouth with tea, ginger ale or salt water before and after meals • Cold foods may be better tolerated • Season foods with herbs, spices, sauces, marinades • Supplement zinc if deficiency diagnosed or suspected • Aversion to meats common; consume other high-protein foods (e.g. eggs, dairy, nuts) • Metallic taste common with some medications; use plastic utensils, avoid canned foods
Difficulty swallowing	• Alter food consistency and beverage thickness as recommended by SLP • Use swallowing strategies (e.g. chin tuck) as recommended by SLP • Eat and drink only when upright • Drink fluids between each bite of food • Avoid mixed-consistency foods (e.g. dry cereal with milk) • Avoid tough, chewy or fibrous foods

Abbreviation: SLP = speech language pathologist.

interpret due to the heterogeneous nature of study participants, as well as differences in interventions, how malnutrition is defined, and the outcomes measured. Some researchers have studied the use of ONS alone, while others have investigated provision of ONS in conjunction with additional MNT interventions such as EN and PN.[24]

In a 2012 review of 36 randomized controlled trials (RCTs) on patients of varying disease states and healthcare settings, Cawood et al. reported that the use of ONS was associated with improvements in total protein and energy intake, handgrip strength, hospital readmission rates, and complications in some populations. Although this evidence is stronger than that from other reviews, as only RCTs were included, Cawood's

TABLE 12.6

Strategies to Mitigate GI Symptoms That May Impair Oral Intake[15–17]

Early satiety	• Eat high-calorie / high-protein foods, limit low-calorie foods and beverages • Consume small frequent meals and keep nutrient-dense snacks on hand • Drink fluids between meals • Low-fat foods and liquids may be better tolerated • Chew thoroughly and eat slowly • Maintain light daily exercise regimen and remain active, if possible • Take medications between or after meals if possible
Nausea	• Eat high-calorie / high-protein foods and small frequent meals • Drink liquids between meals • Avoid foods with strong odors (cold or room-temperature foods may be better tolerated) • Avoid strongly seasoned, high-fat and excessively sweet foods • Eat dry foods (e.g. crackers, toast, dry cereal) every 2 to 3 hours • Take prescribed anti-nausea medications (i.e. scheduled, not as needed)
Diarrhea	• Avoid high-fat and high-fiber foods, alcohol, caffeine • Eat small frequent meals • Maintain hydration; drink oral rehydration solution to replace lost electrolytes • Eat high-soluble fiber foods (e.g. banana, applesauce, white rice, pasta) • Consider limiting high-lactose foods, even if not normally lactose-intolerant • Consider probiotic if altered gut flora suspected • Avoid foods and medications with sugar alcohols (e.g. sorbitol, mannitol, xylitol, malitol, lactilol, isomalt) • Avoid high-osmolarity foods (e.g. juice, concentrated sweets) • Avoid high-osmolarity medications (i.e. many liquid medications) • Take prescribed anti-diarrhea medications • Take prescribed pancreatic enzyme replacements
Constipation	• Eat high-fiber foods and/or take fiber supplement • Maintain adequate hydration • Maintain light daily exercise regimen and remain active, if possible • Avoid medications that can cause constipation, if possible (e.g. opioids, non-steroidal anti-inflammatories, antihistamines, iron supplements) • Use prescribed medications to maintain bowel regimen

Abbreviation: GI = gastrointestinal.

review did include research on both well-nourished and malnourished patients, which may have confounded results.[25]

Conversely, reviews by Baldwin and Lee did not show a benefit of ONS use on malnourished patients. Both reviews concluded that patients who received registered dietitian nutritionist (RDN) counseling showed improved outcomes, regardless of if the patient received ONS or not.[24,26] The review conducted by Lee concluded that the results of ONS consumption alone, without RDN counseling, were inconclusive.[26] Baldwin et al. analyzed the effect of ONS on patients who were malnourished or at risk of malnutrition. Some reviews reported ONS consumption was associated with improvements in energy intake, weight, mortality and complications. However, the

TABLE 12.7
Strategies to Mitigate Constitutional Symptoms That May Impair Oral Intake[18-20]

Anorexia	• Eat high-calorie / high-protein foods, limit low-calorie foods and beverages
	• Consume small frequent meals and keep nutrient-dense snacks on hand
	• Drink fluids between meals
	• Create pleasant eating environment: set table, play music, eat with others
	• Maintain light daily exercise regimen and remain active, if possible
	• View food as medicine and part of a required treatment regimen
	• Consider appetite stimulant (e.g. megace 800 mg/d, marinol 5–20 mg/d)
Fatigue	• Eat high-calorie / high-protein foods, limit low-calorie foods and beverages
	• Consume small frequent meals and keep nutrient-dense snacks on hand
	• Consume main/larger meal when energy levels highest
	• Purchase pre-prepared or pre-cooked items
	• Use meal or grocery delivery or pick up services
	• Prepare/cook multiple servings to be frozen and consumed later
Shortness of breath	• Eat high-calorie / high-protein foods, limit low-calorie foods and beverages
	• Consume small frequent meals and keep nutrient-dense snacks on hand
	• Eat slowly
	• Eat after breathing treatments
	• Eat foods that require little chewing (e.g. pudding or puree consistency)

authors cited poor quality of reviews and heterogeneity as significant study limitations, and when only high-quality studies were analyzed, there was still significant discordance in the results. Baldwin et al. concluded that the benefit of consuming ONS in malnourished patients remains unclear.[24]

When recommending or prescribing ONS, several variables should be considered. Of primary concern is compliance – many patients may not like the taste of the products, thus consumption can be poor. Many products are very sweet, which can be problematic for some patients, especially those who have altered taste perception. Further, in the outpatient or community setting, intake may be constrained by the patient's inability to purchase ONS, due to either costs or limited access to the products. Also of concern is that ONS may replace food in the patient's diet, resulting in little net increase in nutritional intake.

Many clinicians advocate for the "food first" approach, in which the RDN focuses on MNT that helps the patient make dietary changes, such as fortifying foods and offering nourishing beverages and snacks, instead of providing ONS.[27] Benefits to this approach include improved taste and thus compliance with diet changes, avoiding taste fatigue, and cost-effectiveness.[28]

3 Enteral Nutrition

Oral nutrition, including the use of ONS, is usually considered the first line of therapy in managing malnutrition; however, when oral intake remains inadequate, or when swallowing function is unsafe or impaired, an individual may require EN. Enteral nutrition is the preferred method of nutrition support in the setting of a functioning

GI tract because it is necessary to maintain gut function, thus preventing bacterial translocation and supporting immune health; it is a more physiological approach to feeding and is less expensive than PN. Most patients on EN are EN-dependent for less than one month, in which case a nasoenteric tube is the preferred method of delivery.[29] If oral intake is anticipated to be inadequate for more than four to six weeks, a gastrostomy tube should be considered.[30]

In patients with chronic disease, EN is most commonly prescribed for patients with dysphagia due to stroke, oropharyngeal or esophageal malignancy, and chronic neurodegenerative conditions such as ALS and Parkinson's disease. A recent review concluded that the nutritional benefits derived from gastrostomy feeding are not clearly established, likely owing to the heterogeneity of the populations studied, the paucity of data on long-term nutritional outcomes and varied nutrition assessment tools.[31] Another explanation for the lack of demonstrated benefit is inconsistent provision of support services for patients with long-term feeding tubes. One study found only 64% of patients received assistance from home EN support professionals, a service that has been shown to reduce costs and morbidity.[32]

4 Parenteral Nutrition

For patients who do not have a functional GI tract, PN is indicated if the decision has been made to provide nutrition support. In addition to short-term PN provided in the acute care setting, long-term PN may also be infused at home. Published guidelines from the European Society for Clinical Nutrition and Metabolism (ESPEN) indicate the primary requirement for home parenteral nutrition (HPN) in patients without malignancy is "transient or permanent chronic intestinal failure due to non-malignant disease".[33] Intestinal failure is defined as the reduction of gut function below the minimum necessary for the absorption of macronutrients and/or water and electrolytes, such that intravenous supplementation is required to maintain health and/or growth.[34] Intestinal failure in non-malignant disease is most commonly seen in patients with short bowel syndrome, Crohn's disease, mesenteric ischemia and radiation enteritis. These patients often have limited inflammation and may require HPN for months or years; in this setting the therapy has been shown to prolong and improve quality of life.[34]

ESPEN suggests that HPN should be considered for those with chronic intestinal failure due to malignant disease. The prognosis or life expectancy of the patient is an essential part of the decision-making process as well as consideration of existing antineoplastic therapy options, as PN has not been shown to improve overall outcomes in oncology patients.[34] It is used most often in this setting for preoperative nutrition support in severely malnourished patients and for those patients with a bowel obstruction or graft vs. host disease.[34] Lastly, HPN can be considered for patients without intestinal failure who are not able to or do not want to meet their nutritional requirements via the oral or enteral route. Examples include patients with dysphagia who decline a feeding tube or their medical condition precludes the placement of a tube, and patients with cancer who have an indwelling central venous access device.[34]

In a meta-analysis that reviewed research on the effects of nutrition support on cancer patients, the authors found no difference in rates of infection and other complications, as well as mortality, in malnourished patients fed EN vs. PN.[35]

However, in any setting where PN is used, the patient should be reassessed periodically to evaluate if EN or oral intake may be initiated, as absence of nutrients in the GI tract results in atrophy of mucosal villi, further worsening GI function.[34]

B   NUTRITION EDUCATION AND COUNSELING

Nutrition counseling is an ongoing process in which a trained RDN works with an individual to assess their usual dietary intake and identify what changes to the diet are needed. The counselor provides information, educational materials, support and monitoring to help the patient or client make and maintain recommended dietary changes. Nutrition counseling is an integral component of MNT provided by an RDN. Counseling efforts related to malnutrition may include providing patients and their caregivers an assessment of energy and protein needs, and strategies to increase intake, mitigate symptoms that impair adequate intake, and address issues related to the disease process or its treatment.

Evaluating the impact of nutrition counseling on malnourished patients with chronic disease is difficult because of the heterogeneous nature of the populations studied, as well as the fact that nutrition research can be negatively affected by high dropout rates and limited treatment compliance. Baldwin, et al. found that dietary counseling provided by an RDN improved weight, other anthropometric markers and grip strength in people with disease-related malnutrition or those at nutritional risk. No beneficial effect on survival was noted.[24]

In a 2016 review, Lee et al. found that oncology patients who received nutrition counseling had consistent improvements in several nutrition-related outcomes, including energy and protein intake, weight gain and maintenance, and body mass index (BMI). There was also a positive effect on Patient Generated Subjective Global Assessment (PG-SGA) scores and quality of life measures.[26] Similarly, in patients with COPD, an RCT found that tailored nutritional counseling for a period of three months led to significant increases in energy and protein intake, which resulted in improvements in body weight, nutritional status, functional outcomes, and health-related quality of life.[36]

However, in a study by Parsons et al., residents of a care home at risk of malnutrition were randomized to receive either ONS or nutrition education provided twice during the 12-week trial. The investigators found that the ONS group had a significantly higher quality of life and nutritional intake than the dietary advice group, although results should be interpreted with caution due to study limitations, which include a small sample size and the limited number of dietary education sessions provided.[37]

C   COORDINATION OF NUTRITION CARE

No matter the setting, the nutrition professional should communicate the nutrition care plan with other members of the care team. This communication is necessary to ensure that nutrition goals and interventions align with the overall goals of care and medical treatment plans. Communication and collaboration also facilitate referrals to other professionals, organizations, and services that will enable continuation of malnutrition treatments and monitoring at the next level of care.[23]

IV   PHARMACOLOGICAL INTERVENTIONS

As previously noted, anorexia is often a side effect of chronic diseases and/or their treatment, and anorexia of aging has been recognized even in those individuals without comorbidities.[3] Nutrient needs can be difficult to meet on a consistent basis in individuals who struggle to consume more food than their appetite dictates. It is at this point that healthcare providers and patients may consider an appetite stimulant.

Perhaps the most commonly used appetite stimulant is megestrol acetate, as it is FDA approved for the treatment of cachexia, anorexia, or unexplained weight loss in individuals with AIDS and cancer.[38] In a systematic review of its effectiveness and safety, the authors concluded that megestrol acetate did result in increased appetite and slight weight gain of approximately two kilograms. However, several adverse side effects were reported, including thromboembolic events and edema. While 400–800 mg/d is most typically prescribed,[38] there is insufficient evidence to suggest an ideal dosage, although weight gain appeared to be associated with higher doses more than lower doses.[39] These factors should be considered when decisions are made regarding the use of this medication.

Dronabinol, a synthetic tetrahydrocannabinol, similar to the active ingredient of cannabis, has also been used for its appetite-stimulating effects, and is approved for anorexia in AIDS patients, and nausea and vomiting in cancer patients.[38,40] Mirtazapine is an antidepressant medication, but also has the side effect of increased appetite, as well as weight gain in approximately 10% of patients.[41] If a patient has both anorexia and depression, mirtazapine may be beneficial, although research supporting its use for this purpose is limited.[38]

Cannabis is well known to encourage oral intake through alterations in hormones that increase appetite.[40] Research on the effect of cannabis use on diseases and nutrition status is limited due to federal US regulations. Medical marijuana has been legalized in many states; however, as of 2022, it is still designated as a Schedule I substance by the federal government; therefore, research on cannabis is tightly regulated.[42] Some studies have shown cannabis to be effective in the management of chronic pain,[43] which can indirectly affect intake and appetite. Anecdotally, cannabis is also reported to be effective in the treatment of nausea and poor appetite. However, research is very limited, thus the effect of cannabis on symptoms associated with specific disease states, as well as its effect on nutritional status parameters such as weight gain, is unknown.[44]

V   CONCLUSION

Considering the wide range of conditions and symptoms which can cause chronic disease-related malnutrition, there are numerous therapeutic approaches for treatment. Medical nutrition therapies include diet modifications to promote increased oral intake, and the use of ONS, EN and PN. Nutrition counseling and coordination of care with the rest of the healthcare team are key to successful implementation of these MNT strategies.

REFERENCES

1. Cederholm T, Jensen GL, Correia MITD, et al. GLIM criteria for the diagnosis of malnutrition – a consensus report from the global clinical nutrition community. *Clin Nutr.* 2019;38(1):1–9.

2. White JV, Guenter P, Jensen G, et al. Consensus statement of the Academy of Nutrition and Dietetics / American Society for Parenteral and Enteral Nutrition: characteristics recommended for the identification and documentation of adult malnutrition (undernutrition). *JPEN J Parenter Enteral Nutr.* 2012;36(3):275–283.

3. Landi F, Picca A, Calvani R, Marzetti E. Anorexia of aging: assessment and management. *Clin Geriatr Med.* 2017;33(3):315–323.

4. Gulati K, Guhathakurta S, Joshi J, Rai N, Ray R. Cytokines and their role in health and disease: a brief overview. *MOJ Immunol.* 2016;4(2):00121.

5. Zhang F, Shen A, Jin Y, Qiang W. The management strategies of cancer-associated anorexia: a critical appraisal of systematic reviews. *BMC Complement Altern Med.* 2018;18(1):236.

6. Itoh M, Tsuji T, Nemoto K, Nakamura H, Aoshiba K. Undernutrition in patients with COPD and its treatment. *Nutrients.* 2013;5(4):1316–1335.

7. Lawrence DP, Kupelnick B, Miller K, Devine D, Lau J. Evidence report on the occurrence, assessment, and treatment of fatigue in cancer patients. *J Natl Cancer Inst Monogr.* 2004;(32):40–50.

8. Sabbouh T, Torbey MT. Malnutrition in stroke patients: risk factors, assessment, and management. *Neurocrit Care.* 2018;29(3):374–384.

9. Escott-Stump S. *Nutrition and Diagnosis-Related Care.* 8th ed. Baltimore, MD: Lippincott, Williams & Wilkins; 2008.

10. Sura L, Madhavan A, Carnaby G, Crary MA. Dysphagia in the elderly: management and nutritional considerations. *Clin Interv Aging.* 2012;7:287–298.

11. Barbe AG. Medication-induced xerostomia and hyposalivation in the elderly: Culprits, complications, and management. *Drugs and Aging.* 2018;35(10):877–885.

12. Narhi TO, Meurman JH, Ainamo A. Xerostomia and hyposalivation. *Drugs and Aging.* 1999;12(2):103–116.

13. Rommel N, Hamdy S. Oropharyngeal dysphagia: manifestations and diagnosis. *Nat Rev Gastroenterol Hepatol.* 2015;13(1):49–59.

14. Wirth R, Dziewas R, Beck AM, et al. Oropharyngeal dysphagia in older persons – from pathophysiology to adequate intervention: a review and summary of an international expert meeting. *Clin Interv Aging.* 2016;11:189–208.

15. Lacy BE, Parkman HP, Camilleri M. Chronic nausea and vomiting: evaluation and treatment. *Am J Gastroenterol.* 2018;113(5):647–659.

16. Corinaldesi R, Stanghellini V, Barbara G, et al. Clinical approach to diarrhea. *Intern Emerg Med.* 2012;7 Suppl 3:S255–S262.

17. Forootan M, Bagheri N, Darvishi M. Chronic constipation: A review of literature. *Medicine (Baltimore).* 2018;97(20):e10631.

18. Dent E, Hoogendijk E, Wright O. New insights into the anorexia of ageing: from prevention to treatment. *Curr Opin Clin Nutr Metab Care.* 2019;22(1):44–51.

19. Finsterer J, Mahjoub SZ. Fatigue in healthy and diseased individuals. *Am J Hosp Palliat Care.* 2014;31(5):562–575.

20. Wahls SA. Causes and evaluation of chronic dyspnea. *Am Fam Physician.* 2012;86(2):173–180.

21. Schiller LR. Nutrition management of chronic diarrhea and malabsorption. *Nutr Clin Pract.* 2006;21(1):34–39.

22. Dorner B, Friedrich EK. Position of the Academy of Nutrition and Dietetics: individualized approaches for older adults: long-term care, post-acute care, and other settings. *J Acad Nutr Diet*. 2018;118(4):724–735.

23. Electronic Nutrition Care Process and Terminology. Accessed October 7, 2021. www.ncpro.org/pubs/2020-encpt-en?.

24. Baldwin C, Smith R, Gibbs M, Weekes CE, Emery PW. Quality of the evidence supporting the role of oral nutritional supplements in the management of malnutrition: an overview of systematic reviews and meta-analyses. *Adv Nutr*. 2021;12(2):503–522.

25. Cawood AL, Elia M, Stratton RJ. Systematic review and meta-analysis of the effects of high protein oral nutritional supplements. *Ageing Res Rev*. 2012;11(2):278–296.

26. Lee JLC, Leong LP, Lim SL. Nutrition intervention approaches to reduce malnutrition in oncology patients: a systematic review. *Support Care Cancer*. 2016;24(1):469–480.

27. Smith H. The importance of a food first approach. Nualtra. Published March 15, 2020. Accessed June 11, 2021. https://nualtra.com/resources/news/the-importance-of-a-food-first-approach.

28. Leading Nutrition – the Dietitian Care Centre. Are you using the food first approach? Accessed June 11, 2021 at www.leadingnutrition.com.au/foodfirst/.

29. Pearce CB, Duncan HD. Enteral feeding. Nasogastric, nasojejunal, percutaneous endoscopic gastrostomy, or jejunostomy: its indications and limitations. *Postgrad Med J*. 2002;78(918):198–204.

30. Kurien M, McAlindon ME, Westaby D, Sanders DS. Percutaneous endoscopic gastrostomy (PEG) feeding. *BMJ*. 2010;340:c2414.

31. Kurien M, Williams J, Sanders DS. Malnutrition in healthcare settings and the role of gastrostomy feeding. *Proc Nutr Soc*. 2017;76(3):352–360.

32. Kurien M, Westaby D, Romaya C, Sanders DS. National survey evaluating service provision for percutaneous endoscopic gastrostomy within the UK. *Scand J Gastroenterol*. 2011;46(12):1519–1524.

33. Pironi L, Boeykens K, Bozzetti F, et al. ESPEN guideline on home parenteral nutrition. *Clin Nutr*. 2020;39(6):1645–1666.

34. Lappas BM, Patel D, Kumpf V, Adams DW, Seidner DL. Parenteral nutrition: indications, access, and complications. *Gastroenterol Clin North Am*. 2018;47(1):39–59.

35. Chow R, Bruera E, Chiu L, Chow S, Chiu N, Lam H, et al. Enteral and parenteral nutrition in cancer patients: a systematic review and meta-analysis. *Ann Palliat Med*. 2016;5(1):30–41.

36. Nguyen HT, Pavey TG, Collins PF, Nguyen NV, Pham TD, Gallegos D. Effectiveness of tailored dietary counseling in treating malnourished outpatients with chronic obstructive pulmonary disease: a randomized controlled trial. *J Acad Nutr Diet*. 2020;120(5):778–791.

37. Parsons EL, Stratton RJ, Cawood AL, Smith TR, Elia M. Oral nutritional supplements in a randomised trial are more effective than dietary advice at improving quality of life in malnourished care home residents. *Clin Nutr*. 2017;36(1):134–142.

38. Levitt A, O'Neil J. Older adults with unintended weight loss: the role of appetite stimulants. *Home Healthc Now*. 2018;36(5):312–318.

39. Ruiz Garcia V, López-Briz E, Carbonell Sanchis R, Gonzalvez Perales JL, Bort-Marti S. Megestrol acetate for treatment of anorexia-cachexia syndrome. *Cochrane Database Syst Rev*. 2013(3):CD004310.

40. Borowska M, Czarnywojtek A, Sawicka-Gutaj N, Woliński K, Płazińska MT, Mikołajczak P, Ruchała M. The effects of cannabinoids on the endocrine system. *Endokrynol Pol*. 2018;69(6):705–719.

41. Montgomery SA. Safety of mirtazapine: a review. *Int Clin Psychopharmacol.* 1995;10 Suppl 4:37–45.

42. United States Drug Enforcement Agency. Accessed October 7, 2021. /www.dea.gov/drug-information/drug-scheduling.

43. National Academies of Sciences, Engineering and Medicine. Health Effects of marijuana and cannabis-derived products presented in a new report. Released January 12, 2017. Accessed Jun 14, 2021 at www.nationalacademies.org/news/2017/01/health-effects-of-marijuana-and-cannabis-derived-products-presented-in-new-report.

44. Santa Cruz J. Cannabis in cancer care. *Today's Dietitian.* 2020;22(9):40–44.

13 Treatment – Social/Environmental-Related Malnutrition

Wendy Phillips and Jennifer Doley

CONTENTS

I INTRODUCTION

Malnutrition related to behavioral or environmental circumstances is not directly associated with disease, thus is not accompanied by acute or chronic inflammation. Malnutrition unrelated to disease is sometimes referred to as starvation-related malnutrition, and generally is caused by inadequate nutrient intake.[1] The behavioral and environmental factors leading to inadequate intake, however, are myriad. Food insecurity is a major contributor, and can be challenging to address, as treatment and interventions often involve development and administration of social programs that rely on charitable donations or government funding.[1] Factors such as income and education level contribute to food insecurity but are difficult to modify. Other behavioral or environmental contributors to inadequate intake resulting in malnutrition include psychological issues such as substance use disorders and eating disorders. This chapter will review treatments for behavioral or environmental malnutrition etiologies, with a focus on food insecurity.

II FOOD INSECURITY

The United States Department of Agriculture (USDA) describes food security as "access by all people at all times to enough food for an active, healthy life". Food security, at a minimum, includes the ready availability of safe, nutritionally adequate,

DOI: 10.1201/9781003177586-13

227

TABLE 13.1

Categories of Food Insecurity Defined by the USDA[2]

Food security category	Description
High	Household had no problems, or anxiety about, consistently accessing adequate food
Marginal	Household had problems with anxiety at times about accessing adequate food, but the quality, variety and quantity of the food was not substantially reduced
Low	Household reduced the quality, variety, or desirability of their diets, but the quantity of food intake and normal eating patterns was not substantially disrupted
Very low	At times during the year, eating patterns of one or more household members were disrupted and food intake reduced because the household lacked money or other resources for food

Abbreviation: USDA = United States Department of Agriculture.

and culturally appropriate foods, and the ability to acquire foods in socially acceptable ways (i.e. without resorting to emergency food supplies, scavenging, etc.). The three pillars of food security are availability, access, and use. Food insecurity is categorized into four levels, as seen in Table 13.1.[2]

Food insecurity is associated with a higher incidence of nutrition-related diseases, such as diabetes and obesity, elevated markers of low-grade inflammation, and a greater incidence of depression and anxiety.[3] Many of these chronic conditions are also associated with an increased risk of malnutrition, and food insecurity is a common underlying etiology for non-severe or severe malnutrition in the context of social/environmental factors.

A   FACTORS ASSOCIATED WITH FOOD INSECURITY

The Healthy People 2020 report stated that food insecurity may be influenced by a number of factors including income, employment, race, ethnicity, and disability.[4] Income factors, including savings and income volatility (i.e. sudden changes in income), have been found to be the strongest predictors of food insecurity in the United States. Groups that are at greater risk of low income include households with children (especially those with a single parent in the home), less formal education, receiving welfare benefits, ethnic minorities, the homeless, and those with substance use disorders or human immunodeficiency virus (HIV) infection. Other financial factors include income spent on housing and medical care, with less money reserved for healthy food.[3]

For research purposes, the USDA defines food deserts as low-income areas with a substantial number of residents with reduced access to retail outlets selling healthy and affordable foods. In order to be considered a food desert, an area must meet both income and access criteria. See Table 13.2. Factors that contribute to food deserts include the location of stores with a wide variety of healthy foods at a reasonable

TABLE 13.2
USDA Food Desert Definition[5]

Category	Criteria
Access	≥ 500 people or ≥ 33% of the population must live more than one mile from the nearest large grocery store in urban areas, or ten miles in rural areas
Income	≥ 20% of the population has an income less than the federal poverty level – *or* – median household income does not exceed 80% of the statewide or metro-area median income

Abbreviation: USDA = United States Department of Agriculture.

cost, and whether residents have reliable and affordable transportation to travel to the stores. Research indicates that food deserts may contribute to food insecurity, although study results are variable.[5]

As the US population has become increasingly diverse, more attention has been paid to the importance of access to culturally appropriate food. For example, food taboos exist in some cultures, and/or food preparation techniques or food choices common with particular groups may not be reflected in the stores to which they have access. Additionally, grocery stores and other retail outlets may be overwhelming to people who do not speak or read English proficiently.[6,7]

B   IDENTIFICATION OF FOOD INSECURITY

The Department of Economic Research Service of the USDA is largely responsible for research and measurement of food insecurity in the United States, which is conducted via surveys. The US Adult Food Security Survey Module is a ten-question survey; an additional eight questions are used for the US Household Food Security Survey Module for households with children. The survey includes questions related to worry about food running out, diet quality and variety, and quantity of food consumed.[8] Of note, in some cases the Six-Item Short Form of the Food Security Survey Module is used to reduce the number of questions that must be answered. These six questions are derived from the longer surveys.[9]

Acute care and rehabilitation hospitals, outpatient clinics, community agencies such as public health clinics, and organizations involved in setting policy and funding programs often conduct food security screening to understand how to better meet the needs of patients, clients, and their communities. The Food Security Survey Modules from the USDA are beneficial for research purposes, but are cumbersome for use as a quick survey tool in other settings. Therefore, the Hunger Vital Signs tool was developed in 2010 as a means to rapidly identify individuals and households at risk of food insecurity.[10] The screening tool was first validated for use among low-income families with young children, and subsequently in other populations.[11]

Ultimately, the presence and risk of food insecurity should be assessed based on each individual's unique circumstances. Screening should occur in a variety of healthcare settings, such as community health programs and acute care hospitals, and assessments should be repeated periodically to determine if interventions that target food insecurity are successful.

C INTERVENTIONS

Interventions to decrease the risk of malnutrition associated with food insecurity are often administered in a community setting with a common objective to increase access to food, accompanied by nutrition education on how to incorporate the food into a healthy diet. Examples include the Supplemental Nutrition Assistance Program (SNAP), the Women, Infants and Children (WIC) program, food banks and pantries, and community food programs.[3] Table 13.3 summarizes three key government funded programs: SNAP, WIC and Meals on Wheels.[12-14]

1 Supplemental Nutrition Assistance Program

The Supplemental Nutrition Assistance Program, formerly known as the food stamp program, is the largest and broadest nutrition-assistance program for low-income seniors, working families, and people with disabilities on a fixed income in the United States. Consistent with the goal of combining access to food with nutrition education, the SNAP program includes an education component called SNAP-Ed that teaches people how to make their SNAP dollars stretch, how to shop for and cook healthy meals, and how to stay physically active. SNAP-Ed partners with state and local organizations for nutrition education classes, social marketing campaigns, and efforts to improve policies, systems, and community food and nutrition environments, such as reducing food deserts and making healthy foods more affordable and readily available.[12]

a Funding

The federal government pays the full cost of the actual food benefits, and splits the costs of administering the program with the states. Consumers apply through their state; eligibility and other program requirements may vary slightly between states.[12]

b Outcomes

Participating in SNAP has been shown to significantly reduce food insecurity and promote better long-term health outcomes.[15-17] Longitudinal studies on children born in the 1960s and 1970s to mothers who received SNAP benefits suggest that these children had lower rates of metabolic syndrome and 25% lower healthcare costs.[18] Children in low-income families who participate in SNAP benefits show improvements in reading and mathematics skills, and are more likely to graduate from high school.[16] Participating in SNAP has also been shown to reduce nursing home and hospital admissions for adults over the age of 65.[19]

2 Women, Infants, and Children

The Special Supplemental Nutrition Program for Women, Infants, and Children (WIC) provides supplemental foods, healthcare referrals, and nutrition education

TABLE 13.3
Government-Funded Food and Nutrition Programs to Address Food Insecurity[12-14]

Government-funded programs	Funding and administration	Participant requirements	Benefits	Duration
Supplemental Nutrition Assistance Program (SNAP)	Federal government pays all benefits; shares administrative costs with the state Managed/administered by the state	Federal government sets participation requirements Gross income < 130% of the US federal poverty level	Monthly financial aid to purchase food, provided on Electronic Benefit Transfer (EBT) card, works like a debit card	Temporary – benefit period ranges one month to three years
Special Supplemental Nutrition Program for Women, Infants, and Children (WIC)	Funded by federal grants	Low-income pregnant and post-partum women Infants and children at nutrition risk	Supplemental foods include infant cereal, baby foods, iron-fortified adult cereal, fruits and vegetables, vitamin C-rich fruit or vegetable juice, eggs, milk, cheese, yogurt, soy-based beverages, tofu, peanut butter, dried and canned beans/peas, canned fish, whole wheat bread and other whole-grain options Healthcare referrals Nutrition education	Women up to 12 months post-partum if breastfeeding; up to six months if not Children up to five years
Meals on Wheels	Supported by Older Americans Act (39%) State and local sources, donations, federal block grants (61%)	Age > 60 yrs (or spouse > 60 yrs) *and* Home-bound (physical or financial challenges affect ability to eat healthy meals or travel to meal site) *and* Risk of malnutrition (may vary by community)	Free or low-cost home-delivered meals, one per day Monday through Friday Home safety check Congregate meal sites (may vary by community)	Temporary or permanent, as long as participant continues to meet requirements

for low-income pregnant, breastfeeding, and non-breastfeeding post-partum women, and to infants and children up to age five who are found to be at nutritional risk. Participants receive regular nutrition education from peer counselors and registered dietitian nutritionists (RDNs) according to a schedule defined by the state. Education includes, but is not limited to, healthy eating and weight gain during pregnancy, breastfeeding, healthy eating during the post-partum period, infant feeding, and healthy eating during childhood. Participants receive advice for health management behaviors, such as immunizations and medical care, and referrals are made to other healthcare providers and social programs as needed. Many WIC programs are located within public health departments or clinics to improve access to a comprehensive array of services.[20]

WIC benefits include money for the purchase of healthy foods like milk, juice, eggs, cheese, cereal, peanut butter, dry beans or peas; other foods may be included as determined periodically by the federal and state governments. Foods are specifically chosen based on the nutrients that are important during pregnancy, lactation, and childhood. Participants may also receive infant formula during the first year of life.[20–21]

a Funding

The WIC program is funded through federal grants to the states. The Food and Nutrition Service, an agency of the USDA, is responsible for administering the program. Unlike SNAP, WIC is not an entitlement program, meaning not all people who qualify may receive benefits, and additional criteria for participation must be met.[12,20] Congress allots a budget each year to provide grants to the states. Organizations providing WIC benefits must stay within their allotted budget, thus there may be insufficient funds to cover everyone applying for WIC benefits.[20]

b Outcomes

Overall diet quality is significantly improved in WIC participants compared with low-income families who do not receive WIC benefits. The USDA reports that children born to mothers who use WIC services during pregnancy have improved vocabulary scores, and children who are enrolled in WIC after the first year of life have significantly improved memory. Women who continue to receive WIC benefits during the postpartum period have a lower risk of anemia and maternal obesity at the onset of the next pregnancy. Participation in WIC has been shown to increase childhood immunization rates, regular medical care visits, and breastfeeding rates, and lower maternal and infant mortality.[22] Furthermore, overall healthcare costs for low-income families who receive WIC benefits are less than for those who do not.[23]

3 Food Banks and Pantries

Food banks are large warehouses that may store millions of pounds of food that is distributed to local community agencies, including food pantries. Food pantries have a more direct connection to clients.[24] Food banks are a widely recognized resource for food-insecure households; however, their benefit in alleviating the problem is limited. Food banks rely on financial donations and volunteer availability, thus the quantity and quality of food may at times be limited, as well as the number of days or hours they are accessible. Moreover, donated foods may be of little practical use or near their expiration date, as well as highly processed. Studies have shown food banks generally distribute insufficient amounts of fruits, vegetables and dairy foods, thus most of the foods provided are low in vitamins A and C as well as calcium.[25] Use of food pantries is low; shame or stigma has been shown to inhibit individuals from relying on this resource. For these reasons, food banks and pantries are considered a last resort for alleviating food insecurity.[3]

4   Food Pharmacies

Food pharmacies started in 2012 in the United States when Wholesome Wave, a non-profit organization, began partnering with healthcare clinics to offer "prescriptions" for healthy foods to people in need.[26] Since that time, different versions of these programs have been developed and are administered by a variety of healthcare and community organizations.[27]

The goal of food pharmacies, like the social programs discussed earlier in this chapter, is to increase access to food for food-insecure individuals. However, food pharmacy programs are also designed to provide only healthy foods specifically tailored to the client's individual nutrition-related disease needs. In this way, food pharmacies complement, but don't replace, programs such as SNAP and WIC. Nutrition education that is provided and the healthy food prescribed differentiate these programs from food banks.[27]

The eligibility criteria, who can refer clients, benefits received, and operational management vary depending on the program. Obesity, hypertension, cardiovascular disease, and diabetes are common nutrition-related diseases often used as program-participation criteria. Referring providers are commonly physicians and RDNs who may identify potential clients while delivering nutrition and/or medical care. The referring provider then writes a prescription for food items that are consistent with the client's medical nutrition therapy plan. For example, a client with cardiovascular disease may be written a prescription for foods that are low in sodium and high in fiber; the client can then choose items from the food pharmacy's list of available foods that meet these criteria.[27]

a   Funding

Most food pharmacies are funded through philanthropy or program administration and food is provided by an individual hospital or healthcare system as part of a comprehensive plan to address their community's social determinants of health. Therefore, funding may be limited and inconsistent.[27]

b   Outcomes

Overall, food pharmacy programs have been shown to improve household food security while also leading to clinically significant reductions in hemoglobin A1C, body mass index (BMI), and blood pressure.[28–30] Furthermore, clients' self-reported moods and confidence to manage their own health are enhanced when they participate in food pharmacies, with improvements in appropriate health-monitoring behaviors such as routine eye and foot exams.[31] More research is needed on a larger scale to understand the cost-benefit return on investment of such programs.[32] Some state Medicaid programs are conducting pilot studies to determine if food pharmacies improve community and individual outcomes and decrease the cost of healthcare.[33]

5 Medically Tailored Meals

Medically tailored meals (MTM) are complete, prepared meals designed to meet the medical nutrition therapy needs for individuals with nutrition-related diseases. For example, a client with kidney failure may receive meals that are low in sodium and potassium. These meals are either delivered to clients' homes or picked up during a medical appointment. Similar to food pharmacies, a prescription from a physician, RDN, or health insurance plan is usually required for an individual to receive services. These meals are provided for individuals with a nutrition-related chronic disease; food insecurity may or may not be an eligibility criterion. The goal is to prevent malnutrition and decrease nutrition-related disease complications, thereby decreasing the overall cost of healthcare and improving the health and quality of life outcomes of participants.[34]

a Funding

As of 2022, Traditional Medicare Part B, which covers two-thirds of Medicare enrollees, does not provide coverage for MTMs. Medicare Advantage and state Medicaid plans are allowed to provide insurance coverage for these meals, but it is unclear how many make the service available, and for what length of time or how many meals. Private insurances may pay for MTMs, but there is limited information on what is actually covered and by whom.[35]

b Outcomes

More research is available about the benefits of MTM programs than food pharmacies, although results are difficult to interpret due to the large heterogeneity of programs. Populations served differ from one program to the next, the number of meals and length of program participation can vary significantly, and some programs include nutrition education whereas others do not. Furthermore, there is very little research on whether recipients consume all of the meals or whether they are simultaneously participating in other programs that address food insecurity. Nonetheless, health outcomes associated with receiving MTMs show promising results.[36–38]

III MENTAL DISORDERS

The *Diagnostic and Statistical Manual of Mental Disorders* (DSM) is published by the American Psychiatric Association (APA) to guide clinicians and researchers to diagnose and classify mental disorders. The 5th edition, updated in 2013, is referred to as the DSM-5 and contains diagnostic and treatment information for recognized and diagnosable mental disorders, including Substance Use Disorders (SUDs) and

Feeding and Eating Disorders (FEDs).[39] SUDs and FEDs can contribute to or increase the risk for social/environmental malnutrition (starvation), and SUDs are often associated with food insecurity.[39,40] Table 13.4 outlines the classification of malnutrition associated with SUDs and three FEDs (discussed below) based on two malnutrition diagnosis constructs.[1,41]

A SUBSTANCE USE DISORDERS

Substance use disorders are diagnosed when recurrent alcohol or drug use significantly and clinically impairs functions of daily living. Risk factors for developing SUDs include adverse events in childhood (e.g. homelessness, placement in foster care, abuse and neglect) and repeated ongoing stressful life events. These traumas have been shown to cause cognitive, neurotransmitter, and neuroendocrine changes which increase predisposition to developing SUDs and other psychiatric disorders. Other risk factors for developing SUDs include genetic predisposition and lack of social or community support.[42,43]

Individuals with SUDs are at increased risk of malnutrition due to food insecurity, often resulting from limited income for individuals who are unable to maintain employment and/or who may choose to spend their money on the addictive substance instead of food. Individuals with SUDs at times may not have the physical or mental capacity to shop for or prepare appropriate and/or adequate amounts of foods.[43,44]

TABLE 13.4
Malnutrition Classification of SUDs, AN, BN and ARFID Based on AAIM and GLIM Criteria[1,41]

Mental disorder category	Common AAIM classification	Common GLIM classification
Substance use disorder (SUD)	Non-severe or severe malnutrition in the context of social or environmental circumstances	Moderate or severe malnutrition related to starvation; moderate or severe malnutrition related to chronic disease with minimal or no perceived inflammation
Anorexia nervosa (AN)	Severe malnutrition in the context of social or environmental circumstances	Severe malnutrition related to starvation
Bulimia nervosa (BN)	Non-severe or severe malnutrition in the context of social or environmental circumstances	Moderate or severe malnutrition related to starvation
Avoidant/restrictive food intake disorder (ARFID)	Non-severe or severe malnutrition in the context of social or environmental circumstances	Moderate or severe malnutrition related to starvation

Abbreviations: AAIM = Academy and ASPEN (American Society for Parenteral and Enteral Nutrition) Indicators to Diagnose Malnutrition; GLIM = Global Leadership Initiative on Malnutrition.

Homelessness is more prevalent in individuals with SUDs, which is a significant contributor to food insecurity.[44]

The physiological and biochemical effects of long-term SUDs can also lead to malnutrition and micronutrient deficiencies. The preferential intake of the addictive substance can affect hormones that alter satiety and thus food intake.[45] People with opioid use disorder can have chronic constipation that can result in inadequate food intake and unhealthy eating patterns leading to malnutrition.[46] Those with drug addictions have been shown to have a preference for high sugar and low nutrient-dense foods.[47,48] Alcohol-dependent individuals have increased intestinal permeability and inflammation, which can contribute to nutrient deficiencies.[49]

In addition to the physiological and metabolic effects of the SUD itself, chronic conditions caused by SUDs can also increase the risk of malnutrition, most notably seen in liver disease caused by alcohol use. Liver disease is associated with higher rates of malnutrition due to a variety of metabolic and physiological side effects.[50] While social/environmental factors such as food insecurity can cause malnutrition, chronic disease related to SUDs further compounds the problem.

Treatment for SUDs often begins with detoxification, during which patients commonly have inadequate food intake due to the nausea, loss of appetite, and gastrointestinal disturbances associated with withdrawal.[51,52] Strategies to address these symptoms are reviewed in Chapter 12. Some patients undergoing withdrawal may experience altered mental status, resulting in an inability to eat safely. Altered food textures and/or thickened liquids may be required; however, mental status may be too impaired to allow the patient to consume any nutrition by mouth. In these cases, especially when symptoms persist, the initiation of enteral nutrition may be required.[51,52] When providing nutrition support to patients with malnutrition or prolonged inadequate intake, it is important to prevent or treat electrolyte imbalances associated with refeeding, as well as micronutrient deficiencies.[53,54]

After detoxification, the best long-term treatment for malnutrition is to treat the SUD itself. Recovery from SUDs may result in improved food security; however, if issues related to food insecurity persist for other reasons, the strategies discussed earlier in this chapter may be utilized. Some patients recovering from SUDs may have developed chronic medical conditions, such as liver disease, in which case any unresolved malnutrition will become primarily chronic disease-related. See Chapter 12 for treatment of chronic disease-related malnutrition.

B   FEEDING AND EATING DISORDERS

Although commonly referred to as "eating disorders", since the DSM-5 was published in 2013, the official name for these disorders is "Feeding and Eating Disorders" (FEDs).[39] Eating disorders can also contribute to malnutrition, as some FEDs are characterized by starvation. Compared to all other mental disorders, FEDs are associated with some of the highest rates of medical and social disabilities.[55] The eight diagnoses included in the FED group of the DSM-5 are described in Table 13.5.

Anorexia nervosa (AN), bulimia nervosa (BN) and avoidant/restrictive food intake (ARFID) are the FEDs most likely to lead to malnutrition and are therefore reviewed in this section. About 30 million Americans suffer from FEDs, and it is the third most common chronic illness among adolescents. The APA guidelines report that physical consequences from FEDs include all serious disorders caused by malnutrition, especially those related to cardiovascular disease.[56]

1 Anorexia Nervosa

Anorexia nervosa is characterized by persistent and significant restriction of energy intake leading to low body weight, an intense fear of gaining weight or fat, and body

---

TABLE 13.5

Feeding and Eating Disorders (FEDs) as Described by the DSM-5[39,40]

Disorder	Description
Pica	• Repeated eating of non-nutritive, non-food substances for at least one month
Rumination disorder	• Regurgitation of undigested food which is either re-chewed, re-swallowed or spat out
	• Symptoms occur up to 120 minutes after a meal, most common range is 30 seconds to one hour
Avoidant/ restrictive food intake disorder (ARFID)	• Disturbance in eating or feeding resulting in:
	○ Substantial weight loss (adults) or absence of expected weight gain (children)
	○ Nutritional deficiency
	○ Dependence on feeding tube or dietary supplements
	○ Significant psychosocial interference
	• Not associated with distorted body image, weight concerns, availability of food, or cultural norms
Anorexia nervosa (AN)	• Restriction of energy intake relative to requirements leading to significantly low body weight: less than minimally normal (adults) and less than minimally expected (children and adolescents) in the context of age, sex development and physical health
	• Suggested BMI scale for severity:
	○ Mild = ≥ 17
	○ Moderate = 16–16.9
	○ Severe = 15–15.9
	○ Extreme = < 15
	• Intense fear of gaining weight or becoming fat, persistent behavior that interferes with weight gain
	• Disturbance in the way weight or body shape is experienced or lack of recognition about risks of low weight
Bulimia nervosa (BN)	• Frequent episodes of binge eating (defined below) followed by inappropriate behaviors such as self-induced vomiting to avoid weight gain
	• Binge eating and compensatory behaviors: one episode per week over three-month period
	• Suggested number of episodes per week to define severity:
	○ Mild = 1–3
	○ Moderate = 4–7
	○ Severe = 8–13
	○ Extreme = ≥ 14

(continued)

TABLE 13.5 (Continued)

Feeding and Eating Disorders (FEDs) as Described by the DSM-5[39,40]

Disorder	Description

Binge eating disorder (BED)	• Recurring episodes of eating significantly more in a short period of time than most people would eat in similar circumstances
	• Episodes marked by feelings of lack of control; may have feelings of guilt, embarrassment, disgust
	• Binge eating: one episode per week for three months
	• Suggested number of episodes per week to define severity:
	  ◦ Mild = 1–3
	  ◦ Moderate = 4–7
	  ◦ Severe = 8–13
	  ◦ Extreme = ≥ 14

Other specified feeding or eating disorder	• Presence of distressful and impairing symptoms but does not meet full criteria for another FED • Specific reasons for behaviors identified
Unspecified feeding or eating disorder	• Presence of distressful and impairing symptoms but does not meet full criteria for another FED • No specific reasons for behaviors identified

Abbreviations: DSM-5 = *Diagnostic and Statistical Manual of Mental Disorders*, 5th edition; BMI = body mass index.

image distortion.[57] Both adults and children may be affected by AN, and 0.3–0.4% of young women and 0.1% of young men are estimated to suffer from AN.[58] AN is often associated with severe blood pressure and cardiovascular complications, which may result in death. Electrolyte imbalances and nutrient deficiencies are also common.[59]

Patients with AN may rapidly deteriorate if acute illness occurs (e.g. trauma or sepsis), as they are unable to withstand the inflammatory state induced by the illness. Patients with AN have the highest risk of medical complications leading to death if they are also severely malnourished. Severely malnourished patients with AN admitted to the hospital have a high risk of medical instability and longer hospitalization due to the risk of refeeding syndrome (i.e. acid/base imbalances and electrolyte disturbances) as nutritional repletion begins.[60]

Treatment for AN includes psychological and nutritional rehabilitation; there are no medications that have been shown to consistently and effectively treat the disorder.[61] Patients with AN who become clinically unstable and/or who have extreme complications such as hypotension and bradycardia are usually admitted to the hospital for careful monitoring during the early stages of nutrition repletion. Recent research has shown that patients should remain hospitalized until clinically stable, not necessarily until weight is restored.[62]

Historically, patients admitted to a hospital with AN were initially fed a small amount of calories (about 500 kcal/day) either orally or through a feeding tube, in order to reduce the risk of refeeding syndrome. However, controlled studies conducted in pediatric hospitals under close monitoring showed that initial provision of more calories per day, individualized to the patient's needs, with a rapid increase in calorie intake can be safe and lead to greater short-term weight gain as well as improvements in heart rate and blood pressure.[59,63] A multicenter trial that tracked end-of-treatment for one year showed that starting initial feeding at 2000 kcal/day and increasing by 200 kcal/day until daily energy goals were reached was safe and led to earlier return of medical stability without electrolyte abnormalities or other adverse events. The hospital stay was four days shorter, leading to treatment-related cost savings.[63] Exact calorie amounts needed for replenishment have not been established, as this can be highly variable and should be tailored to the individuals' goals and overall treatment plan. Regular monitoring during the recovery period is necessary to adjust nutrient goals over time.[59]

Long-term treatment for AN may involve a residential treatment facility, where patients receive psychological therapy and nutritional repletion treatment for several months. These programs usually provide many types of services, including but not limited to behavioral therapy, nutrition education for healthy eating patterns and relationships with food, classes to learn coping skills for life stressors, body image therapy, and medication management as needed. Treatment stays in these facilities can be expensive and a substantial time, effort and financial commitment for the patient and family. There are not enough facilities in the United States to treat all patients with AN; therefore, day treatment programs have been established. Patients attend group therapy, individual therapy sessions, and eat one to three meals a day (depending on the program) in a controlled environment with supervision. Day treatment programs can be a safe, effective, and less costly alternative to inpatient care after medical stabilization.[64]

2 Bulimia Nervosa

Bulimia nervosa is characterized by repeated episodes of binge eating followed by inappropriate compensatory behaviors to purge consumed energy and/or relieve guilty feelings. Recognition of BN is more difficult than AN because most individuals with BN are of normal or overweight status.[55] When combining prevalence data from multiple sources, researchers found that BN is more common than AN, with estimates that between 1.1% and 4.6% of females and 0.1% to 0.5% of males will develop bulimia during their lifetime.[65]

It is important to diagnose and treat BN due to the medical risks associated with the disease, such as electrolyte disturbances and comorbid psychological disorders. Purging by vomiting or laxatives will cause electrolyte depletion that can lead to heart arrhythmias and possibly heart failure and death. Frequent food restriction and/or purging can lead to stomach pain, blood sugar fluctuations, dental decay, and gastroparesis. Laxative abuse can damage nerve endings and weaken the muscles of the intestines, leading to chronic constipation and early satiety. Binge eating can cause the gastrointestinal tract to rupture, which can be immediately life-threatening. Bulimia nervosa with malnutrition can cause pancreatitis, and the loss of muscle mass associated with malnutrition can cause mechanical bowel problems such as severe gastroparesis or intestinal obstruction, alterations in ability to complete activities of daily living, and the inability to fight off infections.[56] These side effects can contribute to inadequate intake or impaired digestion, therefore increasing the risk of malnutrition.

Similar to other FEDs, treatment for BN is multifactorial, and includes psychological and nutrition interventions. Unlike other FEDs, medications are often used in conjunction with psychological and nutritional counseling. To help patients respond to stress without harmful eating disorders and to reduce the binge-purge cycle, antidepressants are often prescribed; tricyclic antidepressants are the least commonly used as they increase the risk of arrhythmias.[66] Nutrition counseling includes healthful eating guidance, with some RDNs using the Intuitive Eating approach to help patients recover from BN.[67] This approach reinforces that food is not a tool for weight management, but rather that one should learn to eat foods in the amounts that make one's body feel healthy without guilt and without influence from diet culture. One of the principles for Intuitive Eating is that foods are not considered "equal" in nutrient content but are equal in their emotional influence.[68] This nutritional therapeutic approach can therefore be appropriate for treating BN and other types of FEDs.

3   Avoidant/Restrictive Food Intake Disorder

Avoidant/Restrictive Food Intake Disorder is more than "picky eating"; it is characterized by highly selected eating habits and disturbed feeding patterns driven by a psychiatric disorder.[69] Common patterns include reported difficulty digesting food; avoidance of certain food textures, colors, or smells; eating abnormally slowly; and having a general lack of appetite. Avoidant/Restrictive Food Intake Disorder often results in persistent failure to meet nutritional needs, leading to nutrient deficiencies and malnutrition. Up to 14% of people diagnosed with another FED will also be diagnosed with ARFID.[70] Children with ARFID may be more likely to develop chronic malnutrition, and are at higher risk of other mental disorders such as mood disorder, anxiety disorder, and an autism spectrum condition.[70,71]

Avoidant/Restrictive Food Intake Disorder that results in malnutrition should be treated aggressively. Due to the relatively recent identification of ARFID as a disorder, there is limited published evidence to guide treatment. Family-based therapy that can effectively treat AN shows the most promising results for ARFID treatment. Registered dietitian nutritionists often work with patients and families to determine underlying causes of the disorder, and address those as needed. For example, if food textures are not tolerated or refused, then new foods may be slowly introduced and a feeding therapist may be a part of the care team. Anti-anxiety medications and/or appetite stimulants may also be trialed depending on the underlying causes of ARFID.[72]

C   Concurrent SUD and FED

People with SUDs are at increased risk of developing an eating disorder. According to the National Eating Disorders Association, up to 35% of people with alcohol or drug dependency also have an eating disorder, a rate eleven times greater than the overall population. Even more telling, according to the National Center on Addiction and Substance Abuse, up to 50% of people with eating disorders have abused alcohol or drugs.[56] Although these statistics are clinically significant, it is not clear if the pathophysiologies for these categories of disorders are linked either genetically or environmentally. FEDs and SUDs share common risk factors, including altered brain chemistry, depression, anxiety, compulsive behavior, social isolation, and risk of suicide.[73]

IV CONCLUSION

Social/environmental or starvation-related malnutrition can be caused by a number of factors, most notably food insecurity. Some risks of food insecurity are not modifiable, such as race, ethnicity or age. Other risks are very difficult to modify, such as income or location of residence. Screening for food insecurity can occur in a number of settings, including community programs and acute care facilities. Food insecurity can be partially mitigated with the use of successful food assistance programs; however, funding and other support for these programs can be limited, which complicates treatment for this type of malnutrition. The most successful interventions are accompanied by a nutrition education component.

Other causes of starvation-related malnutrition include SUDs and FEDs. Malnutrition treatment related to these disorders is challenging, as recovery is generally reliant on successful treatment of the disorder itself. These populations, especially patients with FEDs, are particularly vulnerable to medical complications, thus it is important to diagnose and treat malnutrition properly.

REFERENCES

1. White JV, Guenter P, Jensen G, Malone A, Schofield M. The consensus statement of the Academy of Nutrition and Dietetics/American Society for Parenteral and Enteral Nutrition: characteristics recommended for the identification and documentation of adult malnutrition (undernutrition). *J Acad Nutr Diet*. 2012;112(5):730–738.
2. U.S. Department of Agriculture. Definitions of food security. Updated September 9, 2020. Accessed August 16, 2021. www.ers.usda.gov/topics/food-nutrition-assistance/food-security-in-the-us/definitions-of-food-security/.
3. Loopstra R. Interventions to address household food insecurity in high-income countries. *Proc Nutr Soc*. 2018;77(3):270–281.
4. Healthy People 2020. Food insecurity influences. Accessed August 16, 2021. www.healthypeople.gov/2020/topics-objectives/topic/social-determinants-health/interventions-resources/food-insecurity.
5. Dutko P, Ver Ploeg M, Farrigan T. Characteristics and influential factors of food deserts. USDA. 2012. Economic Research Report Number 140.
6. Moffat T, Mohammed C, Newbold KB. Cultural dimensions of food insecurity among immigrants and refugees. *Hum Organ*. 2017;76(1):15–27.
7. Olum S, Okello-Uma I, Tumuhimbise GA, Taylor D, Ongeng D. The relationship between cultural norms and food security in the Karamoja sub-region of Uganda. *J Food Nutr Res*. 2017;5(6):427–435.
8. Economic Research Service, U.S. Department of Agriculture. U.S. Adult Food Security Survey Module: three-stage design with screeners. Published September 2012. Accessed August 26, 2021. www.ers.usda.gov/media/8279/ad2012.pdf.

9. Economic Research Service, U.S. Department of Agriculture. U.S. Household Food Security Survey Module: six-item short form. Published September 2012. Accessed August 26, 2021. www.ers.usda.gov/media/8282/short2012.pdf.

10. Hager ER, Quigg AM, Black MM, et al. Development and validity of a 2-item screen to identify families at risk for food insecurity. *Pediatrics.* 2010;126(1):e27–e32.

11. Gattu RK, Paik G, Wang Y, Ray P, Lichenstein R, Black MM. The Hunger Vital Sign identifies household food insecurity among children in emergency departments and primary care. *Children.* 2019;6(10):107.

12. Center on Budget and Policy Priorities. Policy basics: the Supplemental Nutrition Assistance Program (SNAP). Updated June 25, 2021. Accessed August 18, 2021. www.cbpp.org/research/food-assistance/the-supplemental-nutrition-assistance-program-snap.

13. Women, Infants and Children. WIC at a glance. Updated October 10, 2013. Accessed August 18, 2021. www.fns.usda.gov/wic/about-wic-glance.

14. Meals on Wheels. Accessed August 18, 2021. www.mealsonwheelsamerica.org/.

15. Coalition on Human Needs. Outcomes: Supplemental Nutrition Assistance Program. Updated October, 2016. Accessed August 16, 2021. www.chn.org/wp-content/uploads/2016/07/SNAP-Outcomes-2016-Update.pdf.

16. Carlson S, Rosenbaum D, Keith-Jennings B, Nchako C. SNAP works for America's children. Center on Budget and Policy Priorities. Published September 29, 2016. Accessed August 16, 2021. www.cbpp.org/research/food-assistance/snap-works-for-americas-children.

17. Ettinger de Cuba S, Chilton M, Bovell-Ammon A, et al. Loss of SNAP is associated with food insecurity and poor health in working families with young children. *Health Aff.* 2019;38(5):765–773.

18. Carlson S, Keith-Jennings B. SNAP is linked with improved nutritional outcomes and lower health care costs. Center on Budget and Policy Priorities. Published January 17, 2018. Accessed August 16, 2021. www.cbpp.org/sites/default/files/atoms/files/1-17-18fa.pdf.

19. Szanton SL, Samuel LJ, Cahill R, et al. Food assistance is associated with decreased nursing home admissions for Maryland's dually eligible older adults. *BMC Geriatrics.* 2017;17(1):162.

20. Women, Infants and Children. WIC fact sheet. Published February 14, 2019. Accessed August 18, 2021. www.fns.usda.gov/wic/wic-fact-sheet.

21. Women, Infants and Children. Food packages. Updated October 15, 2015. Accessed August 18, 2021. www.fns.usda.gov/wic/wic-food-packages-maximum-monthly-allowances.

22. Women, Infants and Children. How WIC helps. Updated October 10, 2013. Accessed August 18, 2021. www.fns.usda.gov/wic/about-wic-how-wic-helps.

23. United States General Accounting Office. Federal investments like WIC can produce savings. GAO/HRD-92-18. Published April 1992. Accessed August 18, 2021. www.gao.gov/assets/hrd-92-18.pdf.

24. Waite T. What is the difference between a food bank and a food pantry? Feeding America. Published February 20, 2019. Accessed August 18, 2021. https://www.feedingamerica.org/hunger-blog/what-difference-between-food-bank-and-food-pantry

25. Simmet A, Depa J, Tinnemann P, Stroebele-Benschop N. The nutritional quality of food provided from food pantries: a systematic review of existing literature. *J Acad Nutr Diet.* 2017;117(4):577–588.

26. Wholesome Wave. Produce Prescription Programs US Field Scan Report: 2010-2020. Published April 2021. Accessed August 18, 2021. https://static1.squarespace.com/static/5febb5b1df316630764c4dec/t/60d0e873a8100c7ed37499d5/1624303736319/produce_prescription_programs_us_field_scan_report__june_2021_final.pdf.

27. Donohue J, Severson T, Martin LP. The food pharmacy: theory, implementation, and opportunities. *Am J Prev Cardiol.* 2021;5(S2):100145.

28. Bryce R, Guajardo C, Ilarraza D, et al. Participation in a farmers' market fruit and vegetable prescription program at a federally qualified health center improves hemoglobin A1C in low income uncontrolled diabetics. *Prev Med Rep.* 2017;7:176–179.

29. Cavanagh M, Jurkowski J, Bozlak C, Hastings J, Klein A. Veggie RX: an outcome evaluation of a healthy food incentive programme. *Pub Health Nutr.* 2017;20(14):2636–2641.

30. Wetherill MS, McIntosh HC, Beachy C, Shadid O. Design and implementation of a clinic-based food pharmacy for food insecure, uninsured patients to support chronic disease self-management. *Nutr Educ Behav.* 2018;50(9):947–949.

31. Hess A, Passaretti M, Coolbaugh S. Fresh Food Farmacy. *Am J Health Promot.* 33(5):830–832.

32. Swartz H. Produce RX programs for diet-based chronic disease prevention. *AMA J Ethics.* 2018;20(10):E960–973.

33. North Carolina Department of Health and Human Services. Health opportunities pilots. Accessed August 18, 2021. www.ncdhhs.gov/about/department-initiatives/healthy-opportunities/healthy-opportunities-pilots.

34. Food is Medicine Coalition. Accessed August 21, 2021. www.fimcoalition.org/

35. Gerencher K. Health insurers are beginning to include coverage for healthy foods. Could it save lives? Published March 2, 2021. Accessed August 18, 2021. www.goodrx.com/blog/health-insurance-coverage-for-healthy-foods/.

36. Berkowitz SA, Terranova J, Randall L, Cranston K, Waters DB, Hsu J. Association between receipt of a medically tailored meal program and health care use. *JAMA Intern Med.* 2019;179(6):786–793.

37. Rabaut LJ. Medically tailored meals as a prescription for treatment of food-insecure type 2 diabetics. *J Patient Cent Res Rev.* 2019;6(2):179–183.

38. Gurvey J, Rand K, Daugherty S, Dinger C, Schmeling J, Laverty N. Examining health care costs among MANNA clients and a comparison group. *J Prim Care Community Health.* 2013;4(4)311–317.

39. American Psychiatric Association (APA). *Diagnostic and Statistical Manual of Mental Disorders.* 5th ed. American Psychiatric Publishing; 2013.

40. Lessa N. DSM-T update: substance-related and addictive disorders. Updated November 1, 2013. Accessed August 18, 2021. www.slideshare.net/chat2recovery/dsm-5-update-p-p-revision.

41. Jensen GL, Cederholm T, Correia MITD, et al. GLIM criteria for the diagnosis of malnutrition: a consensus report from the global clinical nutrition community. *JPEN J Parenter Enteral Nutr.* 2019;43(1):32–40.

42. Moss HB, Ge S, Trager E, et al. Risk for Substance Use Disorders in young adulthood: Associations with developmental experiences of homelessness, foster care, and adverse childhood experiences. *Compr Psychiatry.* 2020;100:152–175.

43. Cadet JL. Epigenetics of stress, addiction, and resilience: therapeutic implications. *Mol Neurobiol.* 2016;53(1):545–560.

44. Strike C, Rudzinski K, Patterson J, Millson M. Frequent food insecurity among injection drug users: correlates and concerns. *BMC Public Health.* 2012;12:1058.

45. Mahboub N, Rizk R, Karavetian M, de Vries N. Nutritional status and eating habits of people who use drugs and/or are undergoing treatment for recovery: a narrative review. *Nutr Rev.* 2021;79(6):627–635.

46. Chavez MN, Rigg KK. Nutritional implications of opioid use disorder: a guide for drug treatment providers. *Psychol Addict Behav.* 2020;34(6):699–707.

47. Kampov-Polevoy A, Garbutt JC, Janowsky D. Evidence of preference for a high-concentration sucrose solution in alcoholic men. *Am J Psychiatry.* 1997;154(2):269–270.

48. Neale J, Nettleton S, Pickering L, Fischer J. Eating patterns among heroin users: A qualitative study with implications for nutritional interventions. *Addiction.* 2012;107(3):635–641.

49. Leclercq S, Cani PD, Neyrinck AM, et al. Role of intestinal permeability and inflammation in the biological and behavioral control of alcohol-dependent subjects. *Brain Behav Immun.* 2012;26(6):911–918.

50. Ghufran A. Nutrition in chronic liver disease: a point-of-care review. *Nutr Clin Pract.* 2020;35(2):211–217.

51. Dasarathy S. Nutrition and alcoholic liver disease: effects of alcoholism on nutrition, effects of nutrition on ALD and nutritional therapies for ALD. *Clin Liv Dis.* 2016;20(3):535–550.

52. Chao A, Waitzberg D, Passos de Jesus R, et al. Malnutrition and nutritional support in alcoholic liver disease: a review. *Curr Gastroenterol Rep.* 2016;18(12):65.

53. Rossi RE, Conte D, Massironi S. Diagnosis and treatment of nutritional deficiencies in alcoholic liver disease: Overview of available evidence and open issues. *Dig Liver Dis.* 2015;47(10):819–825.

54. Sanvisens A, Zuluaga P, Pineda M, et al. Folate deficiency in patients seeking treatment of alcohol use disorder. *Drug Alcohol Depend.* 2017;180:417–422.

55. Klump KL, Bulik CK, Kaye W, Treasure J, Tyson E. Academy for Eating Disorders position paper: eating disorders are serious mental illnesses. *Int J Eat Disord.* 2009;42(2):97–103.

56. National Eating Disorders Association. Accessed August 18, 2021. www.nationaleati ngdisorders.org/health-consequences.

57. Cuerda C, Vasiloglou MF, Arhip L. Nutritional management and outcomes in malnourished medical inpatients: Anorexia nervosa. *J Clin Med.* 2019;8:1042–1059.

58. Keski-Rahkonen A, Hoek HW, Susser ES, et al. Epidemiology and course of anorexia nervosa in the community. *Am J Psychiatry.* 2007;164(8):1259–1265.

59. Resmark G, Herpertz S, Herpertz-Dahlmann B, Zeeck A. Treatment of anorexia nervosa—new evidence-based guidelines. *J Clin Med.* 2019;8(2):153.

60. Davies JE, Cockfield A, Brown A, Corr J, Smith D, Munro C. The medical risks of severe anorexia nervosa during initial re-feeding and medical stabilisation. *Clin Nutri ESPEN.* 2017;17:92–99.

61. Brockmeyer T, Friederich H-C, Schmidt U. Advances in the treatment of anorexia nervosa: a review of established and emerging interventions. *Psychol Med.* 2018;48(8):1228–1256.

62. Madden S, Miskovic-Wheatley J, Wallis A, et al. A randomized controlled trial of in-patient treatment for anorexia nervosa in medically unstable adolescents. *Psychol Med.* 2015;45(2):415–427.

63. Garber AK, Cheng J, Accurso EC, et al. Short-term outcomes of the study of refeeding to optimize inpatient gains for patients with anorexia nervosa: a multicenter randomized clinical trial. *JAMA Pediatr.* 2021;175(1):19–27.

64. Herpertz-Dahlmann B. Adolescent eating disorders: update on definitions, symptomatology, epidemiology, and comorbidity. *Child Adolesc Psychiatr Clin N Am.* 2015;24(1):177–196.

65. Stice E, Bohon C. Eating disorders. In: *Child and Adolescent Psychopathology.* 2nd ed. Wiley; 2012.

66. Israel M. Should some drugs be avoided when treating bulimia nervosa? *J Psychiatry Neurosci.* 2002;27(6):457.

67. Koller KA, Thompson KA, Miller AJ, Walsh EC, Bardone-Cone AM. Body appreciation and intuitive eating in eating disorder recovery. *Int J Eat Disord.* 2020;53(8):1261–1269.

68. Tribole E, Resch E. *Intuitive Eating: A Revolutionary Program that Works.* St Martin's Griffin; 2012.

69. American Psychiatric Association. Accessed August 18, 2021. www.psychiatry.org/patients-families/eating-disorders/what-are-eating-disorders.

70. Nicely TA, Lane-Loney S, Masciulli E, Hollenbeak CS, Ornstein RM. Prevalence and characteristics of avoidant/restrictive food intake disorder in a cohort of young patients in day treatment for eating disorders. *J Eat Disord.* 2014;2(1):21.

71. Fisher MM, Rosen DS, Ornstein RM, et al. Characteristics of avoidant/restrictive food intake disorder in children and adolescents: a "new disorder" in DSM-5. *J Adolesc Health.* 2014;55(1):49–52.

72. Walden Behavioral Care. Avoidant/Restrictive Food Intake Disorder. Accessed August 18, 2021. www.waldeneatingdisorders.com/what-we-treat/arfid/.

73. The National Center on Addiction and Substance Abuse (CASA) at Columbia University. *Food for Thought: Substance Abuse and Eating Disorders.* New York: 2003.

14 Healthcare Payment Systems

Wendy Phillips

CONTENTS

I INTRODUCTION

There are many ways that healthcare facilities receive payment for services rendered. Payers can be broadly categorized as governmental payers such as Medicare and Medicaid, private payers such as insurance companies, and self-pay. Many private payers create payment policies that are the same as or similar to those enacted by Medicare or Medicaid. Since the advent of the Affordable Care Act and Reconciliation Act in 2010[1] it is not very common to find individuals who choose to pay out of pocket for healthcare services rather than enroll in an insurance plan. Therefore, this chapter will focus on payment policies promulgated through the Centers for Medicare & Medicaid Services (CMS), which administers Medicare and Medicaid, and review CMS payment methodologies that are effective in fiscal year (FY) 2022 for these types of facilities:

- Inpatient – acute care
- Skilled nursing facility
- Outpatient care clinics

DOI: 10.1201/9781003177586-14

CMS pays the service provider based on reimbursement rules created for that facility or provider type. These methodologies and payment rates can be updated each year, with effective dates to mirror CMS's FY of October 1 through September 30 of the following year.

II   BACKGROUND INFORMATION

ICD-10-CM, the International Classification of Diseases, 10th Revision, Clinical Modification, is used to translate documentation of medical diagnoses into numerical codes.[2] Procedures and outpatient services are translated into numerical codes using Current Procedural Terminology (CPT) codes. This translation helps to standardize medical record documentation and contribute towards a large data set that is easily extractable for use in large research studies. The ICD system is mainly used to document and research mortality and morbidity. The United States also uses ICD-CM and CPT codes for billing purposes and has been using the 10th edition since October 1, 2015.[2]

As discussed throughout this chapter, Medicare uses claims data that include billing codes to easily obtain large amounts of extractable data for quality improvement and research purposes. This data set is used to determine which diseases, conditions, and surgeries/procedures are the most likely to increase resource intensity in a given care setting.[3] That information is used to further inform future changes in payment methodologies and classification rates. Therefore, all conditions, including those that are nutrition-related such as obesity and malnutrition, should be diagnosed, documented, treated, coded and added to the claim whenever they exist.

This chapter contains many commonly used abbreviations and terminology. See Table 14.1 for definitions.

III   INPATIENT – ACUTE CARE

Hospitals are rarely reimbursed for costs incurred by patients enrolled in Medicare or Medicaid on a fee-for-service basis. Instead, Medicare uses the Inpatient Prospective Payment System (IPPS), which includes the Medicare Severity-Diagnosis Related Groups (MS-DRGs) classification system.[3] Also funded by CMS, most state Medicaid programs use a similar classification system titled All Patient Refined DRGs (APR-DRGs).[4] Many private insurance companies also use APR-DRGs to determine hospital payments for their beneficiaries. The underlying premise of these payment systems is that patients admitted to the hospital for the same diagnosis, with similar complications and comorbidities, will require about the same amount of resources and have the same length of stay (LOS) if high-quality care is provided efficiently. Hospitals are paid more to care for sicker patients, because these patients are more likely to require higher costs of care (known as resource intensity). The lump-sum payment that hospitals receive under the IPPS encourages them to ensure that patients have good outcomes without utilizing unnecessary hospital resources.

In order to determine payment amounts, each hospital is assigned its own Medicare payment rate based on two national base payment rates for operation and capital expenses (called a blended rate).[3] This blended rate is also influenced by several other

TABLE 14.1

Definition of Terms Commonly Used in Hospitals Related to Medicare and Medicaid Reimbursement[5]

Terminology	Abbreviation	Explanation or definition
International Classification of Diseases, 10th Revision, Clinical Modification	ICD-10-CM	System used by the World Health Organization and adapted for use in the US by the National Center for Health Statistics to classify and code all diagnoses, symptoms, and medical procedures.
Centers for Medicare & Medicaid Services	CMS	A governmental agency that is part of the US Department of Health and Human Services. It is responsible for funding and overseeing Medicare and Medicaid insurance on behalf of the federal government.
Inpatient Prospective Payment System	IPPS	Hospital payment system for inpatient stays under Medicare Part A based on set rates which are updated yearly. Each diagnosis is categorized into a diagnosis-related group (DRG). Each DRG has a payment weight assigned to it, based on the average amount of resources used to treat Medicare patients in that DRG.
Complication or Comorbidity	CC	Secondary diagnoses can be complications (conditions that developed after admission) or comorbidities (conditions present on admission).
Major Complication or Comorbidity	MCC	Similar to CCs, secondary diagnoses that are considered MCCs are more likely to cause severe disease or complications. MCCs are a higher severity level and therefore increase the relative weight (RW) of the MS-DRG.
Major Diagnostic Category	MDC	Defined by Medicare, each principal diagnosis is classified into one of 25 available MDCs. The diagnoses in each MDC correspond to a single organ system or etiology.
Diagnosis Related Group	DRG	Defined by Medicare, groups based on the principal diagnosis causing hospital admission.
Medicare Severity – Diagnosis Related Group	MS-DRG	Each MS-DRG is defined by certain patient attributes, including the principal diagnosis, specific secondary diagnoses (coded as a CC or MCC – see above definitions), medical procedures, sex, and discharge status.
All Patient Refined – Diagnosis Related Group	APR-DRG	The APR-DRG system is similar to the MS-DRGs, and was developed to better reflect the problems and resource utilization of non-Medicare populations, specifically pediatric, neonatal, and obstetric patients.

(continued)

TABLE 14.1 (Continued)

Definition of Terms Commonly Used in Hospitals Related to Medicare and Medicaid Reimbursement[5]

Terminology	Abbreviation	Explanation or definition
Relative Weight	RW	A value assigned by Medicare to each MS-DRG to reflect the expected severity level and calculate hospital payments for patients assigned to that MS-DRG.
Case Mix Index	CMI	The CMI is the average of the RWs for MS-DRGs for all patients admitted to the hospital in that year. It is a measure of the acuity level of the patient population served at that hospital.
Present on Admission	POA	Medical record documentation needs to identify if the diagnosis was POA. Only diagnoses that are POA will influence the MS-DRG assignment, and new diagnoses that develop after admission may be considered hospital-acquired conditions.
Length of Stay	LOS	The number of days a patient spends in the hospital.
Severity of Illness	SOI	The extent of physiological decompensation of an organ system or disease state. It can be categorized as minor, moderate, major, or extreme, and is meant to provide a basis for evaluating hospital resource use or establish patient care guidelines.
Risk of Mortality	ROM	Medicare's estimate of the likelihood of dying from being treated in a particular hospital for a particular condition.
Resource Intensity	- Not commonly abbreviated -	A measure of the resources required to produce a good or service, or for the completion of a process or activity; it measures the efficiency of resource use. In healthcare settings, it refers to the relative volume and types of diagnostic, therapeutic, and bed services needed to manage an illness.

factors, including but not limited to geography, resident and medical education costs, overhead costs, and average case mix index (CMI), which indicates the acuity level of patients cared for at that institution. This payment rate is also known as the Medicare standardized payment rate. This rate is used in the payment calculation for every Medicare beneficiary who receives care at that hospital during that year. Each patient is then assigned to a MS-DRG based on unique characteristics of that hospital stay. Both the hospital's blended rate and the patient's MS-DRG assignment are used in the calculation to determine the payment the hospital will receive.

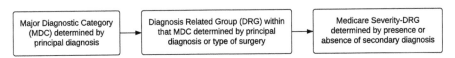

FIGURE 14.1   Steps involved to assign the Medicare Severity – Diagnosis Related Group once the principal diagnosis has been determined prior to discharge.[3]

A   MS-DRG ASSIGNMENT

The principal diagnosis necessitating hospital admission decides the Major Diagnostic Category (MDC) assigned to the patient for that hospital stay.[3] Within this MDC, the individual Diagnosis Related Group (DRG) is determined based on details of the patient's diagnosis and hospital treatment. If the patient is managed medically, the principal diagnosis determines the DRG assignment; if the patient is primarily managed surgically, then the type of surgery will determine the DRG assignment. Secondary diagnoses, known as Complications or Comorbidities (CCs) and Major Complications or Comorbidities (MCCs), can increase the cost of care above what would have been required if the patient only needed treatment for the principal diagnosis. When these secondary diagnoses are documented, treated, and coded, the patient may be assigned to a different severity level within the DRG grouping; this is then known as the Medicare Severity – DRG (MS-DRG). See Figure 14.1. A higher payment is given to hospitals for MS-DRGs associated with a CC, and an even higher payment for MS-DRGs associated an MCC.[3]

Some DRGs are considered triplets, others are doubles, and the remaining are singles, which are determined by CMS based on a complex data analysis methodology that is updated each year.[3] Triplet DRGs are those that have a higher payment amount if there is one or more CC, and a still higher payment amount if there is one or more MCC. Double DRGs do not have a higher payment amount if only CCs are coded; they require an MCC to be coded as a secondary diagnosis before the payment is increased. Admissions associated with a single DRG will be paid the same amount regardless of whether secondary diagnoses that are CCs or MCCs are coded (See Table 14.2).

Patients with secondary diagnoses are sicker and more likely to have poor health outcomes (known as "severity of illness").[5] They are also more likely to die during the hospitalization or shortly thereafter (known as "risk of mortality"). Only one CC is needed to increase the severity level to an MS-DRG with CC, and only one MCC is needed to increase the severity level to the highest level, an MS-DRG with MCC (see Table 14.2). There is no incremental increase in reimbursement provided with the addition of multiple CCs or MCCs as only one CC or MCC is required to impact payment. Each MS-DRG is assigned an associated relative weight (RW) by CMS; this RW can change each FY.[3] CMS publishes the payment tables each year at www.cms.gov/Medicare/Medicare-Fee-for-Service-Payment/AcuteInpat ientPPS/index.

TABLE 14.2

Explanation of Medicare Severity-Diagnosis Related Groups (MS-DRGs) Associated with Secondary Diagnoses with Examples[8]

Explanation type	Triplet DRGs	Double DRGs	Single DRGs
DRG structure	DRG with MCC	DRG with MCC	DRG
	DRG with CC	DRG without MCC	
	DRG without CC/MCC		
Example from Medicare FY 2021	Pneumothorax with MCC	Hypertension with MCC	Psychoses
	Pneumothorax with CC	Hypertension without MCC	
	Pneumothorax without CC/MCC		

Abbreviations: DRG = diagnosis related group; CC = complication or comorbidity; MCC = major complication or comorbidity; FY = fiscal year.

B MALNUTRITION CODING

Patients usually are not admitted to the hospital to treat malnutrition, but malnutrition is often present as a comorbidity that influences the resources required to treat the patient while hospitalized, and it therefore should be coded as a secondary diagnosis. The registered dietitian nutritionist (RDN) needs to document malnutrition as a nutrition diagnosis, and document a nutrition care plan to treat it.[6] In order to be coded using ICD-10-CM codes and added to the claim form, malnutrition must be diagnosed by the licensed independent practitioner (LIP), usually the physician, as a medical diagnosis. Since only one CC or MCC is needed to change the assigned MS-DRG and therefore the RW and payment, a malnutrition diagnosis may not always change the actual payment for a patient's hospital stay. However, the principal and all secondary diagnoses, including malnutrition, need to be documented to be included by the coding department.[6] Malnutrition diagnoses that can be coded are included in Table 14.3.

Although there are ICD-10-CM codes for malnutrition, there is no standardized definition for malnutrition accepted by CMS, the Centers for Disease Control and Prevention or any other agency, nor a universally accepted set of signs and symptoms that indicate the degree of malnutrition.[8] To ensure malnutrition is diagnosed similarly by RDNs and physicians at the same facility, a standard definition for malnutrition should be developed and implemented at each hospital. See Chapter 2 for further discussion on malnutrition diagnosis.

C MEDICARE PAYMENT

The hospital-specific Medicare blended payment rate for that FY is needed to determine the estimated payment for Medicare admissions.[3] This information can usually

TABLE 14.3
Malnutrition Codes That Are Considered MCCs or CCs by CMS[7]

Malnutrition ICD-10-CM codes that are MCCs	Malnutrition ICD-10-CM codes that are CCs
Kwashiorkor (E40)*	Moderate protein-calorie malnutrition (E44)
Nutritional marasmus (E41)*	Mild protein-calorie malnutrition (E44.1)
Marasmic kwashiorkor (E42)*	Retarded development following protein-calorie malnutrition (E45)
Unspecified severe protein-calorie malnutrition (E43)	Unspecified protein-calorie malnutrition (E46)
	Sequelae of protein-calorie malnutrition (E64)

* These conditions rarely occur in developed countries and therefore should only be used with extensive documentation proving the diagnosis.

Abbreviations: CMS = Centers for Medicare & Medicaid Services; ICD-10-CM = International Classification of Diseases, 10th Revision, Clinical Modification; MCC = major complication or comorbidity; CC = complication or comorbidity.

be obtained from the hospital's patient financial services office, the coding department, or administration. Once the hospital rate is known, additional information is needed for each patient. The coding department can provide the assigned MS-DRG and associated RW for each patient's admission. With this basic information, the payment can be estimated (before adjustments as described further in this chapter) as such:

- Relative weight (RW) of the MS-DRG multiplied by Medicare blended rate = payment

For example, a patient's hospital stay is assigned to the MS-DRG 434 (Cirrhosis and Alcoholic Hepatitis without CC/MCC), which has an associated RW of 0.6207 in FY 2022. The hospital's Medicare blended payment rate for 2022 is $6,805. Therefore, the equation would be:

- 0.6207 multiplied by $6,805 = $4,224

Regardless of the costs actually incurred by the hospital to provide services for that patient during that stay, they will receive $4,224 from Medicare (pending adjustments for value-based purchasing, addressed later in this chapter). The hospital accepts this payment structure as a Medicare-approved provider.

This same scenario can be used to demonstrate the higher reimbursement for hospital stays for patients assigned to MS-DRGs associated with CCs or MCCs. In this second example, the patient admitted to the hospital for cirrhosis also has moderate protein-calorie malnutrition, which increases care management needs (i.e. resource intensity) during the hospitalization and is classified by CMS as a CC. This patient would then be assigned to MS-DRG 433 (Cirrhosis and Alcoholic Hepatitis with CC), which has an associated RW of 1.0299 in FY 2022. The same Medicare blended rate of $6,805 would be used. Therefore, the calculation would be:

- 1.0299 multiplied by $6,805 = $7,008

In a third example, the patient admitted for cirrhosis with moderate protein-calorie malnutrition then develops a complication, severe sepsis with septic shock. This secondary diagnosis is classified by CMS as an MCC. This patient would then be assigned MS-DRG 432 (Cirrhosis and Alcoholic Hepatitis with MCC), which has a RW in FY 2022 of 1.8808. The same Medicare blended rate for the hospital would be used ($6,805). Therefore, the calculation would be:

- 1.8808 multiplied by $6,805 = $12,799

This increased payment reflects the increased cost that will likely be required to care for the patient with these additional complications and comorbidities.

D   ALL PATIENT REFINED–DIAGNOSIS–RELATED GROUP (APR-DRG) ASSIGNMENT

The MS-DRG classification system was developed for the Medicare population.[3] Therefore, it does not contain DRGs that are unique to pregnancy, neonatal, or pediatric admissions since these populations are not covered by Medicare. Therefore, the APR-DRG system was developed by a company called 3M™ through a contract with CMS.[4] The software is developed in partnership with the medical community, and is proprietary to 3M™. It is updated annually on the same timeframe as the MS-DRGs.

The underlying principle for assigning a patient's hospital stay to risk-adjusted, severity-level DRGs is the same as with MS-DRGs. Whereas the MS-DRG assignment process has three steps, the APR-DRG assignment is an 18-step process (see Figure 14.2). Therefore, computer algorithms available from 3M™ are the only efficient way to determine APR-DRG assignment. The basic steps for APR-DRG assignment are as follows[4]:

- The patient's hospitalization is first assigned to a "base" APR-DRG according to the principal diagnosis or most important surgical procedure performed in an operating room (as opposed to minor bedside procedures)
- Each base APR-DRG is divided into four subclasses, depending on the severity of illness (SOI) and risk of mortality (ROM) scores. The SOI and ROM scores

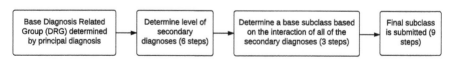

FIGURE 14.2   Steps involved to assign the All Patient Related–Diagnosis-Related Group.[4]

are determined based on the interaction between secondary diagnoses and the principal diagnosis, age, and procedures performed during the hospitalization

- Both an admission and a discharge APR-DRG are assigned, which may differ from one another (in comparison, for Medicare patients only a discharge MS-DRG is assigned). The admission APR-DRG only includes those secondary diagnoses that were present on admission (POA), whereas the discharge APR-DRG will include complications that develop during the admission and any surgeries or procedures performed
- The discharge APR-DRG is the one used for payment purposes, and for risk adjustment in quality-reporting programs

E SEVERITY OF ILLNESS AND RISK OF MORTALITY

The underlying disease state or condition of a patient determines the SOI and ROM scores.[5] Higher SOI and ROM scores are assigned to patients with multiple serious diseases and the interactions between those diseases. Severity of Illness refers to the extent of physiological decompensation or organ damage and loss of function. Risk of Mortality refers to a patient's risk of dying. There are four classifications:

- 1 – Minor
- 2 – Moderate
- 3 – Major
- 4 – Extreme

The SOI and ROM subclasses are calculated independently of each other. For example, a patient may have an SOI score of 3 – Major and an ROM score of 1 – Minor. Since these scores are determined by the interaction of multiple diseases and conditions, a software algorithm is required to perform the calculation.

Most hospital coding departments enter Medicare patients into the APR-DRG computer algorithm in order to obtain the SOI and ROM scores. Even though the SOI and ROM are not used to calculate payment for Medicare patients, they are used for quality-reporting purposes.

F MEDICARE PAYMENT ADJUSTMENTS

Due to annual adjustments by CMS, there are a number of factors besides the annual Medicare blended rate and the patient's assigned MS-DRG that affect the final reimbursement for each case. Performance on Value Based Purchasing (VBP) metrics reported through the Hospital Inpatient Quality Reporting (IQR) can affect the hospital's Medicare payment by approximately 3% of total payments.[9] Factors that may influence overall hospital payments include, but are not limited to:[9,10]

- Patient satisfaction scores on HCAHPS (Hospital Consumer Assessment of Healthcare Providers and Systems) surveys
- Penalties for excess readmissions compared to other hospitals with a similar proportion of patients who are dually eligible for Medicare and Medicaid

- ◦ Since FY 2017, the penalties have focused on a hospital's readmission rates for patients with acute myocardial infarction, heart failure, pneumonia, chronic obstructive pulmonary disease, elective primary total hip arthroplasty/total knee arthroplasty, and coronary artery bypass graft surgery[11]
- Penalties for hospitals in the worst-performing quartile under the Hospital-Acquired Condition (HAC) Reduction Program
  - ◦ HAC Reduction Program Measures for FY 2022 and subsequent years include the CMS Patient Safety and Adverse Events Composite score, catheter-associated urinary tract infection, hospital-onset *Clostridium difficile* infection, central line-associated bloodstream infection, specific surgical site infection, and hospital-onset methicillin-resistant *Staphylococcus aureus* (MRSA) bacteremia[12]

G   CASE MIX INDEX

In addition to affecting payment rates by changing the patient's assigned MS-DRG, documentation of CCs and MCCs affects the case mix index (CMI). The CMI is the average of the RWs of the MS-DRGs for all patients discharged from the hospital for the studied time period (usually averaged over the preceding year).[13] Hospitals with higher CMIs provide more complex and costly care. The CMI for the preceding year influences the upcoming year's Medicare blended rate for that hospital. In this manner, patients assigned with MS-DRG can affect the current hospital stay payment, as well as influence the new blended rate for that hospital for the next year. The level and complexity of services provided at a hospital can also be estimated by comparing the CMI of one hospital to another. Quality-reporting scorecards are often adjusted based on the CMI. Therefore, anything that can increase the assigned MS-DRG's RW and therefore the CMI, such as malnutrition coding, will be important to hospital administration and the financial team.

H   INFLUENCE OF MALNUTRITION CODING ON HOSPITAL PAYMENT

If malnutrition diagnoses documented by RDNs are not also documented by physicians, they will not be coded and the hospital can lose significant revenue due to missed opportunities to accurately assign the MS-DRG and capture patients' SOI and ROM. In 2015, a retrospective chart review was completed at a major academic medical center for 217 patients with community-acquired pneumonia (CAP) discharged over a one-year period.[14] Of these patients, there was a 58% misdiagnosis rate for severe protein-calorie malnutrition (E43) and lost revenue of $29,813. Similarly, another retrospective chart review at the same institution showed that 39 of 456 patients discharged during April 2015 with chronic obstructive pulmonary disease, CAP, spinal fusion, or chemotherapy were malnourished.[15] Of these patients, 19 were coded with malnutrition appropriately, whereas 20 patients were not, indicating malnutrition coding accuracy of only 50%. Of the 20 patients who were not coded for malnutrition when they should have been, nine would have made a payment difference if they had been coded appropriately, translating to $76,500 in missed revenue.

In a different community hospital, a retrospective chart review was conducted for patients with a nutrition diagnosis of malnutrition between February 2015 and June 2017. Of these 1817 patients, 1171 (64.5%) were not coded for malnutrition. Of those, 475 (41%) patients would have been assigned to an MS-DRG with a higher RW and therefore payment if the malnutrition had been coded appropriately, translating to $2.69 million in missed reimbursement.[16]

When malnutrition is documented, treated, and coded properly, significant payment increases can be realized. For example, after the clinical nutrition team implemented a quality-improvement project in 2017 and 2018 at a community hospital, malnutrition identification increased by 613 cases, or 228%. MS-DRG payment increased by an estimated $470,000 (not considering potential Medicare annual adjustments as described above).[17]

Accurately coding for malnutrition can also influence the CMI. In calendar year (CY) 2018, RDNs at a community hospital with an average census of 180 recorded the 961 patients they diagnosed with malnutrition, and compared that to the list of patients who were subsequently diagnosed by the physician and coded with malnutrition.[18] Of those, 609 (63.3%) were either not coded, or were coded inaccurately; 270 (44.3%) of those cases would have increased the CMI if they had been coded properly for malnutrition. The average difference in actual CMI and potential CMI for this group of 270 patients was 0.9028, which could have a significant effect on the hospital's overall CMI for the following year.[18]

1   Malnutrition Coding Denials

CMS has a responsibility to ensure that high-quality, cost-effective care is provided to Medicare and Medicaid beneficiaries.[3] Therefore, the US Department of Health and Human Services (HHS), Office of Inspector General (OIG) has the authority to protect the integrity of programs run by the HHS and to safeguard the health and welfare of beneficiaries served by those programs.[19] The OIG can audit the medical records of Medicare and Medicaid beneficiaries and/or direct regional Recovery Audit Contractors (RACs) to audit medical records to identify improper payments and verify compliance with payment policies. Results of OIG audits are public record, available on the website https://oig.hhs.gov.

While RAC auditors routinely audit hospitals for all diagnoses, they will periodically choose certain diagnoses for increased scrutiny. These are chosen based on high-volume diagnoses, and/or those with a high likelihood of significantly changing the MS-DRG assignment and increasing hospital payments. Code assignment and therefore payments may be deemed incorrect due to lack of evidence, such as inadequate documentation to support the diagnosis of severe malnutrition, or documentation that is inadequate to demonstrate that the malnutrition diagnosis affects the patient's plan of care or resource intensity.

If RAC auditors decide there is inadequate evidence to support code assignment, the MS-DRG that was assigned upon discharge is reduced in severity level to the MS-DRG that would have been assigned if the diagnosis had not been coded.[19] Correspondingly, the reimbursement to the hospital is reduced; if the hospital has already received the payment then they must repay Medicare.

2   Auditing Severe Malnutrition Codes

In 2014, the OIG began an intensive set of audits focused on claims that included kwashiorkor as a diagnosis.[19,20] For CYs 2010 and 2011, Medicare paid hospitals $711 million for claims that included a diagnosis code for kwashiorkor (E40). This raised red flags for Medicare, because kwashiorkor is a form of severe protein malnutrition that usually affects only children living in tropical and subtropical parts of the world during periods of famine or insufficient food supply. Cases in the United States are rare, and are especially rare in people aged 65 or older (the typical Medicare population). Therefore, the OIG launched a series of reviews of hospitals with claims that included that diagnosis code. One hospital in New Jersey was ordered to repay $375,000 to Medicare, as 197 of 198 of the charts audited did not have enough documentation to prove the diagnosis of kwashiorkor; of those, 48 had resulted in increased payment that had to be repaid.[19] Similarly, a hospital in Ohio had to repay $117,863 for incorrectly coding kwashiorkor for 95 patients, 17 of whom had increased payment.[20] These are two of many examples of hospitals that had to repay Medicare for inaccurately assigned kwashiorkor codes. The OIG stated in their decision that other codes for different types of malnutrition may have been accurate, but did not elaborate.

Due to the increased scrutiny on kwashiorkor codes, RDNs, hospital administrators, coders, physicians, and others placed more attention on accurately identifying and documenting malnutrition. In 2012, the consensus statement from the Academy of Nutrition and Dietetics (Academy) and the American Society for Parenteral and Enteral Nutrition (ASPEN) provided guidance to clinicians for malnutrition clinical characteristics that may indicate severe or non-severe (moderate) malnutrition in adults based on etiology.[8] These guidelines provided structure to more accurately assign malnutrition codes other than kwashiorkor. See Chapter 2 for more information on diagnosing malnutrition. The release of the Malnutrition Quality Improvement Initiative (MQii) in 2013 further enhanced clinicians' focus on comprehensive malnutrition programs in hospitals.[21] See Chapter 15 for more information on the MQii.

The increased attention on identification, documentation, and treatment of malnutrition in hospitals was beneficial for patient care. However, this resulted in a significant increase in malnutrition coding in the following years. Since ICD-10-CM code E43 unspecified severe protein-calorie malnutrition (Severe PCM) and code E41 nutritional marasmus are MCCs with a high SOI and ROM and can therefore greatly influence hospital payments, this gained attention from CMS and the OIG.[21]

As hospitals had successfully eliminated coding for kwashiorkor for inappropriate cases, the OIG turned their attention in July 2020 to claims associated with E41 and E43. The initial audit found Medicare paid US hospitals $3.4 billion for 224,175 claims for patients discharged in FY 2016 or 2017 that contained a severe malnutrition diagnosis code and for which removing the diagnosis code changed the MS-DRG.[22] Since they are unable to audit the high volume of cases, they selected for review a random sample of 200 claims with payments totaling $2.9 million.

The OIG found that hospitals correctly billed Medicare for severe malnutrition diagnosis codes for 27 of the 200 claims, and incorrectly billed for the remaining 173 claims.[22] For nine of these claims, the medical record documentation supported a secondary malnutrition diagnosis code other than severe malnutrition, but the error did not change the DRG or payment. For the remaining 164 claims, hospitals used severe malnutrition diagnosis codes when they should have used codes for other forms of malnutrition or no malnutrition diagnosis code at all, resulting in net overpayments of $914,128. Extrapolating from the sample audits to the full population of claims associated with severe malnutrition in those years, they estimated that hospitals received overpayments of $1 billion for FYs 2016 and 2017.

The OIG recommended that CMS collect the $914,128 for the incorrectly billed hospital claims, and notify hospitals that were not part of the audit but had included severe malnutrition on claims forms to review medical records to identify, report, and return any overpayments related to coding for severe malnutrition.[22] CMS concurred with the OIG recommendations and stated that it would instruct its contractors to recover the overpayments consistent with relevant law and CMS's policies and procedures.

In this July 2020 report describing the audit findings,[22] the OIG did not provide a rationale for each of the claims that were denied. Instead, they provided only two examples of reasons they thought hospitals had overbilled for claims related to severe malnutrition. In August 2020, Dr. James Kennedy filed a Freedom of Information Act request to obtain more details for the reasons the codes were denied.[23] The report shows that the review was thorough, and for most patient cases, the auditors utilized the Academy/ASPEN consensus statement malnutrition clinical characteristics to identify whether severe malnutrition was present. Dr. Kennedy noted the following trends that led to many of the coding denials:[23]

- A nutrition assessment was not documented
- The RDN documented severe malnutrition, while the physician documented the patient(s) were "well-developed and well-nourished". This usually happened in medical records for patients with obesity
- Although the patient met the diagnostic criteria for severe malnutrition, the intervention was deemed not complex enough to warrant inclusion of the code
- Although the patient met the diagnostic criteria for severe malnutrition, there was no documentation on how that diagnosis influenced resources required for care or influenced the LOS

Dr. Kennedy recommends that providers clearly document the patient's progress with nutrition interventions, the nursing time required for monitoring and implementation of the nutrition care plan, inclusion of the malnutrition diagnosis in the discharge summary, and the nutrition plan required to address social determinants of health and malnutrition treatment upon discharge.[23] He also recommends hospital coding departments implement a system to evaluate the medical records of all patients who will be assigned a severe malnutrition code that will make a difference in MS-DRG assignment (and therefore payment) prior to the claim form being electronically submitted to Medicare. RDNs should be involved to help ensure documentation is consistent and thorough to substantiate the claim.

Notably, Dr. Kennedy recommends employing this same strategy for all high-risk diagnoses frequently audited by the OIG. This audit and denial process is not unique to malnutrition diagnoses; many diagnoses are audited on a routine basis. Hospital coding departments frequently file appeals when claims are denied. RDNs should develop relationships with the coding department manager, and assist with the appeal process for malnutrition or other nutrition-related coding denials. This is an opportunity to share relevant hospital-specific information beyond what the auditors would have already found in the medical records, such as hospital policies and procedures identifying malnutrition clinical characteristics that are used and treatment plans that are available.

3 Malnutrition Documentation

The malnutrition documentation strategies discussed in this chapter should be utilized in all care settings. Clinicians need to determine if minimum diagnostic thresholds are met and consistently documented by all providers, whether adequate supporting documentation is present, if treatment fits the diagnosis, and if the impact on care is documented.

The statement "the best defense is a good offense" is true in this situation – medical record documentation needs to be clear, concise, and comprehensive so that it will be more likely to pass an audit if it occurs. The most common reasons that malnutrition codes are denied and recommended strategies to address them are listed in Table 14.4.

IV SKILLED NURSING FACILITIES

Long-term care (LTC) facilities provide skilled-care services by nurses or rehabilitation professionals.[25] These are commonly called skilled nursing facilities (SNF) or nursing homes. A new Medicare payment model for LTC, called the Patient Driven Payment Model (PDPM), began in 2019 and consists of one non-case-mix adjusted component and five case-mix adjusted components. Similar to the MS-DRG and APR-DRG payment systems, payment amounts are increased based on the acuity level of the resident, not based on the total therapy minutes provided.[26] The five categories of case-mix adjusted components include:

- Physical therapy (PT)
- Occupational therapy (OT)
- Speech-language pathology (SLP)
- Nursing
- Non-therapy ancillary (NTA)

The NTA classification assigns points when certain comorbidities are present, or when extensive services such as parenteral nutrition are used.[27] As of FY 2021, Medicare has designated 50 possible comorbidities, including malnutrition, that can influence the NTA classification. Points can range from one to eight depending on expected resource use, and comorbidities are grouped together based on the expected associated costs to provide care. Nutrition-related NTA components include:[26]

- Parenteral IV feeding, level high = 7 points
- Parenteral IV feeding, level low = 3 points
- Nutritional approaches: feeding tube = 1 point
- Active diagnoses: Malnutrition code = 1 point
- Morbid obesity = 1 point
- Active diagnoses: Diabetes mellitus (DM) code = 2 points

Similar to the IPPS, SNF payments are subject to VBP adjustments through the Quality Reporting Program (QRP) measures.[28] The FY 2022 measures most related to nutrition care include:

- Changes in skin integrity post-acute care; pressure injuries
- Application of percent of residents experiencing one or more falls with major injury (long stay)
- Potentially preventable 30-day post-discharge readmission measure for SNF QRP

TABLE 14.4
Strategies to Prevent Malnutrition Coding Denials[17–19]

Challenge encountered	Recommended strategy
Inconsistent use of malnutrition diagnostic clinical characteristics (e.g. Academy/ASPEN consensus statement,[8] GLIM,[20] or WHO[21] criteria)	Implement a policy that defines the criteria used to diagnose malnutrition. Educate all clinicians on the criteria. Audit documentation regularly to ensure consistency in practice.
The RDN documents malnutrition, but LIP (usually the physician) does not	Develop a communication process to ensure malnutrition is consistently documented by all clinicians in a way that is not contradictory.
Clinical significance is not documented	Develop a treatment plan and clearly document why interventions are adequately "aggressive" enough to treat the diagnosis. At each visit, document that the diagnosis continues to be an active problem, and increases the resources required to provide care and/or extends the hospital length of stay.
ICD-10-CM Official Guidelines for Coding and Reporting are not met. Note: "Additional billable conditions must affect patient care in terms of requiring clinical evaluation, therapeutic treatment, or diagnostic procedures or if those conditions extend the length of hospital stay or require increased nursing care or monitoring."[22]	RDNs and other clinicians should document how the malnutrition diagnosis affects each of those categories of patient care. It is acceptable to be explicit and use the wording from the coding guidelines.

Abbreviations: Academy / ASPEN = Academy of Nutrition and Dietetics / American Society for Enteral and Parenteral Nutrition; GLIM = Global Leadership Initiative on Malnutrition; WHO = World Health Organization; RDN = registered dietitian nutritionist; LIP = licensed independent practitioner criteria; ICD-10-CM = International Classification of Diseases, 10th Revision, Clinical Modification.

RDNs should work with the interdisciplinary team to implement care strategies to improve the performance on these measures, and communicate the value of medical nutrition therapy by an RDN in this care setting to facility administrators and medical directors. Similar to other care settings, nutrition diagnoses including malnutrition require complete and concise documentation.

V   OUTPATIENT HOSPITAL-BASED CLINICS

Medicare's VBP program that provides incentives for high-quality and cost-effective healthcare extends to outpatient hospital-based clinics through the use of Hierarchical Condition Categories (HCCs).[29] Medicare uses this type of payment for Accountable Care Organizations, Medicare Advantage plans, and Programs of All-Inclusive Care for the Elderly (PACE) programs. Similar to the other care settings discussed in this chapter, accurate coding of chronic diseases, like obesity and malnutrition, helps forecast expected cost of care. Providers are paid a higher rate if they deliver high-quality care at a more efficient cost. A concern expressed by the healthcare industry is that this could lead some healthcare providers to decide to only care for "healthy" patients – those at lower risk of having poor health outcomes – so that their quality and resource-use scores look better. In order to wash out this difference and encourage healthcare providers to also treat sicker patients, CMS uses a Risk Adjustment Factor (RAF) to enable more accurate quality comparisons across beneficiaries.[29] This risk adjustment concept for outpatient clinics is similar to the Medicare payment strategy for hospitals in the MS-DRG and APR-DRG systems.[3]

The RAF is calculated based on points assigned by Medicare to diseases and conditions that predict disease burden on costs and quality of care.[29] A patient's HCC points accumulate over the CY to determine the RAF. Examples of factors that contribute to HCC points include, but are not limited to:

- Demographic data such as age and gender
- Socioeconomic factors based on zip code information and Medicaid eligibility
- Disability status
- Chronic diseases or conditions that affect how sick a patient is or can become
  - A diagnosis of protein-calorie malnutrition adds points to the HCC, thereby increasing the provider and hospital's payment to care for that patient in the outpatient setting

Since the RAF for each patient is recalculated each year, all chronic conditions must be diagnosed, treated, and coded at least once each CY in order to accurately calculate risk-adjustment and budget the appropriate amount of money to care for that patient in the next CY.[29] All ICD-10-CM billing codes must be supported by documentation of a visit between the provider and patient, and documentation sources can include anything in an inpatient or outpatient visit.

In order to ensure accurate code assignment for inclusion as an HCC diagnosis for risk adjustment, providers, including RDNs, should follow the documentation acronym "MEAT", or "Managed – Evaluated – Assessed – Treated". In order for a chronic disease to be included in the RAF calculation, documenting "history of …" should be avoided, because the chronic disease must currently affect the patient's care and prognosis.

VI   CONCLUSION

Whether working in LTC, outpatient, or inpatient settings, it is important to adequately capture all relevant diagnoses, including malnutrition and other nutrition-related diagnoses, using ICD-10-CM codes and all procedures using CPT codes for every patient regardless of payer source. These coding data can then be used in large-scale research studies and quality-reporting purposes. RDNs should incorporate malnutrition care into every step of the nutrition care process, using clear and concise yet complete documentation. The information provided in this chapter can help RDNs take steps to maximize reimbursement from Medicare, Medicaid, and other insurance companies and avoid payment denials related to malnutrition documentation and coding. RDNs should work with an interdisciplinary care team for appropriate malnutrition interventions to help patients meet their goals for care.

REFERENCES

1. Read the Affordable Care Act. HealthCare.gov website. Accessed November 17, 2020. www.healthcare.gov/where-can-i-read-the-affordable-care-act/.
2. International Classification of Diseases (ICD-10-CM/PCS) Transition – Background. Centers for Disease Control and Prevention website. Updated November 6, 2015. Accessed November 17, 2020. www.cdc.gov/nchs/icd/icd10cm_pcs_background.htm.
3. Acute Care Hospital Inpatient Prospective Payment System. Medicare Learning Network website. Updated March 2020. Accessed November 19, 2020. www.cms.gov/Outreach-and-Education/Medicare-Learning-Network-MLN/MLNProducts/downloads/acutepaymtsysfctsht.pdf.
4. 33M™ All Patient Refined Diagnosis Related Groups (3M APR DRG). Accessed November 19, 2020. www.3m.com/3M/en_US/health-information-systems-us/drive-value-based-care/patient-classification-methodologies/apr-drgs/.
5. Using Severity Adjustment Classification for Hospital Internal and External Benchmarking. AHIMA website. Accessed November 19, 2020. https://library.ahima.org/doc?oid=59268#.X7ccJPlKg2w.
6. Phillips W, Browning M. A clinician's guide to defining, identifying, and documenting malnutrition in hospitalized patients. *Practical Gastroenterology*. 2017;169:19–22, 26–33.
7. 2021 ICD-10-CM. Centers for Medicare & Medicaid Services website. Updated August 19, 2020. Accessed November 19, 2020. www.cms.gov/medicare/icd-10/2021-icd-10-cm.
8. White J, Guenter P, Jenson G, et al. Consensus Statement of the Academy of Nutrition and Dietetics/American Society for Parenteral and Enteral Nutrition: Characteristics recommended for the identification and documentation of adult malnutrition (Undernutrition). *J Acad Nutr Diet*. 2012;112:730–738.
9. The Hospital Value-Based Purchasing Program. Centers for Medicare & Medicaid Services website. Updated January 6, 2020. Accessed November 19, 2020. www.cms.gov/Medicare/Quality-Initiatives-Patient-Assessment-Instruments/Value-Based-Programs/HVBP/Hospital-Value-Based-Purchasing

10. Fiscal Year (FY) 2022 Medicare Hospital Inpatient Prospective Payment System (IPPS) and Long Term Care Hospital (LTCH) Rates Final Rule (CMS-1752-F). Centers for Medicare & Medicaid Services website. Updated August 2, 2021. Accessed May 20, 2022. www.cms.gov/newsroom/fact-sheets/fiscal-year-fy-2022-medicare-hospital-inpatient-prospective-payment-system-ipps-and-long-term-care-0.

11. Centers for Medicare & Medicaid Services. Department of Health and Human Services. Federal Register. September 18, 2020. 85(182): 58436. Accessed May 20, 2022. www.govinfo.gov/content/pkg/FR-2020-09-18/pdf/2020-19637.pdf.

12. Centers for Medicare & Medicaid Services. Department of Health and Human Services. Federal Register. September 18, 2020. 85(182): 58861. Accessed May 20, 2022. www.govinfo.gov/content/pkg/FR-2020-09-18/pdf/2020-19637.pdf.

13. Case Mix Index. Centers for Medicare & Medicaid Services website. Accessed November 19, 2020. www.cms.gov/Medicare/Medicare-Fee-for-Service-Payment/AcuteInpatientPPS/Acute-Inpatient-Files-for-Download-Items/CMS022630.

14. Phillips W, Willcutts K. Reducing missed opportunities for hospital revenue and impacts on the case mix index through a malnutrition coding initiative. Abstract/poster presented at the annual symposium for the Clinical Nutrition Manager's dietetic practice group of the Academy of Nutrition and Dietetics. April 2016. Austin, TX.

15. Suarez J, Phillips W, Willcutts K. Accuracy of malnutrition documentation in the hospitalized adult: a retrospective analysis. *J Acad Nutr Diet.* 2016;116(9):A71.

16. Doley J, Phillips W. Accurate coding impacts the geometric length of stay for malnourished inpatients. *J Acad Nutr Diet.* 2019;119(2):193–197.

17. Oblein J, Doverspike K. Increasing malnutrition identification and coding through process improvement. *J Acad Nutr Diet.* 2019;119(9,S2)S64.

18. Doley J. Impact of accurate coding on Case Mix Index. *J Acad Nutr Diet.* 2019;119(9,S2) S68.

19. Department of Health and Human Services Office of Inspector General. Morristown Medical Center Incorrectly Billed Medicare Inpatient Claims with Kwashiorkor. A-03-13-00036. Published May 6, 2014. Accessed November 30, 2020. https://oig.hhs.gov/oas/reports/region3/31300036.asp.

20. Department of Health and Human Services Office of Inspector General. University Hospitals Case Medical Center Incorrectly Billed Medicare Inpatient Claims with Kwashiorkor. A-03-13-00031. Published March 5, 2014. Accessed November 30, 2020. https://oig.hhs.gov/oas/reports/region3/31300031.asp.

21. McCauley S, Mitchell K, Heap A. The malnutrition quality improvement initiative: A multiyear partnership transforms care. *J Acad Nutr Diet.* 2019;119(9 Suppl 2): S18–S24.

22. Department of Health and Human Services Office of Inspector General. Hospitals Overbilled Medicare $1 Billion By Incorrectly Assigning Severe Malnutrition Diagnosis Codes to Inpatient Hospital Claims. Published July 13, 2020. Accessed November 30, 2020. https://oig.hhs.gov/oas/reports/region3/31700010.asp.

23. Belton P, Kennedy JS. Compliance corner – OIG malnutrition audits confound compliance – time to act. *Health Law Connections.* Published October 1, 2020. Accessed November 17, 2020. www.americanhealthlaw.org/content-library/connections-magazine/article/fff97631-68c6-4de0-934b-3ed40d8d8d04/Compliance-Corner-OIG-Malnutrition-Audits-Confound.

24. ICD-10-CM Official Guidelines for Coding and Reporting. FY 2021. FY 2022 – Updated April 1, 2022. Centers for Disease Control and Prevention website. Accessed May 20, 2022. www.cms.gov/files/document/fy-2022-icd-10-cm-coding-guidelines-updated-02012022.

25. Janowski M. Centers for Medicaid & Medicare Services regulation changes for long term care. *Support Line*. 2019;41(4):4–9.

26. Patient Driven Payment Model: Frequently Asked Questions. Centers for Medicare & Medicaid Services. Updated August 30, 2019. Accessed November 13, 2020. www. cms.gov/Medicare/Medicare-Fee-for-Service-Payment/SNFPPS/PDPM#faq.

27. Department of Health and Human Services Centers for Medicare & Medicaid Services. State Operations Manual, Appendix PP – Guidance to Surveyors for Long Term Care Facilities. 2017. Available at www.cms.gov/Regulations-and-Guidance/ Guidance/ Manuals/downloads/som107ap_pp_guidelines_ltcf.pdf. Accessed November 13, 2020.

28. Skilled Nursing Facility Quality Reporting Program Data Collection and Final Submission Deadlines for the FY 2021 SNF QRP. Centers for Medicare & Medicaid Services website. Updated November 22, 2017. Accessed November 13, 2020. www. cms.gov/Medicare/Quality-Initiatives-Patient-Assessment-Instruments/NursingH omeQualityInits/Downloads/SNF-QRP-Data-Collection-and-Final-Submission-Deadlines-for-the-FY-2021-SNF-QRP_Revised.pdf.

29. Risk Adjustment. 2016 QRURs and the 2018 Value Modifier. Centers for Medicare & Medicaid Services website. Updated August 2017. Accessed November 19, 2021. www.cms.gov/Medicare/Medicare-Fee-for-Service-Payment/PhysicianFeedbackProg ram/Downloads/2016-RiskAdj-FactSheet.pdf.

15 Tying Things Together

Ainsley Malone

CONTENTS

I INTRODUCTION

Malnutrition in adult hospitalized patients has been recognized as an issue for well over five decades. Pioneering efforts by Stanley Dudrick and others in the 1960s led to the development of parenteral nutrition, a therapy born from the recognition that individuals who were unable to eat or receive enteral nutrition due to intractable intestinal dysfunction often died of malnutrition.[1] In 1974, Charles Butterworth brought the topic of malnutrition to clinicians and healthcare practitioners by his landmark article "The Skeleton in the Hospital Closet".[2] Early leaders of the American Society for Parenteral and Enteral Nutrition (ASPEN) also recognized the problem by publishing a position statement on addressing malnutrition in hospitalized patients.[3] These were the beginning efforts to address hospital malnutrition.

Despite these early achievements, malnutrition continues to be problematic in healthcare systems and communities worldwide.[4–7] In the United States, it is estimated that as many as one in three patients admitted to the hospital are at high nutrition risk or malnourished.[8,9] In addition, it is well known that nutrition status can decline during hospitalization due to inadequate nutrition care during the hospital course.[10,11] The impact of malnutrition on health outcomes is significant. Malnutrition has been shown to be adversely associated with several functional, clinical, and economic outcomes including elevated risk of comorbid complications, longer length of hospital stay, more frequent readmissions, higher mortality and increased healthcare costs when compared to patients who are adequately nourished.[4,12–14] (See Chapter 1.)

DOI: 10.1201/9781003177586-15

II   REGULATORY EFFORTS TO ADDRESS MALNUTRITION

Regulation in the acute care setting is an important element to safeguard patient care. At the time of this writing, regulatory efforts to address malnutrition throughout a patient's hospital course have not been fully embraced in the United States. One success in 1995 was the introduction of a standard by the United States Joint Commission that required all patients to undergo nutrition screening within 24 hours of hospital admission.[15] In 2016, the specific requirement for nutrition screening was enveloped into a more generic standard in which hospitals will define when nutrition screening is to be performed, and, when applicable for the patient's condition, must be completed within 24 hours of admission. No additional requirements from an accreditation or regulation perspective for inpatient hospital care have been enacted to date.

In 2015, an appeal was made to the Joint Commission, highlighted by Guenter et al. in their publication "Addressing Disease-Related Malnutrition in Hospitalized Patients: A Call for a National Goal" in the *Joint Commission Journal on Quality and Patient Safety*, to consider disease-related malnutrition as a National Patient Safety Goal (NPSG).[16] NPSGs are defined as "goals to improve patient safety and focus on problems in healthcare and how to solve them".[17] NPSGs released in 2016, as well as others to date, have not included the problem of malnutrition.

Numerous organizations including the Academy of Nutrition and Dietetics (Academy) and ASPEN have worked cooperatively since 2010 to address this lack of regulation regarding hospital malnutrition. In 2014, stakeholder organizations convened and produced the "Dialog Proceedings: Measuring the Quality of Malnutrition Care in the Hospitalized Elderly Patient", whose goals included, among others, to "gain consensus on specific quality measure focus areas".[18] Since that time, ongoing work by the Academy, as measure stewards, has focused on adoption of malnutrition clinical quality measures (CQMs) into the Centers for Medicare & Medicaid Services' (CMS) Inpatient Quality Reporting Program. This program collects quality data from hospitals with the goal to drive quality improvement.[19] Including malnutrition CQMs in this program would elevate the role of the healthcare team in addressing malnutrition to promote optimal outcomes for malnourished patients. In 2016 and 2018, the Academy submitted four malnutrition CQMs to CMS: (1) malnutrition screening within 24 hours of admission, (2) nutrition assessment of patients identified as at risk of malnutrition within 24 hours of a malnutrition screening, (3) nutrition care plan for patients identified as malnourished after a completed nutrition assessment and (4) appropriate documentation of a malnutrition diagnosis. These four CQMs have not been adopted by CMS as measures. More recently, the Academy submitted to CMS a "global malnutrition composite score" measure combining the above four CQMs. In December of 2020, this composite score was included in the "Measures Under Consideration" list;[20] a final ruling is pending at the time of this publication. The inclusion of a malnutrition quality measure in hospital CMS reporting requirements would be a significant advance in addressing malnutrition beyond the singular role of the registered dietitian nutritionist (RDN), as hospitals would need to develop malnutrition care processes involving the entire healthcare team.

Other countries have adopted a focused regulatory approach to address malnutrition, more specifically within hospital accreditation systems.[21,22] A current example of

TABLE 15.1

Key Areas Addressed by the Canadian *Malnutrition Prevention, Detection and Treatment Standard 2021*[22]

- Identify patients at risk of malnutrition at admission.
- Diagnose malnutrition.
- Implement an integrated nutrition care plan to prevent and treat malnutrition.
- Provide nutritious and culturally acceptable food and reduce barriers to food intake for patients.
- Monitor nutrition intake and nutrition status changes for patients.
- Provide treatment for malnourished patients throughout their hospital stay
- Facilitate organizational changes to implement and sustain improved nutrition management.
- Focus on nutrition care in the discharge plan when patients are transferred to other care and community settings.

this is the *Malnutrition Prevention, Detection and Treatment Standard* developed by Canada's Health Standards Organization/Standards Council of Canada, the equivalent to the US Joint Commission. This standard outlines requirements and guidance for hospitals to provide best practices in key areas, as highlighted in Table 15.1.[22] It is hopeful that more global healthcare accrediting bodies will include malnutrition in their standards, including the US Joint Commission.

Regulatory requirements addressing malnutrition also exist outside the acute care setting. The minimum data set (MDS) is an assessment required by CMS as well as Medicaid-certified long-term care facilities for all residents.[23] The MDS is completed by various members of the interdisciplinary team, including the RDN. Nutrition-specific information in the MDS includes swallowing function, weight loss or gain, and nutrition interventions.[23] In the community setting, an addition to the Older Americans Act (OAA) in 2020 specifically addresses malnutrition. Malnutrition reduction is a focus of OAA nutrition programs with nutrition screening included as a routine part of program participation.[24]

III   IMPLEMENTING A MALNUTRITION PROGRAM

If healthcare regulation addressing malnutrition, as previously described, is enacted, it will be critical for hospitals to implement quality-focused malnutrition programs. Fortunately, multiple reports have been published describing the development of successful facility or system-wide malnutrition programs.[25-28] Reported programs have varied widely in terms of scope and content but all provide common key contributors.

A critical component of successful malnutrition programs is administrative and medical staff support.[26,29] This can be a member of an institution's medical leadership, a specific nutrition department's administrator or both. Full institutional support will enhance malnutrition program development, which requires integration with other departments and/or divisions. Table 15.2 outlines key team members and the overall contributions they can provide to the malnutrition program.

TABLE 15.2

Malnutrition Program Team Members and Their General Contributions[26–28]

Team member	Contribution
Administrator (medical or administrative)	• Overall program support • Direct and/or assist with financial and labor support
Nursing leadership and staff	• Coordinate nutrition screening and compliance with its use • Ensure practices are in place to support implementation of nutrition intervention
RDN	• Provide nutrition expertise and leadership to all health team members • Conduct nutrition assessments • Diagnose and document malnutrition • Implement nutrition interventions
Physician or provider	• Incorporate nutrition status as an essential component of medical assessment, treatment and monitoring
Clinical documentation specialist	• Provide guidance on process for capturing malnutrition diagnosis from RDN and other providers • Educate other documentation specialists on malnutrition diagnostic methodology • Assist RDNs in provider education
Information technology / clinical informatics	• Assist in EHR structure to optimize malnutrition documentation • Develop structure for data reports and analysis

Abbreviations: RDN = Registered Dietitian Nutritionist; EHR = electronic health record.

Development of a successful malnutrition program involves reviewing current processes and workflow to identify gaps and areas where improvements can be made. Table 15.3 outlines key questions to address in this review. Answers will identify process gaps and areas for improvement and will guide overall program development. Baseline data analysis is an important strategy to evaluate program outcomes over time, and to facilitate initial and ongoing administrative support. Data evaluation can be performed in any one of the process areas. Table 15.4 highlights useful data points for both baseline analysis and for measuring post-program implementation outcomes.

As hospitals begin development of a malnutrition program, the outcomes of an initial review of processes and workflow will identify process gaps and areas where improvements can lead to program success. The following details key malnutrition processes where gaps can occur, and enhancements that may assist in closing those gaps.

A   Nutrition Screening Process

Screening for malnutrition risk is essential to identify those patients who may be malnourished and will likely need nutrition intervention. Many screening approaches or tools have been implemented in a variety of healthcare settings, including tools that are not validated, and specific to that facility.[30] The use of a validated screening tool

TABLE 15.3

Key Questions for Malnutrition Process and Wordflow Assessment[18,21,25]

Process area	Questions
Nutrition screening	• Who performs nutrition screening? • Is nutrition screening performed accurately? • Is a validated screening tool in use? • Is nutrition screening completed within 24 hours of admission? • How is a positive nutrition screen communicated to the RDN?
Nutrition assessment	• Is a standardized assessment methodology in use throughout the healthcare facility? • Is the RDN competent to perform a nutrition assessment? • What is the time frame from receiving a positive nutrition screen until the nutrition assessment is completed by the RDN?
Malnutrition diagnosis	• Are providers educated on the malnutrition diagnostic criteria? • How is malnutrition, as a nutrition diagnosis, documented in the EHR? • How is the malnutrition diagnosis communicated to the provider? • How is malnutrition, as a medical diagnosis, documented in the EHR? • Is the malnutrition diagnosis captured by the correct ICD code at patient discharge?
Intervention to treat malnutrition	• Does the RDN develop and document a malnutrition plan of care? • Is the nutrition intervention ordered by the RDN and/or provider? • Is the nutrition intervention appropriate to treat the patient's malnutrition?
Transition of malnutrition care	• Is the malnutrition diagnosis communicated upon discharge? • Is a nutrition care plan ordered for implementation in the alternate site or home care settings?

Abbreviations: RDN = Registered Dietitian Nutritionist; EHR = electronic health record; ICD = International Classification of Diseases.

is imperative to reduce false positive or negative results. False positive results lead to the inefficient use of RDN time while false negative results may miss patients who are malnourished. (See Chapter 4.)

B NUTRITION ASSESSMENT METHODOLOGY

Multiple nutrition assessment methodologies are in use globally. Important considerations when developing a malnutrition program involve these nutrition assessment components:

- Selection of nutrition assessment methodology
- Selection of malnutrition diagnostic criteria and subsequent hospital/medical staff approval
- Training and education of all RDNs in chosen methodology/diagnostic criteria
- Initial and ongoing RDN competency assessment

TABLE 15.4
Data Analysis Options for Baseline and Post-Malnutrition Program Assessment

Process area	Data points
Nutrition screening	• Percentage of patients with completion of nutrition screening within 24 hours of admission • Percentage of positive nutrition screens communicated to the RDN within 24 hours of screening
Nutrition assessment	• Number of hours between receiving a positive nutrition screen and completion of the nutrition assessment by the RDN
Malnutrition diagnosis	• Percentage of malnutrition diagnoses correctly documented by the RDN in the EHR • Percentage of malnutrition documented by the medical provider in the EHR • Percentage of patients with a nutrition diagnosis of malnutrition and a correct ICD code at patient discharge • Percentage of patients with a medical diagnosis of malnutrition and a correct ICD code at patient discharge
Intervention to treat malnutrition	• Percentage of malnourished patients receiving a nutrition intervention as documented by the RDN in the nutrition plan of care • Percentage of malnourished patients receiving nutrition intervention to provide > 75% of their estimated nutrient requirements
Transition of malnutrition care	• Percentage of malnourished patients with their malnutrition diagnosis communicated on discharge documentation • Percentage of malnourished patients who have a nutrition care plan ordered for implementation in the alternate site or home care settings

Abbreviations: RDN = Registered Dietitian Nutritionist; EHR = electronic health record; ICD = International Classification of Diseases.

Factors to assist in selecting the nutrition assessment methodology include, among others, its usability, familiarity, and validity. Subjective global assessment (SGA) is a highly validated assessment tool used widely throughout the world.[31] The 2012 Academy/ASPEN Malnutrition Consensus Characteristics[32] methodology in 2017 was reported to be in use by over 71% of US hospitals.[33] Most recently in 2019, the Global Leadership on Malnutrition (GLIM) consensus criteria for the diagnosis of malnutrition were published as a framework for diagnosing malnutrition worldwide, especially in settings where experienced nutrition professionals are lacking.[34] While it is beyond the scope of this chapter to discuss validation processes, the Academy/ASPEN consensus characteristics have demonstrated predictive validity in multiple studies and validation studies are continuing at the time of this publication[35,36] (see Chapter 2).

Once a specific assessment methodology / diagnostic criteria are chosen, education and training of all RDNs is essential. Regardless of the method/criteria utilized, the importance of standardization cannot be overemphasized. For a malnutrition program to be successful, it is important that nutrition assessment is performed in a standardized approach, meaning all RDNs in a system or facility follow the same methodology. Lack of standardization can lead to misdiagnosis, inappropriate or lack of nutrition intervention and risk of payer denials.[28,37-39] Nutrition assessment and diagnosis training can be accomplished using a variety of methods including traditional didactic teaching, hands-on approaches, simulation and observation followed by performance.[25,40]

If the Academy/ASPEN, SGA or GLIM is the chosen methodology, the nutrition-focused physical examination (NFPE) is an essential component (see Chapter 6). Performance of an NFPE may be new for some RDNs, although the Commission on Dietetic Registration added an NFPE practice competency for entry-level practitioners in 2014.[41] NFPE performance by RDNs has increased over time.[33] In surveys conducted in 2014 and 2017 totaling 1821 RDNs in the United States, NFPE performance increased from 26.8% to 48.6%. Barriers to performance, including "inadequate training" and "not feeling comfortable touching patients", decreased substantially, which was felt to contribute to the overall performance increase.[33]

Competency evaluation is critical to ensure RDNs are able to correctly perform a nutrition assessment, resulting in the successful outcome of diagnosing malnutrition. Competency assessment can be achieved through a variety of methods including an observed performance using a competency checklist tool[42] or through a formalized observation structured exam.[28] The Academy includes a competency assessment tool in their NFPE Hands-on Training Program[43] which can be used by trainers to assess competency of RDNs in NFPE performance. Clinical peer review audits are another method to assess malnutrition diagnostic competency.[44]

C   DOCUMENTATION AND COMMUNICATION OF NUTRITION DIAGNOSIS

Once the RDN has diagnosed a patient with malnutrition, the next critical step is for that diagnosis to be documented in the health record and communicated to the provider and healthcare team. The essentiality of this step cannot be overemphasized. Without adequate documentation and communication, there is less likelihood the appropriate nutrition intervention will be implemented.[45,46] Adequate nutrition therapy for malnourished individuals can impact outcomes,[47,48] so timely initiation is critical. In addition, the need for comprehensive documentation of malnutrition diagnostic criteria is essential. Providing specific clinical details delineating the criteria will help minimize any possible confusion. Failure to include adequate malnutrition diagnostic criteria and severity details may lead to payment denials.

RDNs, using the nutrition care process, will identify a "nutrition diagnosis" of malnutrition following the nutrition assessment.[49] The diagnostic terminology from both the Nutrition Care Process and Terminology (eNCPT) and the Academy/ASPEN Consensus Malnutrition Characteristics[32] are based on etiology: "Acute Illness or Injury Related Malnutrition", "Chronic Disease or Condition Related Malnutrition" and "Starvation Related Malnutrition" (eNCPT) and "Social/Environmental Related Malnutrition" (Academy/ASPEN). The diagnostic severity (moderate or severe) is delineated by the specific criteria thresholds (see Chapter 2).[32] As highlighted in Chapter 14, a lack of alignment exists between coding nomenclature required by CMS and other insurers and the diagnostic terminology described above. Malnutrition, as a medical diagnosis, does not have the same language as a malnutrition "nutrition diagnosis" (Table 15.5). A need exists to align or link the malnutrition diagnosis identified by the RDN with that documented by the patient's primary medical provider. This step involves communication with the provider, which can be achieved verbally and/or electronically.[27,28] Some hospital systems permit the RDN to add the "nutrition diagnosis" of malnutrition to the patient's problem list;[50] however, the provider must then "activate" the diagnosis for it to be coded as a medical diagnosis. The acceptance by the provider of the RDN's malnutrition diagnosis requires clear documentation by the RDN of the patient's malnutrition assessment including the specific criteria and their severity threshold. Lack of alignment between the primary medical provider and the RDN in malnutrition documentation increases the risk of coverage denials by payers (see Chapter 14).

D LEVERAGING THE ELECTRONIC HEALTH RECORD

The electronic health record (EHR) is the link to many of the critical process steps within a successful malnutrition program. Challenges can exist with EHR systems resulting in breakdowns or gaps in key processes which can impact how well malnourished patients are identified and treated.[51] Including Information Technology and Clinical Informatics specialists in the early stage of developing a malnutrition program will help address these potential gaps.[26–28] Nutrition screening, often performed by nurses during the hospital admission process,[52] can easily be completed within the EHR. Clinical decision support, a health information technology component, should be built within the EHR to improve efficiency in workflow, such as an alert or other

---

TABLE 15.5

Alignment of Nutrition Malnutrition Diagnosis and ICD-10 Malnutrition Terminology[49,62]

Nutrition diagnosis terminology	ICD-10 Code	MS-DRG ICD-10 Terminology
Moderate malnutrition related to acute illness or injury	E44	Moderate protein-calorie malnutrition
Severe malnutrition related to acute illness or injury	E43	Unspecified severe protein-calorie malnutrition
Moderate chronic disease- or condition-related malnutrition	E44	Moderate protein-calorie malnutrition
Severe chronic disease- or condition-related malnutrition	E43	Unspecified severe protein-calorie malnutrition
Moderate starvation-related malnutrition	E44	Moderate protein-calorie malnutrition
Severe starvation-related malnutrition	E43	Unspecified severe protein-calorie malnutrition

Abbreviations: ICD-10 = International Classification of Diseases, 10th Revision; MS-DRG = Medicare Severity Diagnosis Related Group.

automatic reporting mechanism for the RDN to identify those patients who have a positive nutrition screen and therefore need to undergo a nutrition assessment.[52] Automating this process can ultimately lead to improved identification of malnourished patients.[53]

One key component in a successful malnutrition program, as previously mentioned, is the standardization of the nutrition assessment methodology. How this standardized nutrition assessment methodology is built into the EHR will impact ease and efficiency of documentation. Allowing entry of structured data via "drop down" or "bulleted" entry options, rather than "free text", is a more efficient documentation approach.[52,53] In addition to ease of use, having structured data will permit the generation of reports for tracking malnutrition metrics over time. Incorporation of the Academy's eNCPT for malnutrition, its etiology and signs and symptoms (clinical indicators) is one option to ensure all clinicians document malnutrition diagnostic criteria consistently and comprehensively.

As outlined previously, accurate documentation of a patient's malnutrition diagnosis is a critical step in the malnutrition care process. An important partner in this effort is the clinical documentation improvement specialist (CDIS). The CDIS serves as an essential resource to the clinical team and ensures that all relevant conditions requiring healthcare resources throughout the patient's hospitalization are accurately captured.[54] In the context of a malnourished patient the CDIS will often serve as bridge between the RDN and the provider to ensure accurate documentation supporting the malnutrition diagnosis is present. The CDIS creates diagnosis documentation queries to the provider, which can be built into the EHR framework to assist with confirming and documenting the diagnosis.

A critical step in the malnutrition process flow, one that is often omitted, is the transfer of nutrition diagnostic information and the nutrition plan of care with transitions of care.[55] Malnourished patients discharged to an alternate care setting or to home with healthcare without accurate nutrition documentation are at risk of their nutrition status worsening, accompanied by its associated complications, including hospital readmission.[56] Leveraging the EHR to facilitate this information transfer can assist to ensure malnourished patients receive their appropriate nutrition intervention and follow-up care.

E   EDUCATION OF HEALTHCARE TEAM MEMBERS

Perhaps one of the most important questions to ask when developing a malnutrition program is "How will the healthcare team members be educated on the importance of identifying and treating malnutrition?" As described by Tappenden et al., in 2013, "All healthcare professionals involved in patient care must be empowered to influence nutrition decisions".[29] Nurses and physicians often receive limited formal nutrition education during training and may not prioritize nutrition among the competing patient care priorities. Malnutrition care processes encompass all aspects of a patient's hospital course and as such all team members must recognize the role they play in that process. Specific education topics for healthcare team members are outlined in Table 15.6. Education can be formal via didactic lectures such as a medical "grand rounds" or very informal, for example, during a daily "huddle". The key

TABLE 15.6

Topics for Education of Healthcare Team Members on Malnutrition Care Processes

Team member	Strategy
Nurse	• Describe importance of performing nutrition screening and identifying the "at risk" patients
	• Outline malnutrition diagnostic criteria
	• Outline evidence and documentation of hospital patients who do not consume adequate nutrients
Nurse and provider	• Outline key clinical outcomes associated with malnutrition
	• Explain the benefits of treating malnourished patients with nutrition interventions (oral supplements, enteral and/or parenteral nutrition)
	• Outline malnutrition diagnostic criteria
Provider and CDIS	• Outline malnutrition diagnostic criteria

Abbreviation: CDIS = clinical documentation improvement specialist.

is to offer multiple opportunities for education throughout the implementation and continuation of a malnutrition program.

IV EVIDENCE SUPPORTING QUALITY IMPROVEMENT IN MALNUTRITION CARE

Provision of high-quality care is a mission for all healthcare systems. Malnutrition care and its processes certainly fall under the umbrella of quality care. A malnutrition program developed by a specific healthcare system as outlined in this chapter can be broad-based or focused on a single component, e.g. improving documentation of malnutrition in the EHR. A more formalized quality-improvement program addressing malnutrition has been developed and is available for any hospital or healthcare system to participate. The Malnutrition Quality Improvement Initiative (MQii) was developed from 2013 to 2019 by key stakeholders including the Academy, Avalere Health and Abbott Nutrition to address malnutrition in the older adult, specifically for those ≥ 65 years.[57] The goal for this quality program is to support achievement of malnutrition standards of care through measuring and improving care processes.[57] In 2015 the MQii developed and launched a malnutrition toolkit, a collection of evidence-based malnutrition care practices to achieve high quality malnutrition care. The toolkit includes multiple implementation resources and offers participants an opportunity to engage with others via a learning collaborative.[58] Studies published by MQii participants have demonstrated improvements in malnutrition processes and outcomes including reductions in hospital length of stay, improved malnutrition documentation and improved initiation of nutrition interventions.[59–61] As of September 2019, over 265 sites in the United States currently participate or have previously participated in the MQii. Hospitals participating in data collection through the MQii contribute to the assessment of malnutrition care gaps in older adults within the United States, which will assist in the development of quality programs for other patient populations including beyond the hospital setting.[58]

V CONCLUSION

Despite widespread recognition, malnutrition continues to be an issue in hospitals worldwide. However, since the 1970s when nutrition support leaders guided initial efforts to address malnutrition, today much more is known. Improved efforts with identification and treatment can result in reduction of negative clinical outcomes. As regulatory initiatives come closer to realization, it will befit hospitals to develop and maintain programs to address malnutrition processes and care. It is this approach that will help not only advance patient outcomes but hopefully lead to significant improvements overall such that in the future hospital malnutrition no longer remains a substantial healthcare issue.

REFERENCES

1. Wilmore DW, Dudrick SJ. Growth and development of an infant receiving all nutrients exclusively by vein. *JAMA.* 1968;203(10):860–864.
2. Butterworth CE. The skeleton in the hospital closet. *Nutr Today.* 1974;9(2):4–8.
3. Stefee WP. A Statement by the ASPEN Board of Directors, Special Communication. *JPEN J Parenter Enteral Nutr.* 1983;7(3):219–220.
4. Barrett ML, Bailey MK, Owens PL. Non-maternal and non-neonatal inpatient stays in the United States involving malnutrition, 2016. August 30, 2018. US Agency for Healthcare Research and Quality. Accessed February 4, 2021. https://hcup-us.ahrq. gov/reports/HCUPMalnutritionHospReport_083018.pdf.
5. Correia MI, Perman MI, Waitzberg DK. Hospital malnutrition in Latin America: a systematic review. *Clin Nutr.* 2017;36(4):958–967.
6. Marinho R, Pessoa A, Lopes M, et al. High prevalence of malnutrition in internal medicine wards – a multicentre ANUMEDI study. *Eur J Intern Med.* 2020;76:82–88.
7. Allard JP, Keller H, Jeejeebhoy KN, et al. Malnutrition at hospital admission - contributors and effect on length of stay: a prospective cohort study from the Canadian Malnutrition Task Force. *JPEN J Parenter Enteral Nutr.* 2016;40(4):487–497.
8. Barker LA, Gout BS, Crowe TC. Hospital malnutrition: Prevalence, identification and impact on patients and the healthcare system. *Int J Environ Res Public Health.* 2011;8(2):514–527.
9. Sauer AC, Goates S, Malone A, et al. Prevalence of malnutrition risk and impact of nutrition risk on hospital outcomes: results from nutritionDay in the U.S. *JPEN J Parenter Enteral Nutr.* 2019;43(7):918–926.
10. Braunschweig C, Gomez S, Sheean PM. Impact of declines in nutritional status on outcomes in adult patients hospitalized for more than 7 days. *J Am Diet Assoc.* 2000;100(11):1316–1322.
11. Chambers R, Bryan J, Jannat-Khah D, Russo E, Merriman L, Gupta R. Evaluating gaps in care of malnourished patients on general medicine floors in an acute care setting. *Nutr Clin Pract.* 2019;34(2):313–318.

12. Lim SL, Ong KCB, Chan YH, Loke WC, Ferguson M, Daniels L. Malnutrition and its impact on cost of hospitalization, length of stay, readmission and 3-year mortality. *Clin Nutr.* 2012;31(3):345–350.

13. Correia M. The impact of malnutrition on morbidity, mortality, length of hospital stay and costs evaluated through a multivariate model analysis. *Clin Nutr.* 2003;22(3):235–239.

14. Hiller L, Shaw R, Fabri P. Difference in composite end point of readmission and death between malnourished and nonmalnourished veterans assessed using Academy of Nutrition and Dietetics/American Society for Parenteral and Enteral Nutrition clinical characteristics. *JPEN J Parenter Enteral Nutr.* 2017;41(8):1316–1324.

15. Comprehensive Accreditation Manual for Hospitals. Chicago, IL: Joint Commission on Accreditation of Healthcare Organizations; 2007.

16. Guenter P, Jensen G, Patel V, et al. Addressing disease-related malnutrition in hospitalized patients: a call for a national goal. *Jt Comm J Qual Patient Saf.* 2015;41(10):469–473.

17. The Joint Commission. 2021 hospital national patient safety goals. Accessed February 15, 2021. www.jointcommission.org/-/media/tjc/documents/standards/national-pati ent-safety-goals/2021/simplified-2021-hap-npsg-goals-final-11420.pdf.

18. Mitchell K, Jones K. Dialogue proceedings: measuring the quality of nutrition care. May 6, 2014. Avalere Health. Accessed February 15, 2021. https://avalere.com/insig hts/dialogue-proceedings-measuring-the-quality-of-malnutrition-care.

19. Centers for Medicare & Medicaid Services. Hospital Inpatient Quality Reporting Program. Accessed May 23, 2021. www.cms.gov/Medicare/Quality-Initiatives-Pati ent-Assessment-Instruments/HospitalQualityInits/HospitalRHQDAPU.

20. Centers for Medicare & Medicaid Services. List of measures under consideration for December 21, 2020. Accessed February 15, 2021. www.cms.gov/files/document/ measures-under-consideration-list-2020-report.pdf.

21. National policy for effective screening implementation. Accessed February 20, 2021. https://european-nutrition.org/good-practices/national-policy-for-effective-screening-implementation/.

22. CAN/HSO 5066:2021 – Malnutrition Prevention, Detection, and Treatment. Accessed May 20, 2022. https://healthstandards.org/standard/malnutrition-prevention-detect ion-and-treatment/.

23. Centers for Medicare & Medicaid Services. Minimum Data Set. Accessed May 3, 2021. www.cms.gov/Medicare/Quality-Initiatives-Patient-Assessment-Instruments/ NursingHomeQualityInits/Downloads/Archive-Draft-of-the-MDS-30-Nursing-Home-Comprehensive-NC-Version-1140.pdf.

24. Supporting Older Americans Act of 2020. Public Law 116–131. March 25, 2020. Accessed May 3, 2021. www.congress.gov/116/plaws/publ131/PLAW-116publ 131.pdf.

25. Malone A, Hamilton C. The Academy of Nutrition and Dietetics/The American Society for Parenteral and Enteral Nutrition consensus malnutrition characteristics: application in practice. *Nutr Clin Pract.* 2013;28(6):639–650.

26. Groch N, Bacon S. A community hospital's journey in implementing a comprehensive malnutrition program in adults. *Support Line.* 2020;42(4):2–10.

27. Phillips W, Whiddon C, Wehausen D. A step-by-step guide to implementing a malnutrition coding program for adult inpatients. *Support Line.* 2017;39(3):2–9.

28. Doley J, Phillips W, Talaber J, Leger-LeBlanc G. Early implementation of malnutrition clinical quality metrics to identify institutional performance improvement needs. *J Acad Nutr Diet.* 2019;119(4):547–552.

29. Tappenden KA, Quatrara B, Parkhurst ML, Malone AM, Fanjiang G, Ziegler TR. Critical role of nutrition in improving quality of care: an interdisciplinary call to action to address adult hospital malnutrition. *JPEN J Parenter Enteral Nutr.* 2013;37(4):482–497.

30. Patel V, Romano M, Corkins M, et al. Nutrition screening and assessment in hospitalized patients: a survey of current practice in the United States. *Nutr Clin Pract.* 2014;29(4):483–490.

31. Fink JS, de Mello PD, de Mello ED. Subjective global assessment of nutritional status – A systematic review of the literature. *Clin Nutr.* 2015;34(5):785–792.

32. White JV, Guenter P, Jensen GL, Malone A, Schofield M. Consensus statement: Academy of Nutrition and Dietetics and American Society for Parenteral and Enteral Nutrition: characteristics recommended for the identification and documentation of adult malnutrition (under-nutrition). *JPEN J Parenter Ent Nutr.* 2012;36(3):275–283.

33. Modarski BA, Hand RK. Patterns in adult malnutrition assessment and diagnosis by Registered Dietitian Nutritionists: 2014–2017. *J Acad Nutr Diet.* 2018;119(8):1243–1249.

34. Jensen GL, Cederholm T, Correia MITD, et al. GLIM criteria for the diagnosis of malnutrition: a consensus report from the global clinical nutrition community. *JPEN J Parenter Enteral Nutr.* 2019;43(1):32–40.

35. Mogensen KM, Malone A, Becker P, et al. Academy of Nutrition and Dietetics/American Society for Parenteral and Enteral Nutrition Consensus Malnutrition Characteristics: usability and association with outcomes. *Nutr Clin Pract.* 2019;34(5):657–665.

36. Hand RK, Murphy WJ, Field LB, et al. Validation of the Academy/ASPEN malnutrition clinical characteristics. *J Acad Nutr Diet.* 2016;116(5):856–864.

37. Dobak S, Peterson SJ, Corrigan ML, Lefton J. Current practices and perceived barriers to diagnosing, documenting, and coding for malnutrition: a survey of the Dietitians in Nutrition Support dietetic practice group. *J Acad Nutr Diet.* 2018;118(6):978–983.

38. Tobert CM, Mott SL, Nepple KG. Malnutrition diagnosis during adult inpatient hospitalizations: analysis of a multi-institutional collaborative database of academic medical centers. *J Acad Nutr Diet.* 2018;118(1):125–131.

39. Buecheler K, Igel A. Training your staff to perform nutrition-focused physical exams. *Future Dimensions in in Clinical Nutrition Practice*, Fall 2017. Clinical Nutrition Management Dietetic Practice Group of the Academy of Nutrition and Dietetics.

40. Accreditation Council for Education in Nutrition and Dietetics. Future education model standards for accredited graduate programs in dietetics. Accessed May 23, 2021. www.eatrightpro.org/acend/accreditation-standards-fees-and-policies/future-education-model.

41. Commission on Dietetic Registration. Essential Practice Competencies 2014. Accessed May 23, 2021. www.cdrnet.org/educator-toolkit-for-guiding-students.

42. MacQuillan EL, Ford J, Baird K. Clinical competence assessed using simulation: development of a standardized tool to assess nutrition-focused physical exam skill competence for registered dietitian nutritionists. *J Nutr Educ Behav.* 2021;53(2):174–182.

43. Nutrition Focused Physical Exam Hands-on Training Workshop, The Academy of Nutrition and Dietetics. Accessed February 25, 2021. www.eatrightpro.org/practice/professional-development/face-to-face-learning/nfpe-workshop#Details.

44. Deyo-Svendsen ME, Phillips MR, Albright JK, Schilling KA, Palmer KB. A systematic approach to clinical peer review in a critical access hospital. *Qual Manag Health Care.* 2016;25(4):213–218.

45. Gout BS, Barker LA, Crowe TC. Malnutrition identification, diagnosis and dietetic referrals: Are we doing a good enough job? *Nutr Diet.* 2009;66(4):206–211.

46. Phillips W. Accurate documentation of malnutrition diagnosis reflects increased healthcare resource utilization. *Nutr Clin Pract.* 2015;30(5): 604–608.

47. Schuetz P, Fehr R, Baechli V, et al. Individualised nutritional support in medical inpatients at nutritional risk: a randomised clinical trial. *Lancet.* 2019;393(10188):2312–2321.

48. Kaegi-Braun N, Mueller M, Schuetz P, Mueller B, Kutz A. Evaluation of nutritional support and in-hospital mortality in patients with malnutrition. *JAMA Network Open.* 2021;4(1) doi:10.1001/jamanetworkopen.2020.33433.

49. Nutrition Care Process and Terminology, The Academy of Nutrition and Dietetics. Accessed February 26, 2021. www.ncpro.org/modules/portal/web_site_search. cfm?web_site_id=103&keywords=malnutrition.

50. Nepple KG, Tobert CM, Valladares AF, Mitchell K, Yadrick M. Enhancing identification and management of hospitalized patients who are malnourished: a pilot evaluation of electronic quality improvement measures. *J Acad Nutr Diet.* 2019;119(9 Suppl 2):S32–S39.

51. Kight CE, Bouche JM, Curry A, et al. Consensus recommendations for optimizing electronic health records for nutrition care. *Nutr Clin Pract.* 2020;35(1):12–23.

52. Mogensen K, Malone AM, Bouma S, et al. Nutrition Assessment Survey 2016. *Nutr Clin Pract.* 2018;33(5):711–717.

53. Vivanti A, Lee HC, Palmer M. Capitalising on opportunities: Malnutrition coding in hospital before and after the introduction of electronic health records with an embedded malnutrition screening tool. *Clin Nutr ESPEN.* 2021;41:193–197.

54. The Association of Clinical Documentation Integrity Specialists Position Paper; Defining the CDI specialist's roles and responsibilities. Accessed March 1, 2021. https://acdis.org/system/files/resources/define-cdi-specialist-role-responsibilities_0.pdf.

55. Jones K, Mitchell K. Dialogue proceedings / advancing patient-centered malnutrition care transitions. Avalere Health. Accessed May 23, 2021. https://avalere.com/insights/dialogue-proceedings-advancing-patient-centered-malnutrition-care-transitions.

56. Fingar KR, Weiss AJ, Barrett ML, et al. All-cause readmissions following hospital stays for patients with malnutrition, 2013: Statistical Brief #218. Healthcare Cost and Utilization Project (HCUP). PMID: 28125197. Accessed May 23, 2021. www.ncbi.nlm.nih.gov/books/NBK410088/.

57. Malnutrition Quality Improvement Initiative MQii. Accessed March 1, 2021. http://malnutritionquality.org.

58. McCauley SM, Mitchell KM, Heap A. The malnutrition quality improvement initiative: a multiyear partnership transforms care. *J Acad Nutr Diet.* 2019;119(9 Suppl 2):S18–S24.

59. Silver HJ, Pratt KJ, Bruno M, Lynch J, Mitchell K, McCauley SM. Effectiveness of the Malnutrition Quality Improvement Initiative on practitioner malnutrition knowledge and screening, diagnosis, and timeliness of malnutrition-related care provided to older adults admitted to a tertiary care facility: A pilot study. *J Acad Nutr Diet.* 2018;118(1):101–109.

60. Sriram K, Sulo S, VanDerBosch G, et al. Nutrition-focused quality improvement program results in significant readmission and length of stay reductions for malnourished surgical patients. *JPEN J Parenter Enteral Nutr.* 2018;42(6):1093–1098.

61. Danis K, Kline M, Munson M, et al. Identifying and managing malnourished hospitalized patients utilizing the malnutrition quality improvement initiative: the UPMC experience. *J Acad Nutr Diet.* 2019;119(9 Suppl 2):S40–S43.

62. ICD-10-CM/PCS MS-DRG v37.0 Definitions Manual. Accessed February 26, 2021. www.cms.gov/icd10m/version37-fullcode-cms/fullcode_cms/P0242.html.

Index